Integrated Diabetes Care

David Simmons
Helmut Wenzel • Janice C. Zgibor
Editors

Integrated Diabetes Care

A Multidisciplinary Approach

Springer

Editors
David Simmons
School of Medicine
Western Sydney University
Sydney, NSW, Australia

Helmut Wenzel
Health Economist
Konstanz, Germany

Janice C. Zgibor
Department of Epidemiology
and Biostatistics, College
of Public Health
University of South Florida
Tampa, FL, USA

ISBN 978-3-319-13388-1 ISBN 978-3-319-13389-8 (eBook)
DOI 10.1007/978-3-319-13389-8

Library of Congress Control Number: 2016955045

Printed on acid-free paper

This Springer imprint is published by Springer Nature
The registered company is Springer International Publishing AG Switzerland

Foreword

If one wished to choose a health condition that requires an integrated multidisciplinary approach to management, then you cannot go past diabetes. And given the spectacular growth of diabetes over the last 20 years, the number of people with diabetes worldwide has more than doubled. The International Diabetes Federation (IDF) today estimates there are at least 415 million people with diabetes. The IDF also estimates there will be over 620 million with diabetes by 2040. Concerning features in relation to the current epidemic are the increases in both type 1 and 2 diabetes, gestational diabetes, and the emergence of type 2 diabetes in children and adolescents. This scenario poses huge social, public health, and economic problems to most nations and stretches their capacity for optimal diabetes care.

The very nature of diabetes—with its issues relating to day-to-day management and the risk and burden of future complications such as cardiovascular disease, retinopathy, and kidney disease and comorbidities which include liver disease and obstructive sleep apnoea—raises huge issues for an integrated approach to management.

People with diabetes often have multiple comorbidities and see a number of different health professionals across primary, community, and specialist care services. This is where integrated care may have an important "game-changing" role. It has been demonstrated that best-practice, high-quality diabetes care can only be achieved when healthcare professionals work seamlessly. This involves partnerships across primary healthcare, community care, and specialist care services delivering integrated diabetes care to the consumer, the person with diabetes.

Establishing an effective, integrated system will require a transformation in the way care is delivered, making it more consumer focused and team based. The person with diabetes may be looked after in primary, secondary, and also tertiary care. Their healthcare team includes the general practitioner, the diabetologist, diabetes educator, the dietician, and other healthcare providers. There is a requirement for coordination across the relevant agencies, encompassing the whole diabetes care pathway. Consumer engagement, self-management, and empowerment will be major contributing factors in achieving this goal.

Unless we embrace this approach to management of diabetes, health systems in both developed and developing countries will be swamped by the numbers of people with diabetes. This will be associated with the increased direct cost of diabetes, and it also has indirect costs nationally in terms of premature morbidity and impacts on the workforce.

So this brings us to this timely book *Integrated Diabetes Care: A Multidisciplinary Approach*. It addresses integrated care and also the many barriers for improving diabetes care across the globe. So, what do we really need to understand about integrated care and how to overcome these hurdles? This excellent book edited by David Simmons, Helmut Wenzel, and Janice C. Zgibor gives comprehensive coverage of these issues and provides examples of approaches that could improve care while reducing costs. *Integrated Diabetes Care: A Multidisciplinary Approach* collates worldwide evidence of how integrated care works both across disciplines and across organisations to improve diabetes care.

The integrated approach prioritises the needs of the individual and recognises the many interactions required between the person with diabetes, the range of health professionals needed for their care, and the various levels of the health system. Diabetes is for life, and this book provides guidance for all those involved in diabetes to bring seamless and optimal care for the person with diabetes.

Professor Paul Zimmet, AO MD PhD FRACP FRCP (London) FTSE
Honoris Causa Doctoris (Complutense University, Madrid)
Doctor of Laws Honoris Causa (Monash University, Melbourne)
Doctor Philosophiae Honoris Causa (Tel Aviv University, Tel Aviv)
Professor, Department of Medicine, Monash University
Honorary President of International Diabetes Federation
Formerly Director, International Diabetes Institute, and Director Emeritus,
Baker IDI Heart

Preface

Why a book on integrated diabetes care? Over the last 20–30 years, there have been a plethora of projects and policies putatively designed to bring together all the different health workers and health services for defined groups of people with diabetes. Some have sat behind grandiose broader integrated care initiatives. Others have sat within a single health service. Over this time, there have been enormous improvements in the way we can manage type 1 and type 2 diabetes. There has been the growing recognition of the importance of personalised medicine including the ability to diagnose rare forms of diabetes (such as monogenic diabetes). Behind this diabetes clinical evolution has been, perhaps, an even greater revolution in the work behind the scenes, especially in the way we handle health data and clinical governance, and in our understanding that there is a chasm behind what we can do and what is actually happening. Why is care not as good as we know it can be? Why do avoidable complications still happen? It is clear that there is much more that can be done to facilitate and enable those with diabetes: right care, right time, and right place.

This book came about to provide greater depth than possible in academic publications on what worked and what did not from the clinicians' and developers' points of view. This in turn can inform future developers, managers, and clinicians on how best to structure their next attempt to move towards a more united and seamless approach to the way that those with diabetes receive their care.

Sydney, Australia — David Simmons
Konstanz, Germany — Helmut Wenzel
Tampa, FL, USA — Janice C. Zgibor

Contents

Contributors

Heather Bird Diabetes UK, London, UK

Thomas Bodenheimer Department of Family and Community Medicine, University of California, San Francisco School of Medicine and San Francisco General Hospital, San Francisco, CA, USA

Michael A.J. Brown Centre for Diabetes and Endocrinology (Pty) Ltd, Johannesburg, South Africa

Juliana C.N. Chan Department of Medicine and Therapeutics, The Chinese University of Hong Kong, Hong Kong, China

Hong Kong Institute of Diabetes and Obesity, The Chinese University of Hong Kong, Hong Kong, China

International Diabetes Centre of Education, The Chinese University of Hong Kong, Prince of Wales Hospital, Satin, Hong Kong, China

Harold W. de Valk Internist-endocrinologist, Department of Internal Medicine, University Medical Center Utrecht, Utrecht, The Netherlands

Larry A. Distiller Centre for Diabetes and Endocrinology (Pty) Ltd, Johannesburg, South Africa

Anne Dornhorst Department of Diabetes and Endocrinology, Imperial College Healthcare NHS Trust, Hammersmith Hospital, London, UK

Helmut Hildebrandt OptiMedis AG, Hamburg, Germany

Stefan Jansson Department of Family Medicine, Brickebacken Primary Health Care Center, Örebro, Sweden

Elisa A.M. Kern Gesundes Kinzigtal GmbH, Haslach, Germany

Paromita King Department of Diabetes and Endocrinology, Medical Specialties, Derby Teaching Hospitals NHS Foundation Trust, Royal Derby Hospital, Derby, UK

Sudhesh Kumar Warwick Medical School, The University of Warwick, Coventry, UK

University Hospitals Coventry and Warwickshire NHS Trust, Coventry, UK

Mona Landin-Olsson Department of Endocrinology, Lund University Hospital, Lund, Sweden

Caroline Lang Department of Internal Medicine, Prevention and Care of Diabetes, University Hospital Carl Gustav Carus at the Technische Universität, Dresden, Dresden, Germany

Joseph Paul O'Hare Warwick Medical School, The University of Warwick, Coventry, UK

University Hospitals Coventry and Warwickshire NHS Trust, Coventry, UK

Vinod Patel George Eliot Hospital NHS Trust, Coventry, UK

Warwick Medical School, The University of Warwick, Coventry, UK

Peter Perreiah Sapience Technologies, Alpharetta, GA, USA

R. Harsha Rao VAPHS-UD, University Drive, Pittsburgh, PA, USA

Ponnusamy Saravanan George Eliot Hospital NHS Trust, Coventry, UK

Warwick Medical School, The University of Warwick, Coventry, UK

University Hospitals Coventry and Warwickshire NHS Trust, Coventry, UK

Timo Schulte OptiMedis AG, Hamburg, Germany

Linda Siminerio Division of Endocrinology, School of Medicine, University of Pittsburgh, Pittsburgh, PA, USA

David Simmons School of Medicine, Western Sydney University, Sydney, NSW, Australia

Francis X. Solano Community Medicine Inc, University of Pittsburgh Medical Center, Pittsburgh, PA, USA

Physician Services Division, University of Pittsburgh Medical Center, Pittsburgh, PA, USA

Division of General Internal Medicine, School of Medicine, University of Pittsburgh, Pittsburgh, PA, USA

David H. Thom Department of Family and Community Medicine, University of California, San Francisco School of Medicine and San Francisco General Hospital, San Francisco, CA, USA

Bridget Turner Diabetes UK, London, UK

Helmut Wenzel Health Economist, Konstanz, Germany

Roseanne O. Yeung Department of Medicine, Division of Endocrinology, University of Alberta, Edmonton, Alberta, Canada

Hong Kong Institute of Diabetes and Obesity, The Chinese University of Hong Kong, Hong Kong, China

Junmei Yin Department of Medicine and Therapeutics, The Chinese University of Hong Kong, Hong Kong, China

Dahai Yu Research Institute for Primary Care and Health Sciences, Keele University, Newcastle Under Lyme, UK

Janice C. Zgibor Department of Epidemiology and Biostatistics, College of Public Health, University of South Florida, Tampa, FL, USA

An Introduction to Integrated Care and Diabetes Integrated Care

1

Helmut Wenzel and David Simmons

Background

Modern health care is a wonderful thing. We have medications, investigations, procedures, equipment and health-care approaches that can do more than ever before. Half of the "years of life" gained 1950–1995 were due to medical [1] intervention, and benefits have continued further over the last two decades. However, the knowledge and expertise required to provide these interventions is so vast, that it requires different degrees of specialisation, increasingly grouped into a range of "services." Efficiencies have been introduced through the centralisation of the more expensive equipment and expertise into dedicated buildings including hospitals. Access to such facilities has been limited through a range of mechanisms including out of pocket expense, distance, patient knowledge, capacity/waiting times and a variety of gatekeeper functions (e.g., primary care in the UK NHS). The way such services have developed, and the mechanisms for health-care access, has varied between nations, but it is clear that in general, wherever you are in the world, service delivery is now fragmented [2]. Such fragmentation is a manifestation of organisational and financial barriers, which divide providers at the boundaries of primary and secondary care, physical and mental health care, and between health and social care. Diverse specific organisational and professional cultures, and differences in terms of governance and accountability also contribute to this fragmentation [2].

Evaluation demonstrates suboptimal care processes resulting in both poorer health and financial outcomes. Many of these deficiencies are caused by organisational problems (barriers, silo thinking, accountability for budgets) and are often to the detriment of all of those involved: patients, providers and funders – in extreme cases – leading to lose-lose-lose-situations [3]. Patients observe "missing coordination," "random care," "chaotic care" – or even "negative coordination" and state:

> *We are sick of falling through gaps. We are tired of organisational barriers and boundaries that delay or prevent our access to care. We do not accept being discharged from a service into a void. We want services to be seamless and care to be continuous.* [4, p. 11]

"Negative coordination" is characterised by participants caring solely for their own interests. They do not see the common goal and they do not work jointly for an optimal solution. Negative coordination can result from specialisation and a lack of orientation across the broader population, its health and social care and to some extent

H. Wenzel (✉)
Health Economist, Konstanz, Germany
e-mail: hkwen@aol.com

D. Simmons
School of Medicine, Western Sydney University, Sydney, NSW, Australia
e-mail: Da.simmons@westernsydney.edu.au

D. Simmons et al. (eds.), *Integrated Diabetes Care*, DOI 10.1007/978-3-319-13389-8_1

reflects a problem with the division of labour. One important aspect, particularly within a competitive health economy, that must not be underestimated, is an unfavourable organisational culture [5]. Negative Coordination only allows policy changes that are pareto-superior to the status quo, i.e., there will be no losers. If disadvantages occur, the existence of negative coordination prevents new policies as long as there are still parties who are better off without the changes [6]. Some call it "coordination by avoidance," a kind of self-protection where conflicting rules and excessive regulation exists [7]. Negative coordination exists in vertical and horizontal structures and it applies to both civil society and governmental units [8].

Politicians and governments criticise the widening gap between expenditure and available financial resources. The discussions centre on expenditure drivers like the ageing population and medical progress. Governments try to close the gap between rapidly increasing demand and slower growth in financing opportunities, by applying four classical administrative measures:

1. cutting down expenditure (various budgets),
2. excluding services from being reimbursed (a problem for patients), thus increasing the size of the patient's contribution, i.e., out-of-pocket payments,
3. by raising the contribution fees from the insured, and
4. last but not least, by bargaining with providers and forcing the setting of fixed prices.

Of course, there is some variation, depending on the health-care model – tax financed vs contribution fee financed. Rationing of services is also an option. This situation has been aggravated by the recent so-called global financial crisis. However, it is unlikely that there will be a "change for the better" in the budgeting and global economic situations in the near future. From an economic viewpoint the efficient use of resources has to be a major focus for any future health system changes [9].

Of course, the rising burden of chronic disease is about the lives of millions of people, not just an economic or financial issue. Such a large number of people needing complex care calls for appropriate delivery systems that bring together professionals and skills from both social and health-care sectors. There is some evidence that integrated care does improve the quality of patient care and leads to improved health or patient satisfaction [10, 11], but evidence of economic benefits remain an issue for further research [10].

Failure to improve integration and coordination of services along a "care continuum" can result in suboptimal outcomes (health and cost), such as potentially preventable hospitalisation, avoidable death, medication errors and adverse drug events [3, 12, 13]. Clearly, if our health systems are currently fragmented, and, as a result, are not delivering the best care using the resources that are available, care processes and the associated organisational principles of care need to be reappraised and restructured. A broad spectrum of instruments and organisational options are now available for application to facilitate care provision [14] in a more integrated way, but first-what is "integrated care"?

What Is Integrated Care?

Integrated care may be described best by "... *involves the provision of seamless, effective and efficient care that responds to all of a person's health needs, across physical, social and mental health, in partnership with the individual, their carers and family*" [15, p. 1]. Or, like the WHO put it another way: *"The organization and management of health services so that people get the care they need, when they need it, in ways that are user friendly, achieve the desired results and provide value for money"*[10, p. 5].

Nolte et al. [10] point out that "integrated care" is often used in the context with concepts or terms like "case management", "care coordination," "collaborative care" or combinations of these. However, "Integrated health services" means different things to different people [16]. From the patient's perspective it is primarily "continuity of care." In a survey with 254 health expert and 670 patients Juhnke et al. [17] analysed the needs and expectations with regard to patient-centred health care (coordinated care). Coordinated care is made up by seven dimensions: access, data and information, service and infrastructure, professional care, interpersonal care, individualised care, continuity and coordination. For diabetic patients "continuity of care" is a comprehensive and complex concept. The abstract notion comprises five components: access to services, interactions with physician, and interactions with other health-care providers, personal self-responsibility, and communication. This concept exceeds what is traditionally associated with continuity of care and attaches particular importance to personal self-responsibility [18], possibly through patient education and self-management approaches. For example, Haggerty et al. [16] identify three types of continuity: information continuity, management continuity and relation continuity.

From the point of view of providers "provider connectedness" has to be added to Haggerty's concept. Providers felt that the communication was more effective, and it was easier to provide continuity of care, when they already had relationships with other providers [19]. Operationalisation and implementation of continuity of care solutions should therefore consider all perspectives, exploring how these come together to enhance the patient-centredness of care [20].

Typology of Integrated Care Approaches

There have been many proposals on how to structure the various concepts of integrated care. Schrijvers et al. [21] report on classifications according to "target groups" or field of integrated care. However, most of the integrated care literature distinguishes between different ways and grades of working together, depicting a cooperation scale, which is based on three attributes like *autonomy*, *coordination* and *integration*. Autonomy represents the one end of the scale with least cooperation, integration the end with the highest degree of working together. Coordination is somewhat in between and stands for partial cooperation [22]. Nolte et al. [10] report on a more extended analytical grid. Looking closer at possible attributes of the term "integration," three dimensions have been analysed: *the type, the breadth (horizontal, vertical integration), the degree (from full integration to collaboration.), and the process of integration.* For further categorising of the integrated diabetes care projects described in this book, we will apply this typology.

The dimension "types of integration" can be subdivided even further into four categories: Functional, organisational, professional, and clinical [23]. Functional integration means that support functions, such as financial management, information management, strategic planning and human resource management are the target area. "Organisational integration" has to do with the creation of new entities, e.g., mergers or joint ventures, either by the creation of a new organisation or by absorption by one of the others, contracting issues, and creation of networks (aiming at the integration of planning and delivery of services). "Professional integration" deals with strategic alliances of health-care professionals within or between institutions or contracting. "Clinical integration" deals with the level "to which patient care services are coordinated across the various personnel, functions, activities and operating units of a system" [23, p. 71]. With "breadth of integration" a further distinction is made between integration on the same level, e.g., general practices and community care (horizontal integration), and integration at different levels, e.g., primary care, secondary care and tertiary care (vertical integration) [10, 22].

Integrated care is often described as a continuum [10, 24], actually depicting the degree of integration. This degree can range from linkage, to coordination and integration [10], or segregation (absence of any cooperation) to full integration [25], in which the integrated organisation is responsible for the full continuum of care, including funding, to collaboration, which describes separate structures in which organisations retain their own service responsibility and funding criteria [10]. Following Nolte et al. [10] "linkage" works on the basis of the existing separate structures of health and social services systems. See Fig. 1.1. The corresponding organisations preserve their own service responsibilities, way of funding and operating rules. In the case of "coordination," additional structures and processes are added, such as routinely shared information and discharge planning. To coordinate care across the sectors, case management can be implemented. With "full integration" the responsibility for the integrated organisation lies in one place. This applies to all services, resources and funding. This may be incorporated in one managed structure or through contractual agreements between different organisations. Furthermore, this classification of integration degree can be expanded by introducing a second dimension, i.e., the user needs. User need should be defined by criteria, like stability and severity of condition, duration of illness (chronic condition), service needed and capacity for self-direction (autonomy). Accordingly, a low level of need will not require a fully integrated system, then [10, 24].

Kaiser Permanente is a good example of what has been described as a "fully integrated system." According to Goodwin et al. [26] a set of key elements were determined that can characterise such fully integrated delivery systems. This includes *"a population defined by enrolment, contractual responsibility for a defined package of comprehensive healthcare services, financing on the basis of pooling multiple funding streams, a 'closed' network* (i.e., *a selected group of contracted and/or salaried providers), emphasis on primary care and non-institutional services, use of micromanagement techniques to ensure appropriate quality of care and to control costs* (e.g., *utilization review, disease management) and multidisciplinary teams working across the network with joint clinical responsibility for outcomes"* [23, p. 73]. A key element of Kaiser Permanente's approach to chronic care is the categorisation of their chronically ill patients into three groups based on their degree of need [23, p. 73].

Strategies for Successful Implementation

If one asks staff members of care institutions about integrated care and potential hurdles they often mention competing organisational objectives and different employment terms that constitute major barriers to effective care, and as

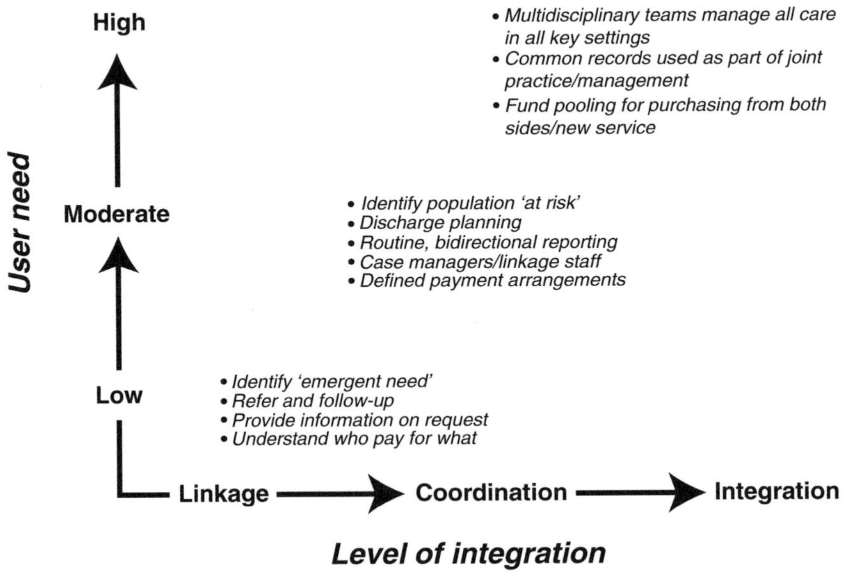

Fig. 1.1 Levels of integration and user needs as defined by Nolte (Used with permission from Nolte and McKee [23])

Britnell states, point to incoherent policy requirements (such as the requirements of collaboration and competition), and leaves the impression that some policy initiatives focus on the means and not the end [27]. This unbalanced attitude towards collaboration and competition was also confirmed in a seminar of The Nuffield Trust, where participants complained that *"policy-makers had given more attention to the development of competition in the NHS than the promotion of collaboration and integration"* [28, p. 2]. This looks very much like "negative coordination" and its related consequences. It would be interesting to further analyse the underlying politics.

With a view to international experiences and research one can identify about ten core ingredients which decide on successful integration efforts [27]: *"a defined and registered population; aligned incentives; shared and joint accountability; seamless IT and information systems; shared clinical protocols and pathways; collaboration between clinicians and managers; authentic patient involvement; relentless focus on quality improvement systems; collaborative organisational cultures; and inspired leadership that endures and is not continually reorganised"* [27, p. 2]. Shortell et al. [29] discuss various organisational models of integrated care delivery. Independent of which particular model is in the focus, information systems are in a central position, as they provide data across the whole care system.

Kodner et al. [30] identified five areas to work on when planning and implementing integrated care projects: funding, administrative, organisational, service delivery, and clinical [31]. Table 1.1 gives an overview. Without consideration of these interdependent areas a successful implementation might fail due to the barriers and bottlenecks which often occur at various levels. The key issues are:

Table 1.1 Continuum of integrated care strategies

Funding:
Pooling of funds (at various levels)
Prepaid capitation (at various levels)
Administrative:
Consolidation/decentralisation of responsibilities/ functions
Intersectional planning
Needs assessment/allocation chain
Joint purchasing or commissioning
Organisational:
Collocation of services
Discharge and transfer agreements
Inter-agency planning and/or budgeting
Service affiliation or contracting
Jointly managed programmes or services
Strategic alliances or care networks
Consolidation, common ownership or merger
Service delivery:
Joint training
Centralised information, referral and intake
Case/care management
Multidisciplinary/interdisciplinary teamwork
Around-the-clock (on-call) coverage
Integrated information systems
Clinical:
Standard diagnostic criteria (e.g., DSM IV)
Uniform, comprehensive assessment procedures
Joint care planning
Shared clinical record(s)
Continuous patient monitoring
Common decision support tools (i.e., practice guidelines and protocols)
Regular patient/family contact and ongoing support

From Open Access Source: Kodner and Spreeuwenberg [30]. Originally adapted from Kodner and Kyriacou [42] and Leutz [24]

- *"Funding: More often than not, form follows financing [sic: not function]. This means that the division, structure and flow of funds for health and social care and related services can affect virtually all aspects of integrated care. The structure, segregation of funds and the flow of money.*
- *Administrative: The manner in which government regulatory and administrative functions are structured and devolved can help eliminate program complexities, streamline eligibility and access, and better manage system resources.*
- *Organisational: Networking, both vertically and horizontally and through formal or informal means, is a major method to improve how*

organisations work together. Collaboration is another important strategy. Joint working relationships within and between agencies in the health and social care sectors can optimise resources, facilitate overall efficiency, and enhance the capacity for 'seamless care,' that is, the smooth and uninterrupted provision of necessary care.

- *Service delivery: The mode of service delivery and management – how staff are trained, perform their responsibilities and tasks, work together, and relate to patients and family carers and their needs – have a major impact on a number of critical variables in integrated care. Such variables include service access, availability and flexibility, continuity and co-ordination of care, consumer satisfaction, and quality and cost outcomes; and,*
- *Clinical: Shared understanding of patient needs, common professional language and criteria, the use of specific, agreed-upon practices and standards throughout the lifecycle of a particular disease or condition, and the maintenance of ongoing patient-provider communication and feedback are essential quality ingredients in integrated care"* [32, p. 4].

Objectives, Expectations, and Evidence

Patients expect seamless care without gaps, and a high quality of care, which is described by access to services, interactions with physician/health-care professional, and interactions with other health-care providers, personal self-responsibility, and communication. Providers expect "provider connectedness." Health insurance managers want expenditure savings due to reduction of redundancies in care, and governments and politicians see an appropriate way of closing the gap between rising expenditures and decreasing financial options. Berwick et al. [33] describe the political position as pursuing simultaneously the triple aim of improving the experience of care, improving the health of populations, and reducing per capita costs of health care. But they also state that the remaining barriers to integrated care are not technical, they are political. Last but not least, staff members hope to improve their job satisfaction.

There is some evidence of a positive impact of integrated care programmes on the quality of patient care [10, 34]. There is also a cautious appraisal that warns that "Even in well-performing care groups, it is likely to take years before cost savings become visible" [35 p. 431]. Based on a literature review from 1996 to 2004 Ouwens et al. [11] found out that integrated care programmes seemed to have positive effects on the quality of care. The most common concepts of integrated care were disease management programmes involving:

- self-management support
- patient education programmes
- Combined with one or more of:
- structured clinical follow-up
- case management
- application of multidisciplinary patient care teams
- multidisciplinary clinical pathways
- Patient feedback, patient reminders
- education for healthcare professionals.

However, disease management programmes focused on approaches that improved the financial balance of the organisation, potentially to the detriment of the patient. In the Netherlands the market power of the care groups, antitrust concerns and possibly limited choices for patients are discussed, since care groups work with preferred providers [36].

Nevertheless, because of the variation in definitions of integrated care programmes and the components used cover a broad spectrum, the results should be interpreted with caution. They also emphasise the relevance of clear and consistent definitions as well as well described interventions in order make reliable comparisons of programmes and to show the efficiency of the integrated care approaches.

Economics and financing issues are important drivers for integrated care approaches [10]. Nevertheless, sound economic evaluations of integrated care approaches are missing. In their systematic review of the effectiveness of integrated care Ouwens et al. [11] could report on only seven (about 54 %) reviews which had included an economic analysis. Four of them showed financial advantages. In their study Powell Davies et al. [34] found that less than 20 % of studies that measured economic outcomes found a significant positive result. Similarly, de Bruin et al. [37] evaluated the impact of disease management programmes on health-care expenditures for patients with diabetes, depression, heart failure or chronic obstructive pulmonary disease (COPD). Thirteen studies of 21 showed cost savings, but the results were not statistically significant, or not actually tested for significance. However, one must bear in mind that important variation was found between the studies with respect to study design, number and combination of components of disease management programmes, interventions within components, and characteristics of economic evaluations [37].

Central criticism comes from Evers [38] who criticises the methods of the available studies. Instead of measuring the relative efficiency (using cost-effectiveness, cost-utility) he wants to see the evidence in terms of absolute efficiency (cost-benefit analyses). Only in the case of absolute efficiency can outcomes be interpreted as if in a business investment calculation. So, well-designed economic evaluation studies of integrated care approaches are needed, in particular in order to support decision-making on the long-term financing of these programmes [30, 39]. Savings from integrated care are only a "hope" as long as there is no carefully designed economic analysis with a kind of full-cost accounting.

The Objectives of Integrated Diabetes Care

Diabetes is a condition in which longstanding hyperglycaemia damages arteries (causing macrovascular, e.g., ischaemic heart, peripheral and cerebrovascular disease, and microvascular disease, e.g., retinopathy, nephropathy), peripheral nerves (causing neuropathy), and other structures such as skin (causing cheiroarthropathy) and the lens (causing cataracts). Different degrees of macrovascular, neuropathic and cutaneous complications lead to the "diabetic foot." A proportion of patients, particularly with type 2 diabetes have metabolic syndrome including central adiposity, dyslipidaemia, hypertension and non alcoholic fatty liver disease. Glucose management can have severe side effects, particularly hypoglycaemia and weight gain. Under-treatment is not only associated with long term complications but infections, vascular events and increased hospitalisation. Absence of treatment in type 1 diabetes can rapidly lead to diabetic keto-acidosis and death. Indeed, a common feature between type 1 and type 2 diabetes is substantial premature mortality, significantly reduced quality of life [40] and increased co-morbid depression. Diabetes doubles the risk for depression, and on the other hand, depression may increase the risk for hyperglycaemia and finally for complications of diabetes [41]. Essentially, diabetes affects every part of the body once complications set in, and the crux of diabetes management is to normalise (as much as possible) the blood glucose and manage any associated risk factors, thereby preventing complications and maintaining the highest quality of life. On the whole, metabolic syndrome responds to oral medications (with lifestyle approaches as a very important component of management). However, glucose management requires minute by minute, day by day management addressing the complexity of diabetes, including clinical and behavioural issues. While other conditions also have the patient as therapist, diabetes requires a fully empowered patient with all of the skills, knowledge and motivation every hour of the waking day. A patient that is fully engaged in self-management, and has support systems, is empowered to manage their diabetes and will likely experience better outcomes compared with those who do not have access to this support. Given the complexity of diabetes treatment and self-management, integrated systems should include a means for diabetes self-management education and support over the life-course of diabetes. Additionally, attention to the psychosocial aspects of diabetes is critically important to consider. Unfortunately, as discussed above, modern health systems do not work in this way for a variety of reasons. As integrated systems become more widespread, consideration of patient-centred care from a variety of sources should be included. Furthermore, in diabetes, the boundaries between primary care and secondary care are blurred. Diabetes specialist services, although secondary care, can provide primary care, and there are GPs, diabetes educators, and other ancillary providers who can provide a level of specialist care. In view of this, another more practical definition of horizontal integration can be "articulation of activities under the same or separate organisations working with different policies/structures" and of vertical integration "articulation of activities under the same or separate organisations working within the same policies/structures."

This book describes different approaches to integrating diabetes care and their outcomes from a range of perspectives including that of a patient organisation (Diabetes UK). The chapters cover different health systems from taxpayer funded and free at the point of care (the United Kingdom National Health Service: three different approaches), Sweden, and United States Veterans, to a range of insurance based systems in the United States (University and Health Management Organisation), Germany, South Africa, and the Netherlands. The final chapter pulls together the common and differing themes to paint a picture of how perhaps, the ideal diabetes integrated care system should be organised.

References

1. Bunker JP. Medicine matters after all. J R Coll Physicians Lond. 1995;29(2):105–12.
2. Glasby J, Dickinson H, Peck E. Guest editorial: partnership working in health and social care. Health Soc Care Community. 2006;14(5):373–4.
3. Simmons D, Wenzel H. Diabetes inpatients: a case of lose, lose, lose. Is it time to use a "diabetes-attributable hospitalization cost" to assess the impact of diabetes? Diabet Med. 2011;28(9):1123–30.
4. National Collaboration for Integrated Care and Support. Integrated care and support: our shared commitment. London: Department of Health; 2013.
5. N.N. Negative Koordination. n.d. Available from: http://www.olev.de/k/koordination.htm
6. Scharpf FW. Coordination in hierarchies and networks. In: Scharpf F, editor. Games in hierarchies and networks. Frankfurt a.M.: Campus-Verl.; 1993: 125–65.
7. Holten Møller NL, Dourish P. Coordination by avoidance: bringing things together and keeping them apart across hospital departments. Proceedings of the 16th ACM international conference on supporting group work. 2010:9.
8. Zingerli C, Bisang K, Zimmermann W. Towards policy integration: experiences with intersectoral coordination in international and national forest policy. Berlin Conference 2004 on the human dimension of global environmental change "Greening of Policies – Interlinkages and Policy Integration". Berlin; 2004.
9. Wenzel H. N 2.10 The global financial crisis and health. South East Eur J Pub Health Spec. vol 2015. A global public health curriculum 1st version. 2015:92–9.
10. Nolte E, Pitchforth E. What is the evidence on the economic impacts of integrated care? Copenhagen World Health Org. 2014;11:478–88.
11. Ouwens M, Wollersheim H, Hermens R, Hulscher M, Grol R. Integrated care programmes for chronically ill patients: a review of systematic reviews. Int J Qual Health Care. 2005;17(2):141–6.
12. Vogeli C, Shields AE, Lee TA, Gibson TB, Marder WD, Weiss KB, et al. Multiple chronic conditions: prevalence, health consequences, and implications for quality, care management, and costs. J Gen Intern Med. 2007;22 Suppl 3:391–5.
13. Committee on Quality of HealthCare in America IoM. Crossing the quality chasm: a new health system for the 21st century. Summary. Washington, DC: National Academy Press; 2001.
14. Laplante A. Integrated systems improve medical care, control costs, according to Enthoven. Stanford report. 26 Oct 2005.
15. New South Wales Government. Info summary – integrated care. n.d.
16. Haggerty JL, Reid RJ, Freeman GK, Starfield BH, Adair CE, McKendry R. Continuity of care: a multidisciplinary review. BMJ. 2003;327(7425):1219–21.
17. Juhnke C, Mühlbacher AC. Patient-centredness in integrated healthcare delivery systems – needs, expectations and priorities for organised healthcare systems. Int J Integr Care. 2013;13(28):e051.
18. Nair KM, Dolovich LR, Ciliska DK, Lee HN. The perception of continuity of care from the perspective of patients with diabetes. Fam Med. 2005;37(2):118–24.
19. Price M, Lau FY. Provider connectedness and communication patterns: extending continuity of care in

the context of the circle of care. BMC Health Serv Res. 2013;13:309.
20. Gulliford M, Naithani S, Morgan M. What is "continuity of care"? J Health Serv Res Policy. 2006;11(4):248–50.
21. Schrijvers G, Goodwin N. Looking back whilst moving forward: observations on the science and application of integrated care over the past 10 years and predictions for what the next 10 years may hold. Int J Integr Care. 2010;10:e057.
22. Gröne O, Garcia-Barbero M. Trends in integrated care – reflections on conceptual issues Copenhagen: World Health Organization, Regional Office for Europe. 2002.
23. Nolte E, McKee M. Integration and chronic care: a review. In: Nolte E, McKee M, editors. Caring for people with chronic conditions: a health system perspective. Maidenhead: Open University Press; 2008. p. 1. online resource (xxi, 259).
24. Leutz WN. Five laws for integrating medical and social services: lessons from the United States and the United Kingdom. Milbank Q. 1999;77(1):77–110. iv–v.
25. Ahgren B, Axelsson R. Evaluating integrated health care: a model for measurement. Int J Integr Care. 2005;5:e01. discussion e3, e9.
26. Goodwin N, Peck E, Freeman T, Posaner R. Managing across diverse networks of care: lessons from other sectors London: report to the National Co-ordinating Centre for NHS Service Delivery and Organisation R & D (NCCSDO). 2004.
27. Britnell M. Patients need to be the focus of integrated care. Healthcare network [internet]. 2013. Available from: http://www.theguardian.com/healthcare-network/2013/jun/04/patients-need-to-be-focus-of-integrated-care
28. Ham C, Smith J. Removing the policy barriers to integrated care in England the Nutfield trust for research and policy studies in health services – briefing. The Nuffield Trust for Research and Policy Studies in Health Services. 2010.
29. Shortell SM, Gillies RR, Anderson DA. The new world of managed care: creating organized delivery systems. Health Aff. 1994;13(5):46–64.
30. Kodner DL, Spreeuwenberg C. Integrated care: meaning, logic, applications, and implications – a discussion paper. Int J Integr Care. 2002;2:e12.
31. Leichsenring K. Developing integrated health and social care services for older persons in Europe. Int J Integr Care. 2004;4:e10.
32. Kodner D. All together now: a conceptual exploration of integrated care. Healthc Q. 2009;13(sp):6–15.
33. Berwick DM, Nolan TW, Whittington J. The triple aim: care, health, and cost. Health Aff (Millwood). 2008;27(3):759–69.
34. Powell Davies G, Harris M, Perkins D, Roland M, Williams A, Larsen K, et al. Coordination of care within primary health care and within other sectors: a systematic review. Research Centre for Primary Health Care and Equity, School of Public Health and Community Medicine, UNSW, 2006.
35. de Bakker DH, Struijs JN, Baan CB, Raams J, Wildt J-E, Vrijhoef HJM, et al. Early results from adoption of bundled payment for diabetes care in the Netherlands show improvement in care coordination. Health Aff (Project Hope). 2012;31(2):426–33.
36. Struijs JN, Baan CA. Integrating care through bundled payments – lessons from The Netherlands. N Engl J Med. 2011;364(11):990–1.
37. de Bruin SR, Heijink R, Lemmens LC, Struijs JN, Baan CA. Impact of disease management programs on healthcare expenditures for patients with diabetes, depression, heart failure or chronic obstructive pulmonary disease: a systematic review of the literature. Health Policy. 2011;101(2):105–21.
38. Evers SM. Value of integrated care: revival of the monetary valuation of health care benefits. Int J Integr Care. 2010;10:e045.
39. Vondeling H. Economic evaluation of integrated care: an introduction. Int J Integr Care. 2004;4:e20.
40. International Diabetes Federation. IDF diabetes atlas. 6th ed. Brussels: International Diabetes Federation; 2013. Available from: www.idf.org/diabetesatlas.
41. Roy T, Lloyd CE. Epidemiology of depression and diabetes: a systematic review. J Affect Disord. 2012;142:S8–21.
42. Kodner DL, Kyriacou CK. Fully integrated care for frail elderly: two American models. Int J Integr Care. 2000;1:e08.

2 Integrating Outpatient Care the Toyota Way: An Individualized Multidisciplinary Team-Care Model for Diabetes Care Delivery

R. Harsha Rao and Peter Perreiah

Introduction

Diabetes mellitus poses unique challenges for both providers and patients – challenges that are arguably more problematic to overcome than those posed by other chronic diseases.

The unique challenge to providers is to satisfy two specific demands in diabetes care. The first is to *anticipate and recognize the onset of complications through comprehensive diabetes care*, which demands meticulous attention to a large number of process-of-care measures at each visit. The second, arguably greater challenge for providers is to *forestall the development of complications through effective diabetes care*, which demands mastery over many different skills in a variety of distinct fields in order to achieve performance goals covering multiple facets of management. Individually and collectively, these dual challenges constitute a virtually unsustainable burden for providers. That is because (a) completing all the mandated process measures for *comprehensive care* requires far more time than is traditionally available in a single patient visit; and (b) most providers do not themselves possess skills in all the ancillary disciplines essential for *effective care*, such as Diabetes Self-Management Education (DSME) or Medical Nutrition Therapy (MNT).

Diabetes presents patients with similarly unique dual challenges in mastering diabetes self-management with self-awareness, self-empowerment and self-confidence. *Comprehensive Diabetes Self-Management* demands the acquisition of a variety of skills in order to fulfil a multitude of tasks in many different areas of daily life. *Effective Diabetes Self-Management*, on the other hand, demands constant vigilance, consistent discipline and persistent attention over a lifetime, without respite, to nutritional self-discipline, monitoring blood glucose levels, and adherence to antidiabetic medication use. Together, they constitute a burden that most patients find difficult to sustain even with expert assistance, and all-but-impossible without it.

Not surprisingly, achieving successful and sustained self-management remains just as elusive for patients as delivering comprehensive and effective care is for many providers. National Health and Nutrition Examination Surveys (NHANES) show that approximately half of diabetic patients in the U.S. fail to reach goals in each of the three major performance (outcome)

R.H. Rao (✉)
VAPHS-UD, University Drive, Room7W-109, Pittsburgh, PA 15240 USA
e-mail: r.rao@va.gov

P. Perreiah
Sapience Technologies, Alpharetta, GA, USA
e-mail: Plp4consult@gmail.com

D. Simmons et al. (eds.), *Integrated Diabetes Care*, DOI 10.1007/978-3-319-13389-8_2

measures in diabetes care (A1c <7 %, BP <130/80, and LDL <100 mg/dl) [1, 2]. Those statistics are disappointing in themselves, given that the development of diabetic complications is closely linked to a failure to attain and maintain each of those three goals. It is even more troubling that just ~19 % of patients are successful in achieving all three goals, which is the hallmark of effective care (i.e., care that forestalls complications).

The inherent complexity of delivering comprehensive and effective diabetes care is not in doubt, but the fact that effective diabetes care remains an exercise in futility in ~80 % of patients suggests that factors other than complexity may be at work. One major contributor, according to Phillips et al, is "Clinical Inertia," which they define as "recognition of the problem, but a failure to act" [3]. Although the term might appear self-explanatory, the authors make it a point to restrict its application to conditions like diabetes, hypertension and hyperlipidemia, for which "goals for management are well defined, effective therapies are widely available, and practice guidelines for each of these diseases have been disseminated extensively." These criteria explicitly exclude a failure to act because the cause or significance of an identified symptom or abnormality is unknown or unclear [3].

A failure to intensify therapy despite clear indication of benefit – the essence of "clinical inertia" – has been ascribed to a widespread tendency of providers to either justify inaction with "soft" reasons (essentially excuses) like "improving control" or "target almost reached" [3], or overestimate the care they provide [4]. According to Philips et al, the root cause is a failure of medical education and training programmes to emphasize the importance of focusing on the achievement of therapeutic goals, or teach practice organization to achieve therapeutic goals [3]. While there is no denying the critical importance of such "provider-driven" factors, attributing a failure to attain therapeutic goals in diabetes to clinical inertia alone runs the risk of oversimplifying a complex problem that may have more than just one layer. The current paradigm of reimbursement for chronic care in the U.S. may be just as culpable as clinical inertia in the furtherance of therapeutic futility, specifically with regard to how that paradigm drives traditional clinical models for diabetes care delivery.

Traditional Clinical Models for Diabetes Care in the US

There are two models currently in use for diabetes care delivery in the US:

1. The "Single Provider-Patient dyad": This model, which is the most widely used method for diabetes care delivery, is predicated on the principle that one provider can cover all aspects of diabetes care and management for a patient with diabetes. The undeniable advantage of this model lies in the intimacy that characterizes one-on-one interactions. Such intimacy becomes the foundation of personalized care that makes it possible to individualize goals selectively and calibrate intensity, depending on patient need. These advantages are offset, however, by the constraints of time-delimited patient visits, which are mandated to meet productivity targets or necessitated by the individual practitioner looking to the bottom line. Such time constraints make it impossible for one provider to cover multiple tasks in a comprehensive manner at any visit, forcing compromises in task selection at any visit. Inevitably patients and providers find themselves prioritizing tasks depending on perceived immediacy and need. These constraints prevent consistent fulfilment of all the process-of-care measures required to detect and prevent complications.

   Another major drawback of the Single Provider-Patient dyad is that most clinical providers cannot fulfil patient needs for integrated care, simply because the skills required for DSME and MNT are outside the domain of most clinical care providers. Even when the importance of these interventions for effective diabetes care is recognized, they require ad hoc referrals to other providers who possess the requisite skill sets. The necessity for such referrals burdens patients with multiple visits, so that their success is subject to the patient determining whether their perceived importance is worth the inconvenience of additional visits. With no assurance of follow-through, comprehensive management becomes hostage to patient discretion.

It is clear, therefore, that the economic costs of additional visits for the patient, provider time constraints and a lack of provider skills in MNT and DSME combine to contribute as much as clinical inertia to the failure of the Single Provider-Patient dyad to deliver comprehensive and effective diabetes care. Care fragmentation with this model is exacerbated further by arcane rules of fee-for-service reimbursement in the US, which disallow reimbursement for some services rendered by more than one provider for the same principal diagnosis (Diabetes, in this case) on the same day (e.g., for Clinical Care and DSME), with the exception of some types of MNT [5, 6]. Since integrated multidisciplinary care, by definition, calls for contemporaneous and synchronized care by more than one provider, each with a different skill set, such care becomes financially unsustainable if only one or two providers (out of three or four) are reimbursed. This is one reason fee-for-service reimbursement can be a prohibitive disincentive to the integration of multidisciplinary care in diabetes.

Another reason is that fee-for-service, the most widespread financial model in U.S. healthcare, adds a layer of particular complexity to chronic disease care. For the most part, fee-for-service reimbursement couples payment to the volume of services provided, not the overall cost or outcomes. Thus, providers are rewarded for increasing volume, which does not necessarily translate into greater value [7]. This model may work for acute care, where treatment is the goal, but not for chronic care, where prevention takes precedence over treatment. Even though reimbursement for chronic care is being increasingly linked to provider performance, diabetes-specific performance is usually measured by global parameters, such as the percentage of all patients above or below some threshold A1c (e.g., <7 % or >9), not from individual patient outcomes. Put another way, at the individual level, the system provides a greater financial reward for treating complications after they occur (downstream revenue generation), rather than preventing them (upstream cost reduction).

The barriers to integrated care delivery in the traditional single patient-provider dyad have led to the development of alternative models for chronic care (including for diabetes) based on the concept of a Patient-Centered Medical Home (PCMH) [8]. At its most fundamental level, the goal of PCMH is to maximize health outcomes by providing comprehensive and continuous medical care led by a healthcare provider through team-based healthcare delivery. The PCMH concept of integrated multidisciplinary care delivery is at the core of the Group Visit model for diabetes.

2. The *Group Visit model*: The inherent inability of the Single Provider-Patient dyad to deliver comprehensive disease management for patients with diabetes has led to the introduction of the Group Visit model to address and overcome the inefficiencies and inadequacies noted above [9]. The Group Visit model is founded on the premise that many facets of diabetes care are repetitive for individual patients and replicative – with relatively small variation – across patients. In this model a group of patients receives serial input from multiple providers covering different prespecified areas in one session. This assures comprehensive coverage of multiple facets of diabetes care (breadth of care) with the added advantage of achieving higher patient throughput (efficiency/volume). The Group model enables multiple providers with different specialized skills to deliver all aspects of diabetes care (MNT and DSME in particular) to a group of patients in a single session. Thus, Group Visits are designed to fulfil – at least in theory – the current definition of Chronic Disease Management (CDM)

as "a group of coherent interventions, designed to prevent or manage one or more chronic conditions using a….systematic and *structured* multidisciplinary approach potentially employing multiple treatment modalities. The goal of *chronic disease prevention and management* is to identify persons with one or more chronic conditions, to promote self-management by patients and to address the illness or conditions *according to disease severity and patient needs and based on the best available evidence*, maximizing clinical effectiveness and efficiency regardless of treatment setting(s) or typical reimbursement patterns. Routine process and outcome measurements should allow feedback to all those involved, as well as to adapt the programme" [10].

The increasing adoption of the Group Visit model in larger healthcare programmes has led to changes in reimbursement rules for Group visits and new billing codes for such visits [6]. This allows for economies of scale that can overcome the fact that per-patient reimbursements for group visits are individually too low to be profitable. Unfortunately, studies show that while the model reliably delivers comprehensive care reflected in *process-of-care* measures (i.e., documentation in identified diabetes care domains), it does not consistently deliver effective care (i.e., achieving BP, lipid or glycaemic goals) [9]. A recent meta-analysis of randomized control trials is more encouraging, with reductions in A1c ~0.5 %, but not blood pressure or cholesterol [11].

The reason why Group Visits fail to consistently achieve performance targets is not clear, but one is left to wonder whether the absence of personalized care might play a role. A key component of CDM, as defined above, is calibration according to disease severity and risk stratification based on patient need. Group visits, by their very nature, are incapable of delivering individualized care calibrated to patient needs and risk stratification. Consequently, a face-to-face visit in a Single Provider-Patient dyad visit, either after the Group Visit, or in a separate visit on another day is required for such calibration and risk stratification.

An additional criticism of the Group Visit model is that achieving the aforementioned economies of scale requires large patient numbers and a significant increase in resource allocation, including-infrastructure changes and manpower commitments. The need for such resources is a stumbling block to the widespread acceptance of this model outside of large organizations like Accountable Care Organizations (ACOs). Recent changes in coding and billing do incentivize ACOs to adopt Group visits for diabetes care. However, such factors provide little incentive for individual practitioners without access to the infrastructure and resources necessary for Group visits. For these reasons the adoption of the Group Visit model remains limited primarily to ACOs.

A Brief Overview of Healthcare Delivery in the VA System

The Veterans Health Administration is in many ways unique (for the U.S.). Run by the Veterans Affairs Department of the Federal Government, it is the largest integrated healthcare system in the U.S., serving 8.76 million Veterans each year through more than 1700 sites of care, including hospitals, community clinics and community living centres, domiciliary units, Vet Centres, and various other facilities [12].

A brief summary of VA healthcare benefits follows for the benefit of readers unfamiliar with the VA's mission and mandate. Even though this summary is excerpted (almost) verbatim from the source document, it must, of necessity, be incomplete, in the interests of brevity. The authors explicitly deny any claim that what follows is a comprehensive or accurate description of the full panoply of federal benefits available to qualifying Veterans. Readers are strongly advised to access the source document from which this summary is excerpted to verify/correct any details that may be vague, incorrect, missing or misleading [12]. The key summary features are:

- *Basic eligibility*: VA healthcare benefits are available to any person who served 24 continuous months or the full period for which he/she was called to active duty in the active military, naval, or air service and who was discharged or released under conditions other than dishonourable. Reservists and National Guard members may also qualify for VA healthcare benefits if they are called to active duty (other than for training only) and complete the full period for which they were called or ordered to active duty by Federal order. This minimum duty requirement may be waived for veterans discharged for hardship, early out or a disability incurred or aggravated in the line of duty.
- *Service connection*: The VA prioritizes healthcare enrolment based on degree of service connected disability, ranging from highest priority (>50 % service connection, Priority Group 1) to lowest (no service connection), and applies geographic mean income threshold tests to further stratify priority in those without service connection (Groups 7–8).
- *Inpatient care*: Copayments for inpatient stays range from zero for the highest priority groups to a maximum of $1216 for inpatient stays up to 90 days for those above the income threshold in the lowest priority group.
- *Copayments for Outpatient Care*: Many Veterans qualify for free healthcare services based on a VA compensable service-connected condition or other qualifying factor, but most are asked to provide a financial assessment to determine if they qualify for free services. Veterans whose income exceeds the established VA Income Thresholds as well as those who choose not to complete the financial assessment must agree to pay required copays to become eligible for VA healthcare services (Primary Care Services: $15; Specialty Care Services: $50). The copay amount is limited to a single charge per visit regardless of the number of healthcare providers seen in a single day, and is based on the highest level of clinical service received. Copays do not apply to outpatient visits solely for preventive screening and/or influenza and pneumococcal vaccinations, or screening for hypertension, hepatitis B, tobacco, alcohol, hyperlipidemia, breast cancer, cervical cancer, Human papillomavirus (HPV), colorectal cancer by faecal occult blood testing, education about the risks and benefits of prostate cancer screening, HIV testing and prevention counselling (including the distribution of condoms), and weight reduction or smoking cessation counselling (individual and group). Laboratory, flat plain film radiology, electrocardiograms, and hospice care and in-home video telehealth are also exempt from copays.
- *Medication Copayments*: While many Veterans are exempt for medication copays, nonservice-connected Veterans in Priority Groups 7 and 8 are charged $9 for each 30-day supply of medication, provided on an outpatient basis for treatment of a nonservice-connected condition. Veterans enrolled in Priority Groups 2 through 6 are charged $8 for each 30-day or less supply of medication; the maximum copay for medications that will be charged in calendar year 2013 is $960 for nonservice-connected medications. Copays apply to prescription and over-the-counter medications, such as aspirin, cough syrup or vitamins, dispensed by a VA pharmacy. Copays are not charged for medical supplies such as syringes or alcohol wipes.
- The preceding paragraphs have been transcribed from the source document (with only minor edits). We add two items to the above that are essential to complete the picture of an integrated healthcare system that has more in common with government-run healthcare systems in other countries (akin to the U.K's NHS), than the indemnity insurance-based healthcare system that predominates in the U.S. The first is that VA employees, including physicians, are either salaried employees of the U.S. government (for the most part) or fee-based contractors compensated by time or patient volume (either way, care decisions are not linked to financial incentives or disincentives). The other is the way in which care is delivered and coordinated within the VA system, with specific relevance to diabetes care

delivery at VAPHS, which we describe briefly in our own words.

- *Primary, Secondary and Tertiary Care Delivery at VAPHS*: The VA system is organized into regional collaboratives called Veterans Integrated Service Networks (or VISNs), usually comprised of one or two tertiary care "Hub" hospitals (the Pittsburgh and Philadelphia VA hospitals are, respectively, the Western and Eastern hubs in VISN4), several feeder "Spoke" hospitals for each hub, which provide both secondary and primary care, and a number of Community Based Outpatient Clinics (CBOCs) devoted to primary care, clustered at varying distances around each spoke and hub hospital, based on geographic location. All patients must have a primary care provider (PCP) who directs and coordinates care, including referrals for specialty care, following the concept of a Patient-Centered Medical Home that emphasizes "care coordination and communication to transform primary care into what patients want it to be" [8]. All documentation is electronic (paperless), through the VA's unique Computerized Patient Record System (CPRS), which allows nationwide access to patient records, regardless of location. Care coordination, with the PCP acting as the gatekeeper, is an integral component of care across the VA, but policies governing how that coordination is achieved are set at the local level, and thus vary by location. At the Pittsburgh VA (VAPHS), all specialty care providers are required to send "Inter-facility Communications" via CPRS to the PCP after any specialty consultation, documenting assessment and management plans (diagnostic and therapeutic).
- Care coordination achieves critical importance for diabetes, in particular, because of the need for management at many different levels and locations. At the most basic level, the symptomatic management of acute hypo- and hyperglycaemia often devolves to the PCP, even when a specialist oversees more advanced strategies for glycaemic management. At another level, the wide variety of chronic complications requires input from many different specialists, whereas hospitalizations for acute emergencies often fall to hospitalists and critical care specialists. Thus, diabetes care is fraught with the potential for sometimes conflicting, even contradictory management strategies, making care coordination mandatory for success. This is an area in which the VA system excels, with its integrated network, common electronic record, and shared responsibility for care.

The Need for a New Model to Deliver Outpatient Diabetes Care

A realization that the traditional Single Provider-Patient dyad used at the Pittsburgh VA was incompatible with delivering both comprehensive and effective diabetes care encouraged us to explore other avenues for diabetes care delivery. We understood, furthermore, that the alternative of Group visits would require major changes to infrastructure that were not practical or financially feasible at our institution. Third, we were emboldened to develop a "third way" by the fact that there would be no financial disincentives to multi-provider visits in an integrated healthcare system like the VA, unlike a fee-for-service system. Lastly, the VA system has the unique ability to integrate and coordinate care across multiple disciplines.

These were the reasons why we explored the feasibility of constructing a chronic disease care model centred on an integrated multidisciplinary team that would deliver diabetes care that was both comprehensive and effective, yet retained the intimacy of the traditional Single Patient-Provider dyad. Critical to the success of that effort was funding through a Physician Champion Award from the Jewish Healthcare Foundation [13], as well as direct advisory guidance during development and implementation from the Pittsburgh Regional Health Initiative (PRHI), one of the nation's first regional collaboratives of medical, business and civic leaders organized to address healthcare safety and quality improvements [14].

We started with the fundamental premise that the model had to satisfy the needs of both comprehensive and effective care without compromising either the personalized one-on-one care of the single patient-provider dyad or the coordinated care of the Group visit model. In other words, the goal was to preserve the advantages of both existing models while eliminating their disadvantages. In order to achieve such a seemingly impossible goal, we turned to industry, specifically the principles of the Toyota Production Systems [15], to develop a model of multidisciplinary outpatient diabetes care that is both comprehensive and effective. In order to understand how concepts developed for industrial manufacturing can be applied to bedside medicine, a brief introduction to the Toyota Way is warranted.

An Introduction to Lean Systems Design

In his book *The Toyota Way*, Jeffery Liker lays out four Core Tenets for achieving efficiency and improving quality based on Toyota's unique management system [15]. These Core Tenets, shown in Fig. 2.1, are (i) a Long-term Philosophy, (ii) the Right Process, (iii) People as Partners, and (iv) Continuous Reflection to Solve Problems. Even though these tenets are principally associated with manufacturing processes, they have been shown by PRHI, a leader in the field of healthcare reform, to hold true for healthcare delivery [16]. Perfecting Patient Care[SM] (or PPC) is PRHI's flagship healthcare process improvement methodology based on the principles of the Toyota Production System. See Fig. 2.2.

Redesigning the Diabetes Clinic at the VA Using Toyota Principles

Our initial purpose in redesigning diabetes management was to simply combine four distinct clinical disciplines in diabetes care (DSME, MNT, Blood Pressure/Lipid Management, and Glycaemic Management) into a single, clinic visit. From such crude and unpolished beginnings – off-handedly referred to in an initial team meeting as "one-stop shopping," our purpose was transformed, thanks to direct engagement by PRHI and funding support from JHF, into a sophisticated application, which we call the "Individualized Multidisciplinary Team-Care Model." The model, as implemented, has a far more ambitious purpose that goes beyond just patient convenience to the delivery of integrated, multidisciplinary care of high quality that not only meets patient needs but achieves better outcomes. (Parenthetically, it may be noted here that our model differs fundamentally from efforts to integrate diabetes care in Health Disparities Collaboratives (HDC) in the US or the Diabetes

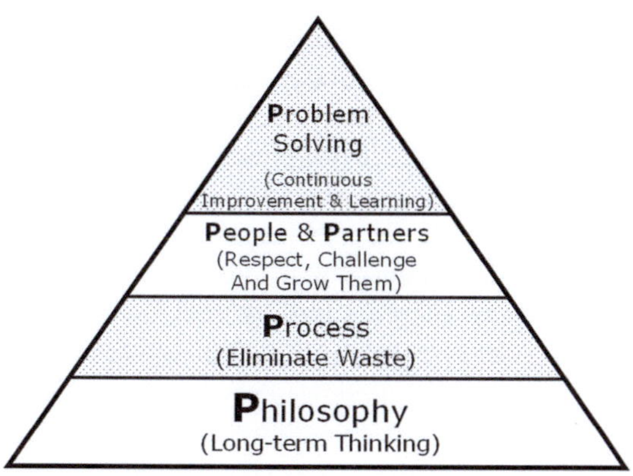

Fig. 2.1 Liker's 4P model (Adapted with permission from Liker [15])

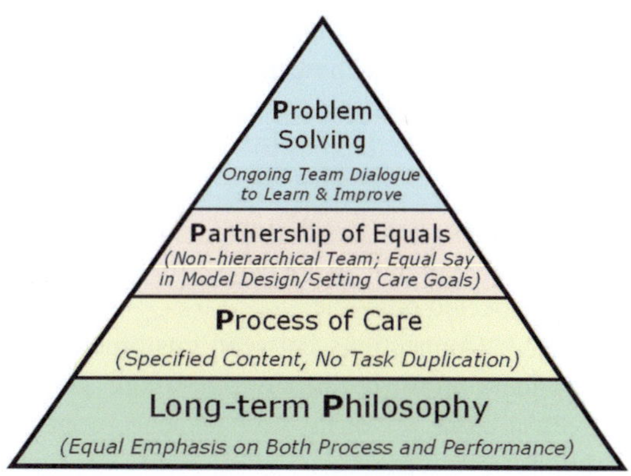

Fig. 2.2 Liker's 4P Tenets adapted to an Individualized Multidisciplinary Team-Care Model for integrated diabetes care delivery

Integrated Care Initiative (DICI) in the U.K) [17, 18]. The "Individualized Multidisciplinary Team-Care Model" integrates multidisciplinary *collaborative outpatient specialist care* (DSME, MNT and clinical) for diabetes in a *tertiary care setting*, whereas HDC and DICI focused on integrating patient education and lifestyle modifications (DSME and MNT) into *primary care* for diabetes in a *community setting* [17, 18].

Our redesign of diabetes care delivery has a direct analogy in manufacturing, where a product manufactured in a traditional "job shop" moves from one functional grouping of machines to another (e.g., stamping, drilling, assembly, painting, etc). Process redesign in manufacturing is often done by regrouping machines around the needs of a product group into a "manufacturing cell." Individual product components enter the cell in a specified order and are rapidly transformed at the cell's stations into a finished product. In industry, transforming traditional production into cellular production often yields dramatic improvements in quality, inventory reduction and efficiency. Distilled to its essence, our redesign of diabetes care delivery is analogous to a cellular manufacturing process, in that it involves the regrouping of specified tasks into "stations" responsible for each care discipline, with the patient moving from one station to the next, accumulating care that is both comprehensive and integrated in the aggregate.

We were guided in our redesign by four principles derived from Spear and Bowen's "Rules in Use" for business, which form the core of PPC^{SM} [19]. Grunden terms these principles "Rules of Work Design that Guide Process Improvement" [16], and describes them as follows:

- *Rule 1*: Activities (work) must be highly specified as to content, sequence, timing, location and expected outcome.
- *Rule 2*: Connections between customers and suppliers must be highly specified, direct, with a clear yes-or-no way to send requests and receive responses.
- *Rule 3*: The pathway for every product and service must be predefined, highly specified, simple, and direct – no loops or forks.
- *Rule 4*: Improvements are made using scientific method, with guidance from a teacher, as close as possible to the work, aiming towards the ideal.

We operationalized these principles in the process of implementing our redesign by, first,

(A) Outlining the actual work required of redesign (in six stages), then,
(B) Constructing and implementing the model and, finally,
(C) Re-evaluating constantly to improve model efficiency and performance (*kaizen*)

(A) **Outline the Actual Work of Redesign for Integrated, Multidisciplinary Care**

This was achieved in six stages, as follows:

1. *Define the Explicit Purpose of Redesign in Relation to Care Delivery*: After extensive discussions, team members reached consensus that any new model for integrating multidisciplinary care in diabetic patients must focus on delivering "*continuing care*," rather than "*initial care*." The reasons for that restriction will become readily apparent when we describe the elements of the model in greater detail, but they can be summarized briefly as follows:
   (a) A focused, time-delimited and structured clinic visit is ideal for implementing and adjusting an established plan of *continuing* care but ill-suited to the elastic and sometimes drawn-out process of evaluating, discussing, and getting patient "buy-in" for an *initial* plan of care and therapeutic strategy, which can vary greatly in both length and complexity, depending on individual patient need.
   (b) An essential precondition, therefore, is to establish an initial plan of care in a traditional Single Provider-Patient dyad visit prior to enrolment in the multidisciplinary clinic for continuing care,
   (c) The only other precondition for enrolment is the patient must have the abil-

ity and motivation to engage in a comprehensive diabetes management strategy, and must possess a basic understanding of DSME and MNT.

2. *Define the Objectives of Care Delivery in Relation to Patient Needs*: The redesign was based on fulfilling specific patient needs, as follows:
   (a) Set individualized clinical goals based on patient need and risk stratification
   (b) Meeting 100 % of all process-of-care measures (HbA_{1c}, LDL, blood pressure, creatinine and urinary microalbumin levels, annual foot and eye exams, and aspirin and statin use/contraindications/alternatives).
   (c) Ordering all necessary lab tests to fulfil process-of-care measures
   (d) Ensuring timely completion (annual at least) of periodic Foot and Eye Exams
   (e) Providing DSME and MNT contemporaneously with clinical care
   (f) Enabling process efficiency to utilize all resources available to care for the assigned patient population.
3. *Document the Current Process for Diabetes Care Delivery*, to identify areas of deficiency/improvement, including:
   (a) A complete description of tasks currently performed by each provider during various patient contacts (i.e., for clinical care, DSME, and MNT)
   (b) The timing and sequence of all provider tasks
   (c) The actual time for completing provider tasks (cycle times) and their variability
   (d) Any shared tasks requiring joint provider participation
   (e) Any potentially duplicative tasks by different providers (i.e., task sharing).
   (f) The current performance relative to patient need and efficiency.
4. *Sort the tasks* as follows:
   (a) Identify essential tasks that must be accomplished in each continuing care visit and which belong in other patient contacts.
   (b) Decide what, if any, remaining tasks can be eliminated or automated.
   (c) Allocate those tasks to team members exclusive to their particular skill set.
   (d) Arrange and assign each team member to "individual stations of care" working in sequence during each visit
   (e) Assess the cycle times for each member of the team to complete their current list of tasks at each station.
   (f) Allocate any tasks that overlap between two or more team members, depending on skill set, with the goal of balancing the work among all stations.
   (g) Continue rearranging station sequencing and/or task lists until all station task lists have about the same cycle time and cycle time variability.
   (h) Set up materials, equipment, information systems and back up assistance to allow providers to accomplish their work without interruption.
5. Run the redesigned process with actual patients:
   (a) Intensively observe whether tasks assigned to each station can be accomplished with high quality and within the targeted cycle times.
   (b) Note any instances where task completion or quality breaks down, and examine individual events for evidence of root causes.
   (c) Measure both quality and efficiency outcomes, based on delivering high quality care that is both comprehensive (i.e., achieves all process-of-care measures) and effective (i.e., meets performance goals for A1c, BP and Lipids) in reducing long term complications.
6. Continuously redesign the process to meet patient, provider and business needs:
   (a) Assess whether patient, provider, and business needs are all met.
   (b) Look to reduce the cycle times of individual tasks.
   (c) Rebalance work between stations.

(d) As the process becomes more stable and efficient, decide by consensus how gains in improvement can be leveraged to enhance care, reduce provider workload, or service more patients.

(e) Call for help outside the team, if additional resources or other enablers are needed to support the process in meeting objectives.

(B) **Construct and Implement a Model of Integrated, Multidisciplinary Care**

The practical aspects of implementing our model of integrated multidisciplinary care for diabetes can now be outlined, keeping in mind that the purpose of the redesign is explicitly restricted to continuing care. The model is organized into "stations of care," each assigned to a single discipline and staffed by a provider with particular skills in that discipline. These stations are setup in a specified sequence, like a manufacturing cell, with individual patients moving through each station and service elements of diabetes care delivered serially to provide multidisciplinary care in the aggregate. Based on this, a model for diabetes care delivery was constructed as follows:

1. *Assemble the essential components of diabetes care into a comprehensive patient visit* involving a team of diabetes care providers assigned to specific "stations of care," each responsible for *explicitly defined work content related to their expertise* (*PPC Rule #1*), covering all aspects of multidisciplinary diabetes care, as follows:
   (i) A Certified Diabetes Nurse Educator (CDE-RN)
   (ii) A Diabetologist/Endocrinologist (Team leader, who oversees/problem solves at all stations)
   (iii) A Nutritionist with CDE certification (CDE-RD)
   (iv) A Clinical Pharmacist (Pharm D)
   (v) A Nurse Practitioner with CDE certification and diabetes management experience (CDE-NP)

2. *Define Work Content across the 4 stations* . The first step was to set Takt time[1] to accommodate a <15 min cycle time at each station (total visit length = 60 min), and assure *unambiguous work flow* (*PPC Rule #2*) *along a highly specified path* (*PPC Rule #3*), in the following sequence:
   (i) *Station 1* ("*DSME*" [*Cycle Time = 13,-2,+4*]): The CDE-RN does the following tasks:
      (a) Collect the home blood glucose log or download from metre or insulin pump
      (b) Measure blood pressure;
      (c) Take a finger-stick blood sample to measure HbA_{1c} and Lipid levels in the clinic (using point-of-care [POC] laboratory equipment);
      (d) Provide diabetes education in one of four predetermined "patient knowledge/skill areas," in a repeating cycle over four visits. It is vital that the patient be familiar with the basics because the purpose is to review and reinforce familiar information, not introduce new information. Thus, the patient must participate in a preliminary DSME session prior to enrolment.

      The four assigned tasks differ, depending on whether the patient needs reinforcement of basic skills or more advanced skills, and are calibrated to patient needs. The four basic skills reviewed are:
      - Metre technique
      - Injection technique
      - Sick-day and hypoglycaemia management, including instruction on glucagon administration by spouse/home caregiver
      - Foot care

[1]Takt time is the maximum amount of time in which a product needs to be produced. Adjustable time unit used in lean production to synchronize the rate of production with the rate of demand.

More advanced skills for patients on an insulin pump include

- priming and refilling the insulin pump
- infusion set insertion technique
- ability to change pump basal rates, and
- familiarity with the pump's bolus administration tool (e.g., Carb Smart or Bolus Wizard)

(e) Work content is designed specifically to assure that the nurse completes tasks a to c (above) plus one of the DSME skill areas in d. within a cycle time of 13 min on average, although that can be as short as 11 min, or as long as 17 min when unexpected delays occur in accessing pump and metre software.

(ii) *Station 2* ("*MNT*" [*Cycle Time*=*11 min*, *−1*,*+3*]): The CDE Nutritionist's tasks include the following:

(a) Weigh the patient, discuss implications of weight gain, or need for weight loss

(b) Review dietary principles in one of four predetermined "patient knowledge areas" over four visits in turn in a repeating cycle. Just as for DSME, the intent is to review and reinforce familiar information, not introduce new information, which is why it is essential for the patient to participate in a preliminary nutrition education session prior to enrolment.

The four assigned tasks differ, depending on whether the patient needs reinforcement of basic skills or advanced skills.

The four basic nutritional skills reviewed

- food groups
- food choice
- hypoglycemia, and
- portion control.

In patients on a Multiple Daily Insulin (MDI) regimen or using an Insulin Pump, the focus of MNT is on more advanced skills, including:

- Carbohydrate counting, including verification by food logs, if necessary
- Effect of dietary fat and protein on carbohydrate absorption
- Dual, extended and square-wave bolus strategies, and
- Hypoglycaemia prevention strategies, e.g., the proactive use of carbohydrate intake before exercise

(c) Work content at this station is designed specifically to assure that the nutritionist weighs the patient and provides one of the MNT skill areas in (b) within a cycle time of 11 min on average, although that can be as short as 10 min, or as long as 14 min

(iii) *Station 3* ("*BP-Lipids*" [*Cycle Time 10 min*, *−4*, *+1*]): The initial configuration of the model had this station manned by a clinical pharmacist who performs the following tasks (this configuration changed subsequently, for reasons we will outline later):

(a) Rechecks BP in those not at goal at initial measurement (Station 1)

(b) Orders labs as needed for annual surveillance

(c) Performs medication reconciliation

(d) Interprets POC Lipid results and reconciles with previous lab results

(e) Adjusts/intensifies/refills BP, lipid, and aspirin therapy, according to patient need, to achieve patient-specific targets (BP <140/90 in all patients, and <130/80; LDL <100 mg/dl or <70 mg/dl, depending on risk stratification).

(f) Work content at the BP/Lipid station varies more than at any other Station, depending on whether or not the patient is at goals for BP and Lipid therapy. Thus, cycle time can be as short as 7 min in patients at goal for both BP and Lipids (which applies to the great majority of patients currently seen in the clinic) up to a maximum of 12 min in the rare patient needing intensification of both BP and Lipid therapy. This assures task completion with a cycle time well within the 15 min Takt time, so that the model is able to accommodate delays (i.e., "make-up" for lost time) at one of the earlier stations.

(iv) *Station 4* ("*Glycaemia*"): A CDE-Nurse Practitioner performs the following tasks:
  (a) A diabetes-focused exam (e.g., injection sites, feet)
  (b) Reviews and records results from Diabetes Retinopathy Surveillance Reports
  (c) Reviews the home blood glucose (or insulin pump) printout
  (d) Adjusts therapy as needed to meet patient-specific glycaemic targets (A1c), calibrated to patient need, based on individual risk stratification.
  (e) Ensures compliance with annual retinopathy surveillance (referral to ophthalmology)
  (f) Work content at this station is predictable for the most part (~14 min) and, while stable, is variable enough that cycle time can extend to as much as 25 min when unanticipated problems or complications are recognized, such as an infected abrasion or ulcer on the foot. In such patients, the Supervising MD enters Station 4 as soon as the problem is recognized, in order to provide input for managing both glycaemia and the unanticipated problem within the allotted Takt of 15 min. The MD then exits allowing the NP to concentrate on providing extended task completion for such patients, while the MD takes the next patient in line for Glycaemic Management, so that there are no hold-ups in patient throughput.

(v) "*Floating Station*" (*Supervising Diabetologist*): Work content at this station consists of the following tasks:
  (a) See all patients at Station 4 to discuss/endorse decisions on glycaemic management
  (b) Sign off on all changes in therapy at Stations 3 and 4
  (c) Provide continuous oversight of work flow across the four stations
  (d) Act as an on-site problem solver for interruptions in work flow
  (e) Function as an extra outlet to maintain work flow when hold-ups occur at any station because of unanticipated complexity (as discussed above).
  (f) Perform medication reconciliation
  (g) Document and send Inter-facility Communication to PCP
  (h) Seek specialist consultation for newly recognized or existing problems (e.g., Cardiology, Nephrology, Podiatry, Vascular Surgery, and Psychiatry etc.)

3. *Ensure Task Completion through Documentation*: Template-based electronic documentation in modular form for each station assures completion of all assigned tasks. Documentation modules for each station were developed by individual team members and only finalized after extensive dialogue among team members to ensure appropriateness and brevity, and to eliminate duplication. Previously documented information in CPRS is imported into a

templated note that mandates completion of all identified tasks in specific fields at each Station, while also allowing for inclusion of free text. Thus, *work content and documentation requirement for each visit and station is explicitly defined* (*PPC Rule #1*). At the end of the visit, the unique capability of CPRS allows the four modules, each individually signed by the assigned provider at each Station, to be combined to appear as a single cohesive and comprehensive note in the electronic record, rather than as four separate notes.

(C) **Re-evaluate constantly to Improve Model Efficiency and Performance (*Kaizen*)**

Team meetings are held regularly *to constantly evaluate performance through problem-solving* (*PPC Rule #4*). The purpose is to engage in team dialogue focused on making sure the model is working for each team member, without finger-pointing or blame (the essence of *kaizen*). We cite three specific examples of how *kaizen* was utilized to make changes in work content, work flow, and model design.

(i) *The reassignment of the task of BP measurement from the "BP/Lipids" Station to its current placement in Station 1, "DSME"*: This represents an early example of how constructive dialogue based on evidence was used to reassign work content in order to improve workflow. Initially, the team assumed that the natural placement of the task of BP measurement would be in the "BP/Lipids" Station. However, it became clear early in implementation that hold-ups at that station were an intermittent but recurring problem. Evidence from time measurements revealed a periodic imbalance in workload because the pharmacist was sometimes compelled to wait as much as 10 min for the patient to reach a resting state for accurate BP measurements, particularly when repeat measurements were called for in patients not at goal on the first measurement. A realization that such hold-ups were of little consequence at the start of the visit prompted a redistribution of the task of initial BP measurement to the "DSME" Station, achieving better work balance and evening out cycle times across stations (*heijunka*).

(ii) *The reordering of station sequence over time*: This constitutes a second example of how evidence from ongoing monitoring was used to make adjustments in work flow (Fig. 2.3a–c). "BP-Lipids" was initially thought to be ideally positioned as Station 2 (Fig. 2.3a. First Iteration), but monitoring showed significant hold-ups in workflow occurring even after it was divested of the task of initial BP measurement. Continued monitoring revealed that the hold-ups occurred because it often took >15 min for the POC-lipids test to result, which meant the pharmacist did not receive those within the 15 min takt, with further delays added on whenever treatment changes were called for. The BP/Lipids Station was therefore moved to what was then though to be its "ideal" position at Station #3 in the visit sequence, exchanging places with "MNT" (Fig. 2.3b Second Iteration). This allowed for an additional 15 min to elapse while the patient received MNT at the newly configured Station #2, before the patient was seen for BP/Lipid management at Station #3, by which time the POC Lipid result was available for any adjustments in therapy.

(iii) *Changing the configuration of the model from its original conception based on changing circumstances.* We have been forced into yet another reconfiguration of the model, which further demonstrates the flexibility of the model. This was prompted by administrative reallocation of manpower resources, which terminated the Clinical Pharmacist's participation in the clinic. Consequently, the

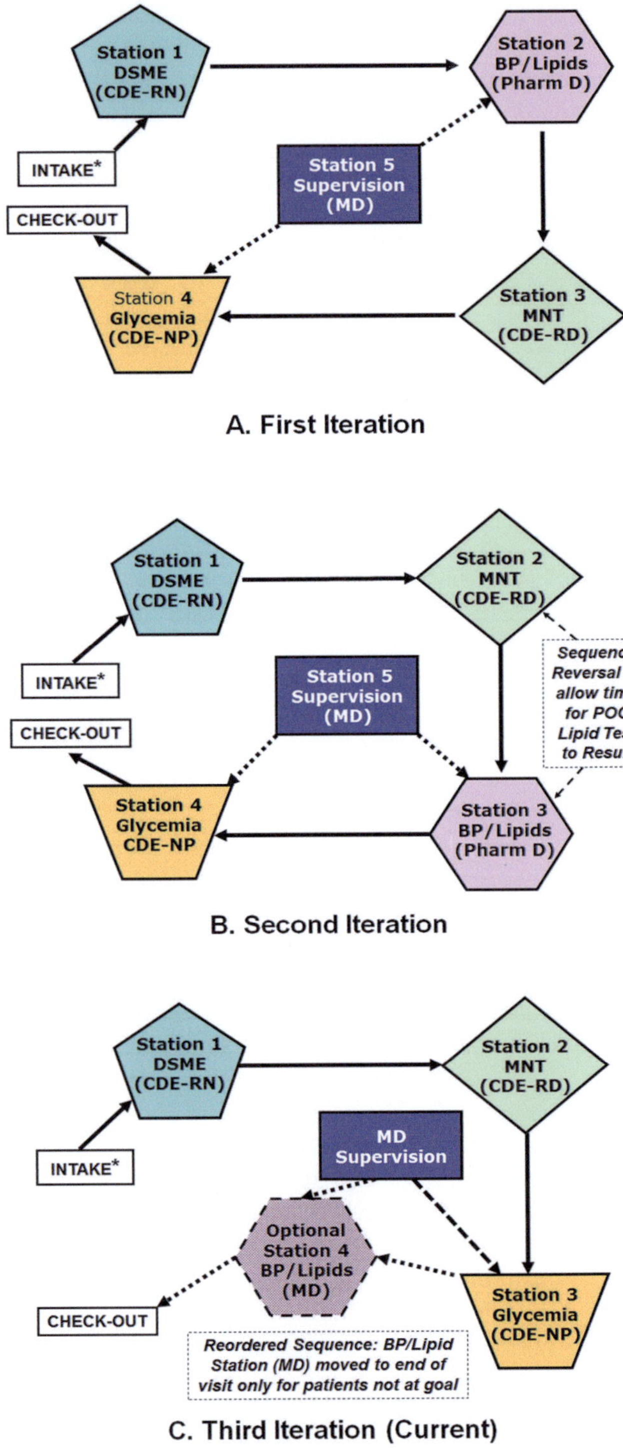

Fig. 2.3 Changes made to Station sequence over time (*kaizen* in practice). (**a**) First iteration: five stations in their original sequence. (**b**) Second iteration: sequence reversal of "BP/Lipids" and "MNT" stations, prompted by hold-ups traced to POC Lipid results taking >15 min to become available. (**c**) Third iteration (current), showing BP/Lipids last in sequence as an "Optional Station." Supervising MD provides one-on-one BP/Lipid management at the end of the visit in patients not meeting goals, and oversees glycaemic management (See text for details). *Intake restricted to Continuing/Established Care, not Initial Care. Key: *CDE* Certified Diabetes Educator, *NP* Nurse Practitioner, *Pharm D* Doctor of Pharmacy, *POC* Point-of-care, *RD* Registered Dietitian, *RN* Registered Nurse

tasks assigned to this station were reassigned, of necessity, to the Supervising Diabetologist, the only team member "free" to engage in completing those tasks. As part of the reconfiguration of task assignment, it was necessary to move "BP-Lipids" to the last Station in line (Station #4), exchanging places with "Glycaemia," which became Station #3. The reconfiguration required the team to accept that the Supervising MD would be, of necessity, unavailable to engage in glycaemic management on the spot. In anticipation of this, it was decided to reserve a 30 min time slot at the end of clinic for specific interactions between the NP and MD regarding glycaemic management. In the event that changes in recommendations became necessary, these would be subsequently communicated to the patient by the NP, and documented by the MD in the "Supervising Diabetologist" component of the composite visit note.

Our expectation of insoluble problems resulting from the potentially crippling loss of what was originally considered a critical component of the model has turned out to be completely unfounded! The keys to such a stress-free turnaround were vigorous team dialogue and evidence-based task monitoring, as soon as it became clear that the loss of the Pharm D's participation was irrevocable. The critical importance of *kaizen* – a combination of dialogue and evidence – is shown in our discovery that cycle time at the BP/Lipids Station could be as low as 4 min in patients at goal for both parameters. (Parenthetically, we must note here – to be revisited later – that the model has been successful in achieving BP/Lipid goals in ~90 % of patients after the second visit, so that visit complexity is drastically curtailed in 90 % of patients receiving ongoing care for BP/Lipid management.) As a result, most patients need only one session – at most, two – of one-on-one intervention for BP/Lipids management to achieve and maintain goal for both measures.

The current configuration (Fig. 2.3c, Third Iteration) makes use of this fact by effectively combining the last two stations in 90 % of patients meeting BP and Lipid goals, so that the patient visit ends after three Stations. The "downtime" afforded by this combination of stations allows the supervising MD to complete documentation tasks for the BP/Lipids Station, including medication reconciliation, and ordering labs in anticipation of the next patient's needs, during the first 5 min of the cycle time at Station 3, while the NP completes a preparatory glycaemic evaluation. The supervising MD then enters Station #3 during the latter half of cycle time, combining endorsement of success in reaching BP/Lipid goals with supervisory functions at the "Glycaemia" station (now Station #3). In the minority of patients who need specific interventions because BP-Lipid goals are not met, the Supervising MD can render those at an "Optional" Station #4 during a truncated visit (~7–8 min) after the completion of the "Glycaemia" visit, which still leaves enough time for the MD to fulfil a glycaemic supervisory role for the next patient at Station 3.

The above examples demonstrate the inherent plasticity of the model, to the extent that we were able to accommodate a loss of manpower with little or no disruption in work flow. That experience further validates the adaptability of the Toyota Way to care delivery in a multitude of chronic disease states. It must be reiterated, however, that the ability to make the BP/Lipid Station optional in the current configuration is critically dependent on the fact that BP/Lipid goals are met in 90 % of patients. This would not be possible in a population in whom these goals are not met in a significant number of patients; in that case, the configuration shown in Fig. 2.3b, Second Iteration, would be mandatory.

Performance and Results

Process-of-Care Measures (Table 2.1)

As part of annual performance reviews at VAPHS over the past 8 years, we are required to show compliance with standards of care in a random sample of ~20 patients each year. These reviews show 100 % documentation in *all* ADA specified domains of diabetes care (HbA$_{1c}$, LDL, blood pressure, creatinine and urinary microalbumin levels, annual foot and eye exams, and aspirin and statin use/contraindications/alternatives). No published diabetic care model approaches, let alone equals, this level of performance.

Performance Measures (Figs. 2.4, 2.5, and 2.6)

To evaluate performance, we secured IRB permission to track surrogate measures associated with better long-term outcomes (A1c, LDL and SBP) in 57 patients who were seen at least three times in the traditional single provider clinic prior to redesign and followed for at least three visits after redesign. Significant improvements were achieved in all three measures compared to prior performance in the same patients who had been attending the traditional single provider-patient clinic prior to redesign.

Figure 2.4 shows that mean HbA$_{1c}$ declined by 0.6 % after redesign (7.4 % compared to 8 % for the same patients before redesign) and that a greater proportion of patients achieved an HbA$_{1c}$ of <8.0 % (a modified care goal driven by the fact that most of our patients are of advanced age and have multiple co-morbidities). Similarly, Fig. 2.5 shows that mean LDL fell by 20 mg/dl (0.5 mmol/l), with a goal LDL of <100 mg/dl (<2.6 mmol/l) being achieved in 90 % of patients, compared to 75 % in the prior clinic, with no patient having an LDL >130 mg/dl (3.4 mmol/l). Finally, as shown in Fig. 2.6, SBP levels fell by 11 mmHg, and SBP <130 mmHg was achieved in almost twice as many patients as before (63 % vs 35 %), with 100 % of patients maintaining goal SBP <140 mmHg. Most importantly, in every instance in which SBP was >130 mmHg, or LDL >100, there was documentation of action taken to intensify therapy, or the reason for a decision not to intervene.

Table 2.1 Fulfilment of 12 process-of-care measures in the Individualized Multidisciplinary Team-Care Model for Integrated Diabetes Care

Process measure	Documentation[b]	Assessment[c]	Intervention[d]
Blood pressure	100 %	100 %	–
A1c (POC testing)	100 %	100 %	–
LDL (POC testing)	100 %	100 %	–
Annual foot exam	100 %	100 %	–
Annual dilated eye exam[a]	100 %	100 %	–
Annual urinary ACR	100 %	100 %	–
Annual creatinine	100 %	100 %	–
Medication reconciliation	100 %	–	–
ASA/contraindications	100 %	–	100 %
Lipid Rx/contraindications	100 %	100 %	100 %
HTN Rx/contraindications	100 %	100 %	100 %
Glycaemia Rx/contraindications	100 %	100 %	100 %

ACR Albumin Creatinine Ratio, *ASA* aspirin, *HTN* hypertension, *POC* Point of Care, *Rx* Treatment
[a]Retinopathy (absent/present and type/severity) documented from Annual Surveillance exams
[b]Documentation that each measure was either performed/resulted or due/ordered
[c]Assessment of each Measure documented as "normal"/"at goal" or "abnormal"/"not at goal"
[d]Intervention (therapy intensification/contraindication) documented in all patients not at goal

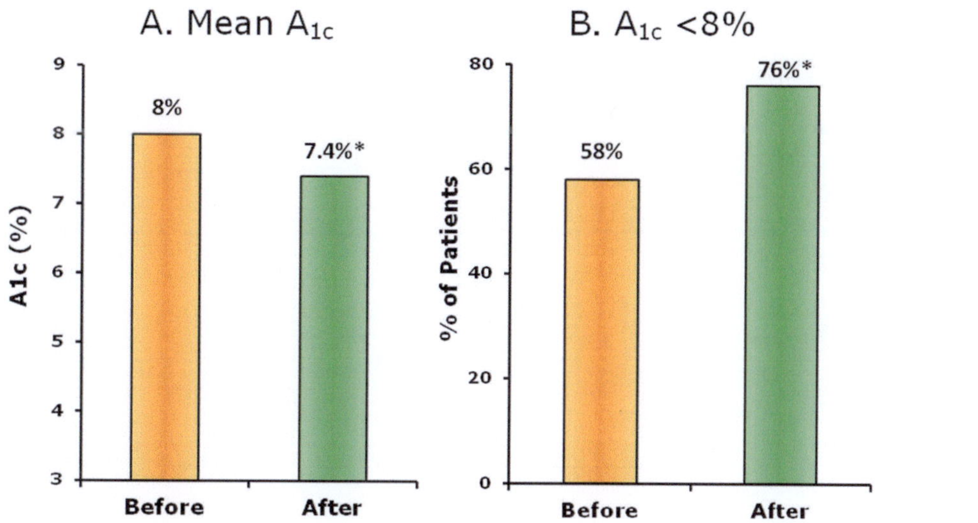

Fig. 2.4 (**a**, **b**) Change in A1c in 57 patients seen for ≥3 visits before and after changing from a traditional Single Patient-Provider Model to an Individualized Multidisciplinary Team-Care Model for Delivering Integrated Diabetes Care (* $p<0.05$)

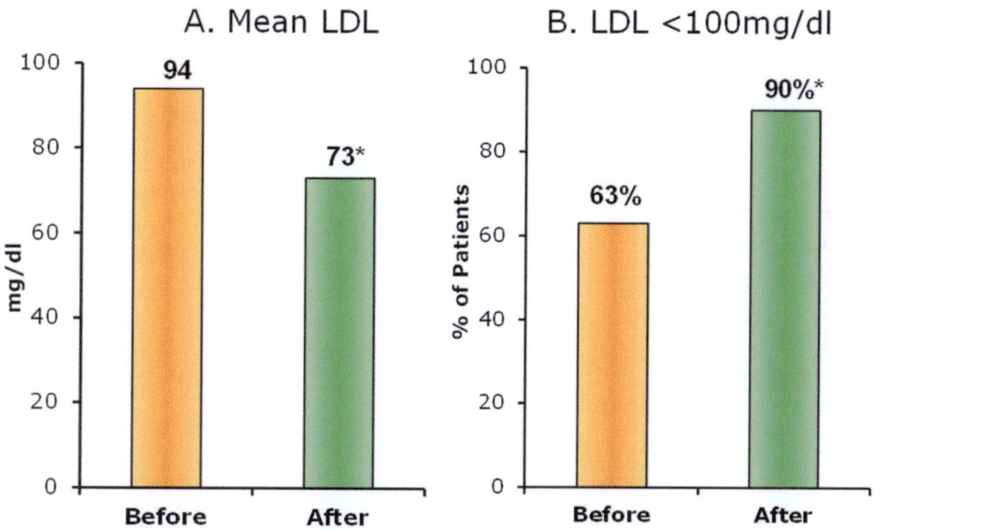

Fig. 2.5 (**a**, **b**) Change in LDL Cholesterol in 57 patients seen for ≥3 visits before and after changing from a traditional Single Patient-Provider Model to an Individualized Multidisciplinary Team-Care Model for Delivering Integrated Diabetes Care (* $p<0.01$)

Provider Patient Interactions in the Individualized Multidisciplinary Team Care Model (Table 2.2)

In the traditional "single provider" clinic that existed prior to redesign, there were ten scheduled appointments, including two overbooks, for a net of eight patient appointments of 30 min each with a Nurse Practitioner in a 4 h clinic session (which included direct supervisory input from a Diabetologist), for a total of 240 min of face-to-face patient contact. In the redesigned clinic, 14 visits are scheduled, with three overbooks, for a net of 11 patient visits, on average, totaling 60 min each (15 min with four provid-

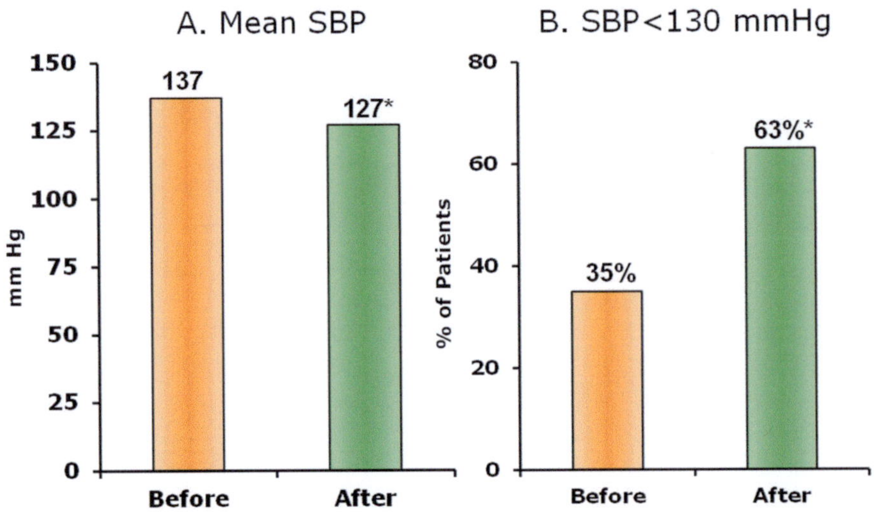

Fig. 2.6 (**a**, **b**) Change in Systolic Blood Pressure in 57 patients seen for ≥3 visits before and after changing from a traditional single patient: provider model to an Individualized Multidisciplinary Team-Care Model for Delivering Integrated Diabetes Care (* p<0.01)

Table 2.2 Patient-provider interactions before and after implementation of the Individualized Multidisciplinary Team-Care Model

Parameter	Before redesign	After redesign	% Change
Number of providers	2	4	100 % ⇑
Daily appointment slots	10	14	40 % ⇑
Average # of patients seen/day	8	11	38 % ⇑
Scheduled clinic duration (min)	240	240	⇔
Scheduled visit duration (min)	30	60	100 % ⇑
Mean time Check-in to Depart (min)	56	63	12 % ⇑
Mean (max) wait time (min)	23 (58)	8 (19)	65 % ⇓
Average face-to-face time (min)	33	55	68 % ⇑
Integrated delivery of DSME calibrated to need	No	Yes	–
Integrated delivery of MNT calibrated to need	No	Yes	–
Fragmented/uncoordinated ancillary care	Yes	No	–

ers). This translates to 660 min of face-to-face patient contact, which represents a 175 % increase in available time for care delivery in the 4 h session.

The inclusion of MNT and DSME in an integrated visit, in particular, represents a major improvement in care that cannot be quantified. In addition, one-on-one interactions at every station ensure patient-centred (individualized) care delivery calibrated to each patient's needs, abilities and goals. Finally, an unexpected benefit from time-constrained visits in the redesigned clinic is a dramatic improvement in punctuality. Average patient-wait time is now 8 min, with a maximum of 19 min, so that 90 % of patients are seen within 5 min of their scheduled appointment time, compared to an average wait time of 23 min previously, when only 30 % were seen within 15 min of their scheduled appointment time.

Conclusions

Krumholz et al. identify eight domains of care that must be covered in any CDM programme [20, 21]. The component interventions encompassing those domains comprise a precise yardstick for measuring the effectiveness of a CDM programme, as follows:

(i) an identified population with specific health and disease conditions;
(ii) the application of evidence-based practice guidelines to treat those patients;
(iii) collaborative practice models that include physician and support-service providers;
(iv) patient self-management education (may include primary prevention, behaviour modification programmes, and compliance/surveillance);
(v) risk stratification to match interventions with need;
(vi) process and outcomes measurement, evaluation, and management (including primary prevention, behavior modification programs, and compliance/surveillance);
(vii) routine reporting and feedback loops that include communication with the patient, physician, health plan, and ancillary providers; and
(viii) appropriate use of information technology (including use of specialized software, data registries, automated decision support tools, and callback systems).

The "Individualized Multidisciplinary Teamcare Model" of Diabetes Care at VA Pittsburgh, which was designed according to PPC^{SM} Principles, derived from the Toyota Production System, has achieved an exceptional level of success in fulfilling all of the above criteria, as follows:

(i) The model is designed for a specific, at-risk population (veterans with diabetes);
(ii) Goals of care are set according to evidence-based practice guidelines;
(iii) It delivers collaborative care through ongoing dialogue between physician and ancillary care providers to set and attain care goals, based on individual patient needs;
(iv) It places equal emphasis on patient self-management (DSME and MNT) and therapeutic management (BP/Lipids, and Glycaemia) for attaining care goals;
(v) Care at each station is calibrated to match interventions to individual patient need, based on proactive risk stratification;
(vi) It meets all process and performance measures;
(vii) It incorporates feedback loops through open communication between all care providers to not only set, achieve and maintain individualized care goals but also to improve care delivery through alterations in the practice model;
(viii) It uses information technology to create a templated note that mandates documentation of all process measures at each station, and to compile notes at each station into a single cohesive visit note.

In addition, the model has proven to be remarkably successful in fulfilling all process-of-care and performance measures. By providing comprehensive and effective diabetes care without compromising individualized attention – the hallmark of patient-centred care – our Individualized Multidisciplinary Team-care Model has achieved a level of success exceeding that in published studies of other models, where documentation in each of the nine ADA-identified domains ranges from 12 % to 70 % individually (and only 10 % for all nine domains collectively), and goal for any one outcome measure (A_{1c}, LDL or SBP) is reached in just 35–60 % of patients and all three in just 19 %.

One source of ongoing disappointment must, however, be mentioned before closing. It is our failure to imbue others with our enthusiasm for changing diabetes care delivery, which means that our success has not been replicated elsewhere in the VA system. That, however, may reflect the inertia that resists any change to a deep rooted tradition. That is what we encountered when we first set out to redesign diabetes care delivery, and our experience shows that the inertia becomes particularly obdurate when faced with a paradigm-shifting change that seeks to replace long-held practices with those based on concepts borrowed from industry! Our experience shows that overcoming the resistance requires unshakeable belief, sustained commitment, and enthusiastic buy-in from all presumptive stakeholders, including (most importantly) decision-makers responsible for allocating resources. If all those prerequisites are marshalled, then it is possible to (a) improve surrogate measures associated with improved outcomes; (b) achieve 100 % performance on all ADA-identified process-of-care measures; and (c) improve punctuality and timeliness in providing patient-centred care for diabetes.

References

1. Centers for Disease Control and Prevention. National diabetes statistics report: estimates of diabetes and its burden in the United States. Atlanta: US Department of Health and Human Services; 2014.
2. Casagrande SS, Fradkin JE, Saydah SH, Rust KF, Cowie CC. The prevalence of meeting A1C, blood pressure, and LDL goals among people with diabetes, 1988–2010. Diabetes Care. 2013;36:2271–9.
3. Phillips LS, Branch WT, Cook CB, Doyle JP, El-Kebbi IM, Gallina DL, et al. Clinical inertia. Ann Intern Med. 2001;135:825–34.
4. Drass J, Kell S, Osborn M, Bausell B, Corcoran Jr J, Moskowitz A, et al. Diabetes care for Medicare beneficiaries. Attitudes and behaviors of primary care physicians. Diabetes Care. 1998;21:1282–7.
5. American Association of Diabetes Educators. Diabetes education services reimbursement tips for primary care practice. Revised May 2009. www.diabeteseducator.org/docs/default-source/practice/Entrepreneurial-DE/reimbursement-tips-2009.pdf?sfvrsn=0. Accessed 21 Sep 2015.
6. Hodorowicz MA. Reimbursement for shared medical appointments incorporating diabetes self-management education/training or diabetes medical nutrition therapy. Diabetes Spectr. 2012;25:84–90.
7. Porter ME, Lee TH. The strategy that will fix health care. Harv Bus Rev. https://hbr.org/2013/10/the-strategy-that-will-fix-health-care. Accessed 3 Dec 2015.
8. American College of Physicians: Guidelines for Patient-Centered Medical Home (PCMH) recognition and accreditation programs. https://www.acponline.org/running_practice/delivery_and_payment_models/pcmh/understanding/guidelines_pcmh.pdf. Accessed 3 Dec 2015.
9. Davis AM, Sawyer DR, Vinci LM. The potential of group visits in diabetes care. Clin Diabetes. 2008;28:58–62.
10. Peytremann-Bridevaux I, Burnand B. Disease management: a proposal for a new definition. Int J Integr Care. 2009;9:e16.
11. Housden L, Wong ST, Dawes M. Effectiveness of group medical visits for improving diabetes care: a systematic review and meta-analysis. CMAJ. 2013;185:E635–44.
12. U.S. Department of Veterans Affairs. Federal benefits for veterans, dependents and survivors. Chapter 1: health care benefits. http://www.va.gov/opa/publications/benefits_book/benefits_chap01.asp. Accessed 2 Dec 2015.
13. Fulton EL. Physician champions awarded grant monies for research. The Bulletin of the Allegheny County Medical Society p 195–197. April 2006. http://elizabethfulton-pr.com/wp-content/uploads/2009/06/feature_champions.pdf. Accessed 21 Sep 2015.
14. Pittsburgh Regional Health Initiative-Perfecting Patient Care. www.prhi.org. Accessed 21 Sep 2015.
15. Liker JK. The Toyota way: 14 management principles from the world's greatest manufacturer. New York: McGraw-Hill; 2004.
16. Grunden N. The Pittsburgh way to efficient healthcare. Improving patient care using Toyota based methods. New York: Productivity Press; 2008.
17. Landon BE, Hicks LS, O'Malley AJ, Lieu TA, Keegan T, McNeil BJ, et al. Improving the management of chronic disease at community health centers. N Engl J Med. 2007;356:921–34.
18. Simmons D, Yu D, Wentzel H. Changes in hospital admissions and inpatient tariff associated with a diabetes integrated care initiative: preliminary findings. J Diabetes. 2014;6:81–9.
19. Spear S, Bowen HK. Decoding the DNA of the Toyota production system. Harv Bus Rev. 1999;77:96–106.
20. Krumholz HM, Currie PM, Riegel B, Phillips CO, Peterson ED, Smith R, et al. A taxonomy for disease management. A scientific statement from the American Heart Association Disease Management Taxonomy Writing Group. Circulation. 2006;114:1432–45.
21. Goetzel RZ, Ozminkowski RJ, Villagra VG. Return on investment in disease management: a review. Health Care Financ Rev. 2005;26:1–19.

3 Approaches to Integrated Diabetes Care: United States: San Francisco

David H. Thom and Thomas Bodenheimer

Introduction

Despite the availability of effective treatment for diabetes and the publication of clear guidelines for diabetes management, 41 % of persons with diabetes in the United States do not have their blood sugar under optimal control as defined by a glycosylated haemoglobin (HbA1c) less than 7 % [1]. This fact suggests that the traditional lone-doctor model for diabetes care – busy doctors seeing patients in rushed 15 min visits without the help of a team – is not working. Over the past 20 years, a new approach – integrated care – has been taking hold in the United States. Non-physicians – nurse practitioners, physician assistants, registered nurses, pharmacists, health educators, nutritionists, medical assistants, health coaches, and community health workers – have become engaged in the care of patients with diabetes. Our group has contributed to several innovations for providing better integrated care to patients with diabetes and other chronic conditions. To understand our approach to integrated diabetes care it is important to know about how our approach was developed within the larger national movements and models for integrated care.

In this chapter, we will briefly review the history of integrated care in the US including the major movements that, in the past two decades, have contributed to current models of integrated care. The chapter will then review the evidence for several approaches to integrated care for patients with diabetes, including emerging areas of telemedicine/digital technology. We will conclude with a description of approaches to integrated care for patients with diabetes at our institution and a note on the issue of paying for integrated care within the US health-care system.

It is worth noting that "integrated care" has generally been used in the US to mean integration of physical and mental health care while the terms "coordinated care" and "team care" more closely approximate the meaning of integrated care used in this book. We will use the term integrated care in its broader sense: bringing together multiple sources and components of care, including primary and secondary care, services provided different professionals and non-licensed health workers, and care delivered in the community as well as through the medical care system. For clarification, the term "clinician" as used in this chapter refers to any health professional who has the authority to order diagnostic studies and prescribe medications and who receives re-imbursement for their services. In the

D.H. Thom (✉) • T. Bodenheimer
Department of Family and Community Medicine, University of California, San Francisco School of Medicine and San Francisco General Hospital, San Francisco, CA, USA
e-mail: david.thom@ucsf.edu; Thomas.Bodenheimer@ucsf.edu

D. Simmons et al. (eds.), *Integrated Diabetes Care*, DOI 10.1007/978-3-319-13389-8_3

US this group typically includes physicians, nurse practitioners and physician assistants.

In addition to definition of integrated care, there is the question of how integrated care is evaluated. The most common measure of success of integrated care, or virtually any intervention for patients with diabetes, is the level of glycosylated haemoglobin (HbA1c). However, there are additional recognized diabetes-related process and outcome measures, including screening for complications of diabetes (retinopathy, renal insufficiency and foot ulcers) and controlling diabetes-associated risk factors (typically hypertension and hyperlipidemia). Moreover, "patient-centred" measures include general quality of life [2], the diabetes distress scale [3], the symptoms of depression [4], and patient satisfaction [5]. Additional measures may include the economic impact of integrated care and the extent to which a model of integrated care is adopted and maintained. Most of the studies reported in the current chapter use HbA1c as their primary, or only, outcome measure; additional measures are included when available.

Integrated Care for Chronic Disease in the United States

Integrated care for diabetes in the US is best understood within the broader context of efforts to improve the coordination of care for patients with chronic disease in general. The movement to provide integrated care is multifaceted and historically complex, reflecting the heterogeneity and changing landscape of health-care delivery in the US. One of the earliest models of publicly available integrated care in the US is that developed by health maintenance organizations. In the 1940s Kaiser Permanente and Group Health Cooperative of Puget Sound pioneered many aspects of integrated care including comprehensive care for patients, shared medical records, partnership between specialists and GPs who were salaried employees, which stood in contrast to the dominant model at the time of solo or small independent, fee for service practices. Prospective funding (capitation) with an emphasis on prevention, also provided a more supportive environment for the incorporation of dieticians, nurse educators, pharmacists and mental health specialists into patient care.

The Chronic Care Model

In 1998 a leader in the care of patients with chronic illnesses, Dr. Ed Wagner, then at Group Health Cooperative of Puget Sound, published an integrated model of patient-centred care known as the Chronic Care Model (CCM) (Fig. 3.1) [6, 7]. The CCM recognizes three spheres of care for patients with chronic conditions: the health-care system as a whole, primary care and specialty practices, and the broader community in which those practices are located. Fundamental to the Chronic Care Model is the necessity to engage patients to be informed, activated partners in the management of their own conditions. Numerous studies have shown the CCM to be effective in improving outcomes [8], including for patients with diabetes [9–17]. The CCM has been the basis for many if not most interventions to improve integrated care.

Care Managers

Multiple studies over the past 20 years have found that care managers (generally nurses or pharmacists) can significantly improve HbA1c levels for patients with diabetes, particularly when given authority to adjust treatment plans using approved algorithms [18, 19]. The importance of care managers being able to adjust medications is illustrated by comparing outcomes from two studies at the same institution [20]. In the study where changes in medication required approval by the primary care physician, there was no change in HbA1c levels over 18 months [21] while in the second study, where medication changes were allowed based on an approved protocol, the HbA1c declined 2.1 % (from 10.1 % to 8.0 %) in the intervention group compared to 0.9 % (from 10.2 % to 9.3 %) in the control group, a significant effect [22] Care management using a

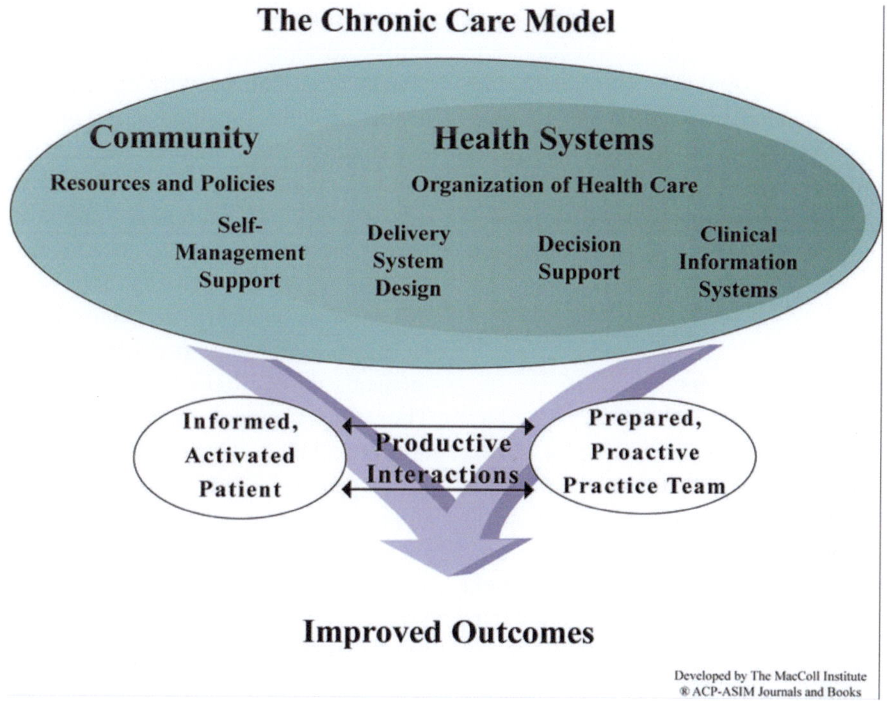

Fig. 3.1 The chronic care model (Used with permission from Wagner [7])

therapeutic algorithm has also been shown to be effective in improving blood pressure control for patients with diabetes [23].

Multiple Interventions

Interventions to improve integrated care for patients with diabetes may combine multiple components. For example care management can be combined with team care, group visits and/or a patient activation intervention. In a randomized controlled trial of group visits with care management by team members including a diabetes nurse educator, a psychologist, a nutritionist, and a pharmacist, HbA1c levels declined by 1.3 % (from 9.5 % to 8.2 %) in the intervention subjects versus 0.2 % (from 9.5 % to 9.3 %), in the control subjects a highly significant difference [24]. The intervention group also showed significant improvements in self-care practices and patients experienced significantly lower utilization of both hospital and outpatient services. In Minnesota, a randomized controlled trial (RCT) compared usual care to a multicomponent intervention that included a site coordinator who facilitated pre-visit planning with patients and a monthly review of performance with a local physician champion at each clinic [25]. At 12 months, intervention practices had significantly greater improvement in achieving recommended clinical values for systolic blood pressure (SBP), HbA1c, and low density lipoprotein (LDL) cholesterol than control clinics. Diabetes process measures also improved significantly more in the intervention group, including increases in the percent of patients receiving annual foot examinations (35 %), eye examinations (26 %); and renal testing (29 %). A cluster RCT of 11 primary care practices in Pittsburgh Pennsylvania comparing a CCM-based multifaceted intervention, a provider education intervention and usual care found a significant improvement in HbA1c in the CCM group (dropping from 7.6 % to 7.0 %) but no improvement in the other groups [11]. A similar pattern was seen for improvement in lipids. The proportion of patients self-monitoring glucose increased from 78 % to 100 % in the CCM group, compared to 84–91 % in the education group with no change in the usual care group. Another

RCT of a Diabetes Outpatient Intensive Treatment (DOIT) programme, a multiday group education and skills training experience combined with daily medical management followed by care management over 6 months, found a significant benefit on patients HbA1c [26]. However, the intervention was resource intensive and depended on multiple contacts with a highly trained nurse care manager.

Organizational Systems

Better health-care delivery organization allows for implementation and maintenance of multiple components to improve care, including use of diabetes registries, care management, electronic health records, patient education, and payment incentives. A study of patients receiving Medicare in 90 managed care organizations (MCOs) in 2001 found strong relationships between better organizational systems and all 6 measures of the quality of care for patients with diabetes (HbA1c and LDL testing, screening for nephropathy and retinal disease, and control of glucose and lipid levels) [27]. For example, 50 % of patients in the bottom quartile of MCO organizational performance had HbA1c levels >9.5 %, compared to 20 % the top quartile. A 2005 Minnesota study of 41 medical groups, ranging in size from less than 10 to more than 200 physicians, created a scoring system based on the presence or absence of 53 systems and process items within five domains: general health system, delivery system redesign, clinician formation system, decision support for clinicians and self-management support [28]. Significant correlations ranging from 0.39 to 0.46 were found between the sum of domain scores and testing of HbA1c, LDL and blood pressure, and for control of diabetes (HbA1c ≤ 8 %) and cholesterol (LDL <130 mg/dL (3.4 mmol/l)).

The Patient-Centered Medical Home

The CCM has been a major impetus to the Patient-Centered Medical Home (PCMH) movement [29, 30]. (A primary principle of the PCMH is that "care is coordinated and/or integrated across all elements of the complex health-care system (e.g., subspecialty care, hospitals, home health agencies, nursing homes) and the patient's community (e.g., family, public and private community-based services)" [31]. To accomplish this, the PCMH encourages the use of clinic based care teams and care coordination [32, 33]. Teams, led by the primary care physician, are tasked with insuring that care is coordinated across specialties and providers with attention to medical, psychological and social needs [34]. The PCMH model includes multiple features aimed at better integrated care, including care managers/coordinators, patient registries, improved access, regular reporting of quality measures, patient access to electronic health information, and payment restructuring to support these activities. The model is being widely implemented across the US with support from payers, policy makers, patient advocacy groups, and professional organizations including the American Academy of Family Medicine and the American College of Physicians. Standards for three levels of PCMH status has been developed by the National Center for Quality Assurance [35]. Recognition by the NCQA can, in turn, be tied to higher payments for services.

The description of the PCMH in shown in Table 3.1 is consistent with the most common versions of the model [2, 31, 36, 37], but is not meant to be complete or definitive as key characteristics and components of the PCMH have been described in slightly different ways at different time by different groups. Some key characteristics overlap or reinforce each other: for example, some level of coordinated care is necessary for care to be comprehensive and accessibility is important for patient safety. The PCMH model also includes each patient having a personal physician or other clinician who is responsible for their care. Use of health information technology, including electronic health records and health information exchanges, is considered necessary to reach the full potential of the medical home. The success of the medical home model depends in large part on realignment of monetary incentives away from the number of patient visits with

Table 3.1 Key characteristics of the Patient-Centered Medical Home

Key characteristic	Description	Components/examples
Comprehensive	Provides for all the patient's health-care needs or taking responsibility for appropriately arranging care with other qualified professionals	Team care
		Practice panels
		Primary care
Patient-centred	Recognizes and respects patients' individual needs, values, preferences and culture and partners with patients and their families	Shared decision-making
		Patient and family engagement
		Patient self-management support
		Continuous relationship with a personal physician or other clinician
Coordinated/integrated	Care is coordinated and/or integrated across all elements of the health-care system, including subspecialty care, hospitals, nursing homes, home health agencies, and community-based services	Health information technology, including health information exchanges
		Care coordinators
		Referral tracking
Accessible	Convenient access to care by in person visits and by other modes of communication	Enhanced clinic hours including evenings and weekends
		24 h telephone access to medical advice from care team
		E-mail communication
		Patient portals
High quality and safety	Provides care that meets nationally recognized measures of quality; engages in continuous quality improvement; has protocols in place protect patients from medical errors	Evidence-based medicine and clinical decision support tools
		Health information technology support
		Measurement of health status and quality indicators
		Electronic prescribing
		Patients participate in quality improvement activities at the practice level

clinicians, to targeted processes and outcomes of the five key medical home characteristics.

It has been recognized that the PCMH exists within a "medical neighbourhood" which refers to health-care entities beyond the primary care clinic (e.g., area hospitals, specialists, home care agencies) as well as community resources [29]. See Fig. 3.2. PCMHs are expected to assume accountability for coordinating their patients' care by establishing relationship and connectivity with members of the "medical neighbourhood" such as specialists, hospitals and community agencies. This role of the PCMH has been further elucidated and expanded in the "Care Coordination Model" (Fig. 3.3) which includes information sharing, care coordination for referrals and transitions in care (e.g., from community to hospital or nursing home), linking patients with community resources to facilitate referrals and respond to social service needs, integrating mental health and specialty care into care delivery through collocation or referral agreements, tracking patients receiving outside services and following up on patients soon after emergency room visit or hospital discharge [33]. Performance measures of the coordinated care function of the PCMH include the Care Coordination Process Measures [38], which is used for PCMH recognition, the PCMH-A [39], a practice self-assessment measure, and the Key Activities for Care Coordination which measures specific actions of key importance for care coordination, such as developing information sharing agreements or tracking systems [33].

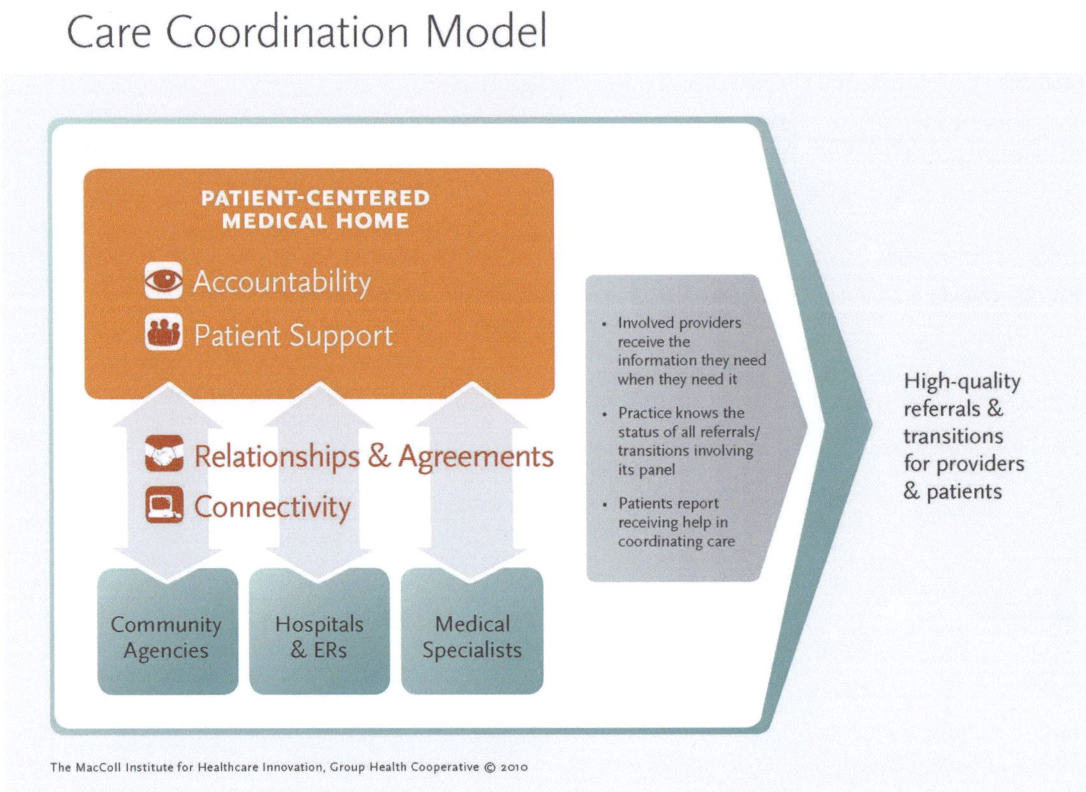

Fig. 3.2 The medical neighbourhood: care coordination model (From Reducing Care Fragmentation: A Toolkit for Coordinating Care. Prepared by Group Health's MacColl Institute for Healthcare Innovation. Supported by The Commonwealth Fund. April 2011)

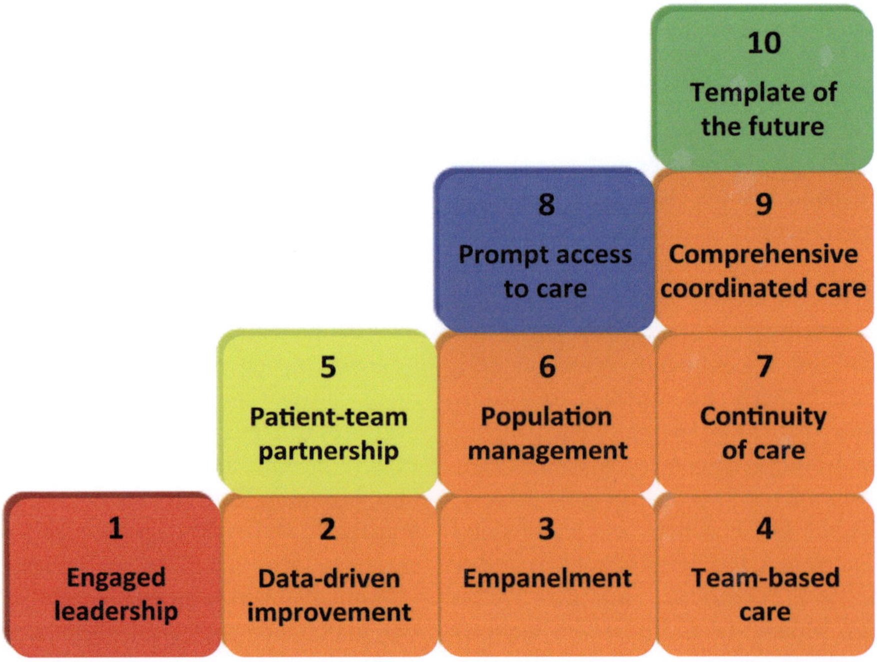

Fig. 3.3 Ten building blocks of high-performing primary care

Because integration of care is fundamental to the PCMH, the PCMH has been touted as a model to provide high-quality integrated care for diabetes [34, 40]. A review of PCMH demonstration project sites, ranging in size from a single clinic to 1200 practices, which have provided outcomes for patients with diabetes, reported improvement in diabetes-related care processes and outcomes at five of the sites and improvement in quality of care from chronic conditions (which included diabetes) in the other three sites [34]. Care coordination was a key feature for all sites. In addition, three sites had performance-based payments or incentives [41–44], two had capitated care [44, 45], one provided support for a care coordinator [46] and two had no change in payment structure [47, 48].

A recently reported study of the Pennsylvania Chronic Care Initiative examined the impact of a 3 year multifaceted intervention that included practice coaching, learning collaboratives, disease registries, payment for care managers and incentives for practice transformation to meet National Committee for Quality Assurance (NCQA) standards as medical homes [42]. Data from the 27 small primary care practices participating in the intervention were compared to 29 similar practices in the area. At 3 years, participating practices significantly outperformed comparison practices on all four screening measures related to diabetes: HbA1c testing, LDL testing, nephropathy monitoring and annual eye examinations. However, only the proportion of patients receiving nephropathy monitoring actually increased in the participating practices, moving from 78 % to 86 %. The percent of patients receiving the other three screening measures actually decreased slightly in the participating clinics, but decreased markedly in the comparison clinics, creating a significant difference in favour of the participating clinics.

The Patient Care Team

The use of patient care teams has been promoted as a means to implement integrated care both in parallel with and as part of the PCMH [32, 49]. Implementation of the team model requires sharing of tasks and responsibilities that have traditionally been the purview of the physician. The term "team care" has traditionally been used to indicate a group of health-care professionals such as physicians, nurses, pharmacists, or social workers, who work together in caring for a group of patients. In a 2006 systematic review of 66 trials testing 11 strategies for improving glycaemic control for patients with diabetes, only team care and case management showed a significant impact on reducing HbA1c levels [18]. Four types of team care were defined (1) the patient seeing a health professional in addition to their primary care clinician; (2) care from a multidisciplinary team of professionals in addition to the primary clinician; (3) "expansion of an existing professional role (e.g., nurse or pharmacist playing a more active role in patient monitoring or adjusting medication regimens)" or (4) "shared care between specialists and primary care clinicians." Based on 26 randomized controlled trials (the majority conducted in the US), team care interventions were associated with a mean decline in HbA1c of 0.33 % independent of any co-interventions. Of the four types of team care intervention, multidisciplinary care, expansion of existing professional roles and "shared care" all had nearly identical effect sizes, while simply having the patient see an additional health professional (which arguably does not constitute team care) had no impact. Studies of patients with baseline HbA1c levels of 8.0 % or higher reported greater effect sizes than studies with patients whose baseline HbA1c levels were less than 8.0 %.

Perhaps the most widely studied addition to the traditional physician care model of patients with diabetes is a pharmacist. In randomized controlled trials conducted in the US, patients randomized to receive diabetes education, medication counselling and adjustment, and instructions by a pharmacist have experienced significantly greater reductions in their HbA1c then control patients, as well as improved process measures and better control of other cardiovascular disease risk factors [22, 50–52].

Expansion of Care Teams to Include Non-licensed Health Workers

Part of the team care model promoted by the PCMH is that all members of the team work at "the top of their licence or certification" through additional instruction or training and wider use of algorithms. For example, medical assistants may assume such responsibilities as checking patient medicines (medication reconciliation), performing diabetic foot exams, screening for depression, providing education, giving navigation assistance for access to resources within the health system, and supporting patient activation, engagement and self-management [34, 53].

Another model using non-licensed health workers is the health coaching model. Health coaching provides in-depth self-management support by assisting patients to gain the knowledge, skills, and confidence to become informed, active participants in their care. Health coaching has several central components: setting agendas to ensure that patients' concerns are discussed in medical visits; ensuring that patients "know your numbers," e.g., know their HbA1c level and goal; "closing the loop" which means checking patients' understanding of the care plan decided on in the medical visit by having the patient repeat the care plan themselves; and action plans which are behaviour-change agreements – including medication adherence – made between health coaches and patients [54, 55]. Action plans have been found in a RCT to improve HbA1c levels more than traditional patient education [56].

In randomized controlled trial, medical assistant health coaching significantly reduced patient HbA1c levels from 9.8 % to 8.6 % compared to a reduction of 9.9–9.4 % for usual care (net difference of 0.6 %) [57]. Training peer supporters can also be effective. In a randomized controlled trial study by Heisler et al., reciprocal peer support was more effective than being assigned a nurse care manager in lowering HbA1c levels for male veterans with diabetes [58]. In another RCT, peer support significantly reduced mean HbA1c by 1.1 % (from 10.1 % to 9.0 %) in the coached group compared to 0.3 % (from 9.9 % to 9.6 %) in the usual care group [59]. Community health workers have also been shown to reduce HbA1c compared to nurse care managers [60]. Project Dulce, a programme targeting Latino immigrants found that peer-led education by community health workers (promotoras) significantly lowered HbA1c, diastolic blood pressure, and lipids compared to usual care [61, 62]. In 2013, diabetes was identified as a top priority area for community health workers [63].

Incorporating Mental Health into the Patient Care Team

The association between depression and diabetes is well established, as are the personal and social stresses for coping with diabetes as a serious chronic disease. However, few studies have examined the impact of a mental health expert into the patient care team. In a clustered RCT of 387 patients with a PHQ-9 score ≥10 and either diabetes or heart disease or both, a multi-method intervention that included up to eight therapy sessions and education of the primary care practitioners found a significant reduction in symptoms of depression [64]. HbA1c was not assessed. Team-based interventions can improve quality of life and reduce depression scores for patients with diabetes even without including mental health expertise [65]. One of the barriers to incorporating mental health care into the patient care team is the difficulty of collocating mental health providers with clinicians. In fact, one qualitative study found that while patients appreciate coordination and communication between their clinicians and their mental health providers, they actually prefer to avoid collocation of the two services [66].

Engaging the Patient as Part of the Integrated Care Team

Fundamental to the Chronic Care Model is the need for patients to be informed, activated partners in the management of their own conditions. In recent years, the concept of integrated care has been expanded to include the patient as a key member of the care team [67, 68]. While patient engagement is most commonly thought of as occurring at the level of direct patient care, engagement can also occur at organizational and policy [69].

Two areas closely related to patient engagement are patient activation and shared decision-making. Patient activation, while sometimes used synonymously with patient engagement, refers to increasing patients' knowledge, confidence, and/or skills for disease self-management, while engagement generally refers to actual patient behaviours [70]. None the less, patient engagement is most often assessed using the widely validated Patient Activation Measure [71]. Patient activation has been associated with higher quality of care for chronic conditions generally and to have a modest association with lower costs [72]. A recent meta-analysis of interventions to increase the activation of patients with type 2 diabetes found modest but significant net improvement in HbA1c (0.4 %), SBP (2.2 mmHg), LDL and weight (2.3 lb) [73].

Shared decision-making has various definitions, but at a minimum seems to require that the patient and physician share information and preferences and engage in a process of coming to a mutually agreeable decision [74]. Ethically, shared decision-making respects a patient's autonomy and right to make an informed choice; pragmatically, shared decision-making allows the patient to contribute information and preferences that will presumably result in a better decision and greater patient participation in implementing the decision [75]. Multiple measures of shared decision-making have been developed [76, 77] and interventions to increase shared decision-making have been tested [78, 79]. Shared decision-making can also include decision-making between the patient and the care team [80].

Practice Transformation and the Ten Building Blocks

A PCMH-related model that may be more transformative of diabetes care is the Building Blocks of High-Performing Primary Care [81, 82]. The building blocks (Fig. 3.3) are characteristics found in primary care practices with excellent patient access, continuity of care, use of data to drive improvement, well-functioning teams, and an orientation towards population-wide care. Blocks in the first row are practice characteristics that support the higher blocks. Block 1, engaged leadership, refers to leadership at all levels of the organization, including clinicians, nursing, medical staff and in some clinics patients as well. Data-driven improvement (block 2) requires systems that can track and feedback "clinical (e.g., cancer screening and diabetes management), operational (continuity of care and access), and patients' experience metrics." Empanelment (block 3) means linking each patient to a care team and a primary care clinician. Many exemplar practices have created teams (block 4) with well-trained non-clinicians who add primary care capacity by "sharing the care" [82, 83]. The patient-team partnership (block 5) recognizes the expertise that patients bring to the medical encounter so that patients are not told what to do but are engaged in shared decision-making that respects their personal goals. Block 6, population management, includes proactively addressing gaps in care, such as screening LDL and foot examinations for patients with diabetes. Health coaching and complex care management are also included in this block. Blocks 7, 8 and 9 are self-explanatory and are considered key characteristics of primary care. The last block, template of the future, refers to a practice which supplements one-on-one clinician visits with group visits, telephone visits, patient-portal e-visits, and visits to non-clinician team members, operating in a payment system that supports this model, rather than simply paying for in-person clinician visits. For patients with diabetes, such high-performing practices closely follow a number of diabetes-related processes of care and outcome metrics drilled down to the level of individual clinicians and teams, and organize diabetes care as a team responsibility rather than the sole province of the clinician. Patients with diabetes may have access to RN or pharmacist care managers, group diabetes visits, and health coaches.

Telemedicine and Digital Health Tools: The Future of Integrated Care for Patients with Diabetes?

The rapidly increasing availability of telecommunication options has recently opened up new opportunities for providing more integrated care. Telemedicine, defined as medical activity using some form of telecommunication, includes telephone, internet and smartphone-based programmes [84]. A recent systematic review and meta-analysis of 13 RCTs of telemedicine for patients with diabetes reported that telemedicine-based interventions resulted in a statistically significant decline in mean HbA1c (difference = 0.44 %) and LDL (difference = 6.6 mg/dL (0.17 mmol/l)) levels compared to controls, with no impact on blood pressure [85]. Specific examples of the application of telemedicine to the management of diabetes are described below.

Automated telephone self-management support (ATSM) uses interactive telephone technology to provide surveillance and patient education which can be combined with nurse care management [86]. In one study, English-, Spanish-, and Cantonese-speaking patients with diabetes seen in community ("safety-net") clinics in San Francisco were randomized to receive usual care, interactive weekly automated telephone self-management support with nurse follow-up (ATSM), or monthly group medical visits with physician and health educator facilitation (GMV). No significant difference in HbA1c levels was found [87, 88]. Only the ATSM group showed improvements in reported interpersonal processes of care. Both intervention arms showed significant improvements in self-management behaviours versus the usual care arm with gains being greater for the ATSM group than for the GMV group. The ATSM group also had fewer bed days per month than the usual care and GMV groups and less interference with daily activities than the usual care group. A follow-up study using waitlist controls found that, compared with waitlisted patients, immediate intervention participants had significantly greater 6-month improvement in overall diabetes self-care behaviours [89].

Another promising use of digital technology is to enhance communication between primary care clinicians and specialist colleagues to improve patient care for a variety of conditions, including diabetes. One such programme, "e-referral" (electronic referral), was developed for use at San Francisco General Hospital to facilitate communication between primary care clinicians and specialists in the context of making an electronic referral or consultation [90, 91]. E-referral documents the pertinent clinical history and reason for the consultation. A designated specialist reviewer then responds, perhaps requesting further information, suggesting additional tests or management strategies, redirecting the referral if indicated, or simply making an appointment for the patient. E-referral been shown to increase access to care and increase the appropriateness of referrals. It can also improve the primary care clinician's capacity for complex decision-making and promote a dialogue between primary care clinicians and specialists [92]. The effectiveness of e-referral has been best documented for rheumatology [93] and gastroenterology [94] and is currently being used for referrals to endocrinologists and diabetes nurse educators at San Francisco General Hospital. Similar systems are being implemented in Los Angeles, Boston, and other sites.

A variety of internet-based programmes have been used to improve patient self-care for diabetes [95] including increasing blood glucose monitoring frequency [96], reducing HbA1c levels [97–104] and increasing self-reported physical activity [99, 102]. An early example from Seattle, Washington provided patients with type 2 diabetes access to their electronic health records, a secure e-mail with providers, diabetes education, feedback on blood glucose readings, and an interactive tool to track exercise, diet and medication; intervention patients demonstrated a greater decline in HbA1c (0.7 %) compared to patients randomized to receive usual care alone [103]. Internet-based programmes may also be used to augment care management [104] and to provide behavioural support [105]. Similar programmes can include a mechanism to upload blood glucose values measured by the patient, of particular importance in type 1 diabetes [106]. Internet-based patient engagement may be effective by itself, even without a care manager [98, 107].

A burgeoning number of mobile phone applications (apps) have been created to improve patient self-management of diabetes and communication between the patient and the health-care team. The simplest technology allows for one way messaging, e.g., for appointment reminders or to take medications. In 2011 Liang et al. reported a meta-analysis of 22 trials investigating mobile phone-based interventions for diabetes [108]. Half the trials were RCTs; approximately half were of patients with type 1, and half with type 2, diabetes. All apps used short messages to support self-monitoring of blood glucose, education, diet, exercise and medication adjustment. Eight studies also included a component of internet support and 14 studies featured downloading or entering daily blood glucose values. The meta-analysis found significant reductions in HbA1c of 0.8 % for patients with type 2 diabetes and 0.3 % for patients with type 1 diabetes compared to usual care controls. Studies with both mobile phone and Internet interventions showed greater reduction in HbA1c than the studies with only a mobile phone intervention and studies with daily intervention reported greater reduction in HbA1c than those with only weekly intervention; however, these differences did not reach statistical significance.

A more recent study enrolled 65 people with HbA1c >8.0 % who were established (>6 months) patients in the endocrinology clinics of the Walter Reed Health Care System. Participants were randomized to receive "usual care" or self-care video messages from their diabetes nurse practitioner [109]. Video messages were sent daily to cell phones of study participants. Participants who received the messages had small but significant improvement in their HbA1c levels compared to those who received usual care (0.2 % difference over 12 months). Haemoglobin A1c decline was greatest among participants who received video messages and viewed more than ten messages a month (0.6 % difference).

More sophisticated mobile phone applications for helping patients are now commercially available [110]. Essentially all allow short messaging from a care provider and entry and retrieval of data such as blood glucose or blood pressure. Many allow two-way communication between the patient and patient care team, can provide targeted educational materials, allow access to personal health information, and can be used to adjust medications. Examples include CarePlanManager™ (CircleLink Health, Stamford, CT, USA) (https://www.careplanmanager.com/), MedAdherence (Norwalk, CT, USA) (www.medadherence.com), CareMessage™ (San Francisco, CA, USA) (http://caremessage.org/), Twine (Twine Health, Cambridge, MA, USA) (http://www.twinehealth.com/), WellDoc DiabetesManager (Baltimore, MD, USA) (http://www.welldoc.com) and CareSmarts (Larkspur, CA, USA) (https://www.mhealth-solutions.com) to name a few. WellDoc DiabetesManager provides three components (1) real-time educational and behavioural messaging to patients based on blood glucose values, medications and lifestyle behaviours plus summary data; (2) a portal where patients and their physicians can access the data; and (3) a data analysis and evidence-based treatment recommendations for physicians [110–113]. A cluster RCT of 26 practices (total of 163 patients) compared usual care to three versions of the intervention: component 1 only, and components 1 and 2, to the full version with all three components [113]. At 12 months, the mean HbA1c had declined 0.7 % (from 9.2 % to 8.5 %) in usual care group, compared to 1.6 % (from in 9.3 to 7.7) in the component 1 group, by 1.2 % (from 9.0 to 7.9) in the component and two group, and by 1.9 % (from 9.9 % to 7.9 %) in the full version, The decline in HbA1c was significantly greater in the full version group compared to usual care (difference of 1.2 % $P<0.001$) but not significantly different compared to the other two intervention groups. There were no appreciable differences between groups for patient-reported diabetes distress, depression, diabetes symptoms, or blood pressure and lipid levels. Another mobile phone-based application, CareSmarts, developed at University of Chicago Medicine, provides automated text messages to provide patient education, support patient self-management and facilitate communication between the patients and members of their health-care team [110, 114]. Patient responses to self-assessment questions are used to monitor patient care and, if outside an established range, can trigger a member of the care team to contact the patient. In a prospective study, patients with diabetes in the University of Chicago's employee health plan were offered the programme; 74 enrolled in the programme and 274 did not [110]. Those enrolled had a higher baseline HbA1c (7.9 vs 7.4 but were similar in demographic characteristics to those not enrolled. Enrolled patients experienced significant improvements in HbA1c (-0.4 %, care utilization, and self-reported healthy eating, glucose monitoring and diabetes medication adherence at 6 months, but outcomes for patients not enrolled were not reported in sufficient detail to provide a meaningful comparison. The website www.diabetesmine.com provides an updated list and evaluations of mobile apps for type 1 and type 2 diabetes. Wider application of mobile or "smart phone" applications in the US will require compliance with requirements for handling personal medical information. It remains to be seen what proportion of the population will adopt such applications and how these applications will be integrated into their medical care.

Integrated Care for the Urban and Rural Underserved

While most studies have found a positive association between characteristics of a Patient-Centered Medical Home and the quality of care for patients with diabetes, it is not clear that this relationship holds among community (safety net) clinics already meeting basic standards of a medical home. A study of 40 community health clinics in Los Angeles, all of whom met the NCQA standards to qualify as a medical home, found that scoring higher on a widely used medical home assessment instrument, the NCQA Physician Practice Connections–Patient-Centered Medical Home tool, was not associated with better diabetes performance on processes of care (e.g., screening for early renal disease) and intermediate outcomes including HbA1c and blood pressure [115].

In contrast, several studies using integrated care models for patients with diabetes living in rural areas have shown improvement in outcomes. In North Carolina, a team-based intervention used a nurse, pharmacist and dietitian to provide point-of-care education, coaching and medication intensification for rural African Americans with diabetes [116]. Patients receiving the intervention had a significantly greater drop in HbA1c compared to usual care patients (0.5 % vs 0.1 %). A significantly higher proportion of intervention patients achieved an HbA1c level <7.5 % (68 % vs 59 %) and a systolic blood pressure <140 mmHg (69 % vs 57 %). A recently published multidisciplinary team care management intervention for 3373 American Indians/Alaska Natives found modest but significant decreases in HbA1c (0.2 %) after 1 year as well as a significant reduction in LDL cholesterol [117].

In the IDEATel study, 1665 Medicare recipients with diabetes, residing in federally designated medically underserved areas of rural New York State, were randomized to receive a home telemedicine unit with nurse care management versus usual care [118]. Patients in the telemedicine group received a web camera that allowed video conferencing with nurse care managers, a home glucose metre and blood pressure cuff that connected to the internet, access to their own clinical data and to an educational webpage. Telemedicine achieved modest though statistically significant net overall reductions over 5 years of follow-up for the primary endpoints of HbA1c (0.3 %), LDL (3.8 mg/dl), systolic and diastolic blood pressure (4.3 and 2.6 mmHg, respectively). In an observational study of telemedicine using touchscreen internet technology and home monitoring of blood glucose and blood pressure in 109 rural patients, significant improvements for baseline were seen for HbA1c which decreased from a mean of 9.7 % to 7.8 %, for systolic blood pressure which dropped from 131 to 123 mmHg, and for LDL which moved from 103 to 93 mg/dl [119].

Project Dulce is a programme, originating in San Diego, which has provided integrated care to low-income people with diabetes since 1997. Project Dulce is a mixed community and primary care-based model, combining RN care management and peer-led education classes. People with diabetes are referred by primary care providers (PCPs) from many community health centres. Patients are linked to a RN care manager in regular contact with the PCP and are encouraged to join a group self-management support class taught by trained community health workers (CHWs) known as "promotoras." The classes, in English, Spanish, Vietnamese, and other languages cover the basic concepts of diabetes, healthy eating, exercise, and medications. The "promotoras" often have diabetes themselves and must complete a 4-month training and mentoring programme. The peer-led classes take place in the community, while visits with the registered nurses (RNs) are performed in the patient's clinic so that the RN can interact with the PCP. RNs travel from one clinic to another on a regular schedule. RNs order and review laboratory studies, do foot exams, refer for eye exams, and manage medications in consultation with the PCP. A study conducted by Project Dulce found that participants in the programme had significant improvements in HbA1c, LDL cholesterol, and diastolic blood pressure compared with controls [62]. A further study looked at patients who attended the peer-led classes but did not engage in RN care management and found that they also had a significant improvement in HbA1c compared with controls [61].

Our Approach to Integrated Diabetes Care

The authors' primary research and practice site is the system of community clinics and hospital outpatient clinics operated by the City and County of San Francisco. This "safety net" system serves a highly diverse population of low-income patients, many of whom face challenges such as being non-English speaking and of low literacy, in addition to economic and social stressors. Many of our patients have current or past problems with drug abuse, alcoholism, and mental health conditions. As in many under-resourced safety net systems in the US, improvement in integrated care for our patients with diabetes and other chronic diseases has taken place in a somewhat piece-meal and opportunistic fashion, in contrast with the more comprehensive forms of primary care transformation promoted by the PCMH movement. Leaders of San Francisco's public safety-net system, tasked with providing care for low-income and uninsured patients, work closely with researchers and clinical leaders in Family and Community Medicine, General Internal Medicine, and other disciplines in the schools of Medicine, Nursing and Pharmacy at the University of California, San Francisco as well as with health-care clinicians, staff and patients. The result has been the development or adoption of several models for integrated care described earlier in this chapter, including automated telephone support [87, 88], electronic referrals [90–92], and patient care teams [53] that include pharmacists, nurses, dieticians and mental health providers. The system has implemented registries of patients with diabetes [120], health coaching [54, 55, 57, 59] and practice transformation using the 10 Building Blocks of High-Performing Primary Care model [82, 83]. Several clinics have mental health professionals on-site in the form of social workers and psychologists, allowing for warm handoffs for patients with diabetes and depression or other mental health issues. Processes have been worked out to allow health coaches access to patients' electronic health records (with patients' permission) and the ability to communicate information to clinicians using the electronic medical record. A patient portal which will initially allow patients access to laboratory results and appointments is being rolled out, with plans to expand allowing secure electronic communication between patients and their care team. We are also looking at ways to include patients in electronic communications between primary care clinicians and subspecialists and to increase patient involvement at the organizational level of care. The potential of many of these approaches has not been fully realized and work is continuing towards the goal of providing better integrated care for all of our patients.

Paying for Integrated Diabetes Care

Integrated care for patients for diabetes has become increasingly common in the US due to consolidation of health care into larger organizational units, recognition of the importance of integrated care, and efforts to organize, support and reward clinical care that is more integrated. These developments have been spearheaded by the PCMH movement and further supported by provisions of the Affordable Care Act of 2010. The PCMH has promoted integrated care by advocating for changes in payment structure to move beyond paying only for face-to-face clinician visits to include payment for care coordination services, improved access and communication, and adoption of health information technology [37]. Financial facilitators of integrated care include support for development and adoption of health information technology, most notably as part of the 2010 Affordable Care Act, and tying higher payment to NCQA certification as a PCMH. In 2015, the Centers for Medicare and Medicaid Services, which administers the federal programmes for health care to elderly and low-income Americans, introduced the first non–visit-based payment for chronic care management [121, 122].

The cost-effectiveness of integrated care for patients with diabetes depends on the model of integrated care used, the system in which it is used, and the time-horizon chosen [123]. Models of cost benefit for using health coaching interventions for patients with poorly controlled diabetes have generally found a benefit in reducing HbA1c levels, but at the cost of paying for the added cost of health coaching which is not offset in the short term by savings from emergency department visits and hospitalizations [124–126]. Costs for medication and numbers of primary care visits may increase as health coaches improve patient adherence to medications and re-engage patients in the health-care system [123, 127].

Another approach to estimating cost-effectiveness is to use models to estimate future cost savings from reduction in HbA1c levels and better management of associated cardiovascular disease risk factors such as hypertension and hyperlipidemia [128]. Adopting such a model of cost-effectiveness assumes that gains in the short run can be maintained over time, and that the party incurring the short term costs will also benefit from any long-term savings.

An important question in assessing the cost of integrated care is whether it needs to be cost-saving or cost-neutral to be adopted, or is it enough to increase quality-adjusted life years (QALYs) at a "reasonable" cost (usually pegged at between $30,000 and $60,000 per QALY saved). Most integrated care programmes for patients with diabetes that have been evaluated for cost-effectiveness would meet this more liberal criterion [124, 126].

In practice, integrated care programmes for patients with diabetes are often part of generalized programmes of care for patients with other chronic medical conditions, making the allocation of costs and savings with respect to integrated care for diabetes difficult to estimate. At this point, integrated care for patients with diabetes appears to be a widely accepted goal. The question becomes: which model of integrated care is most effective at reasonable cost? Answering this question depends both on what costs are included and what outcomes are measured; the answers may vary among different patient populations and different care systems.

Summary and Conclusions

An unacceptably large proportion of patients with diabetes in the US do not meet national guidelines for control of their diabetes and related conditions. The importance of integrated, patient-centred care has long been recognized and was the basis for the development of the Chronic Care Model in the mid-1990s. The CCM in turn has provided a basis for development and testing of new models of care, including care management, care teams, and the Patient-Centered Medical

Home (PCMH). The PCMH has been seen as a strong model for integration in general and for the care of patients with diabetes in particular. In concert with the PCMH movement, a substantial amount of work has taken place to make integrated care more patient-centred, through patient activation, patient education and engagement, shared decision-making, and self-management support including health coaching. Research in these areas has generally supported the view that including patients with diabetes in their care can improve patient care processes and outcomes, including better control of blood glucose, blood pressure and LDL cholesterol. Such interventions do not appear to reduce short-term costs, but most studies have found them to be cost-effective in terms of quality-adjusted life years saved, particularly if the benefits are projected over time to include late complications of poorly controlled diabetes.

Many PCMH-based models now incorporate multiple intervention components with ongoing evaluation. Realizing the potential of these approaches to integrated care is particularly challenging for providing care to patients with diabetes in urban and rural underserved populations. Our work in San Francisco's safety-net system illustrates those challenges and has led to new approaches for providing integrated care. The role of telehealth in providing integrated care will continue to grow. How digital programmes will be incorporated into current models of integrated care, and the balance between digital programmes and personal relationships, will likely be an important area for future research. While the growing support for integrated care has included financial incentives from both public and private payers, the optimal models of integrated care and their cost-effectiveness in both the short- and long-term remains an area of active investigation.

References

1. Selvin E, Parrinello CM, Sacks DB, Coresh J. Trends in prevalence and control of diabetes in the United States, 1988–1994 and 1999–2010. Ann Intern Med. 2014;160(8):517–25.
2. El Achhab Y, Nejjari C, Chikri M, Lyoussi B. Disease-specific health-related quality of life instruments among adults diabetic: a systematic review. Diabetes Res Clin Pract. 2008;80(2):171–84.
3. Polonsky WH, Fisher L, Earles J, Dudl RJ, Lees J, Mullan J, Jackson RA. Assessing psychosocial distress in diabetes. Diabetes Care. 2005;28(3):626–31.
4. Kroenke K, Spitzer RL, Williams JBW. The PHQ-9. J Gen Intern Med. 2001;16(9):606–13.
5. Narayan KM, Gregg EW, Fagot-Campagna A, Gary TL, Saaddine JB, Parker C, Imperatore G, Valdez R, Beckles G, Engelgau MM. Relationship between quality of diabetes care and patient satisfaction. J Natl Med Assoc. 2003;95(1):64–70.
6. Wagner EH, Austin BT, Von Korff M. Organizing care for patients with chronic illness. Milbank Q. 1996;74(4):511–44.
7. Wagner EH. Chronic disease management: what will it take to improve care for chronic illness? Eff Clin Pract. 1998;1:2–4.
8. Coleman K, Austin BT, Brach C, Wagner EH. Evidence on the chronic care model in the new millennium. Health Aff (Millwood). 2009;28(1):75–85.
9. Parchman ML, et al. Risk of coronary artery disease in type 2 diabetes and the delivery of care consistent with the chronic care model in primary care settings: a STARNet study. Med Care. 2007;45:1129–34.
10. DiPiero A, Dorr DA, Kelso C, Bowen JL. Integrating systematic chronic care for diabetes into an academic general internal medicine resident-faculty practice. J Gen Intern Med. 2008;23(11):1749–56.
11. Piatt GA, Orchard TJ, Emerson S, Simmons D, Songer TJ, Brooks MM, Korytkowski M, Siminerio LM, Ahmad U, Zgibor JC. Translating the chronic care model into the community: results from a randomized controlled trial of a multifaceted diabetes care intervention. Diabetes Care. 2006;29:811–7.
12. McCulloch DK, Price MJ, Hindmarsh M, Wagner EH. A population-based approach to diabetes management in a primary care setting: early results and lessons learned. Eff Clin Pract. 1998;1(1):12–22.
13. Smith SA, Shah ND, Bryant SC, Christianson TJ, Bjornsen SS, Giesler PD, et al. Chronic care model and shared care in diabetes: randomized trial of an electronic decision support system. Mayo Clin Proc. 2008;83(7):747–57.
14. Stock S, Pitcavage JM, Simic D, Altin S, Graf C, Feng W, Graf TR. Chronic care model strategies in the United States and Germany deliver patient-centered, high-quality diabetes care. Health Aff (Millwood). 2014;33(9):1540–8.
15. Stellefson M, Dipnarine K, Stopka C. The chronic care model and diabetes management in US primary care settings: a systematic review. Prev Chronic Dis. 2013;10:E26.

16. Sunaert P, Bastiaens H, Nobels F, Feyen L, Verbeke G, Vermeire E, De Maeseneer J, Willems S, De Sutter A. Effectiveness of the introduction of a chronic care model-based program for type 2 diabetes in Belgium. BMC Health Serv Res. 2010;10:207.
17. Nutting PA, Dickinson WP, Dickinson LM, Nelson CC, King DK, Crabtree BF, Glasgow RE. Use of chronic care model elements is associated with higher-quality care for diabetes. Ann Fam Med. 2007;5(1):14–20.
18. Shojania KG, Ranji SR, McDonald KM, et al. Effects of quality improvement strategies for type 2 diabetes on glycemic control: a meta-regression analysis. JAMA. 2006;296:427–40.
19. Pimouguet C, Le Goff M, Thiébaut R, Dartigues JF, Helmer C. Effectiveness of disease-management programs for improving diabetes care: a meta-analysis. CMAJ. 2011;183(2):E115–27.
20. Davidson MB. How our current medical care system fails people with diabetes. Diabetes Care. 2009;32:370–2.
21. Krein SL, Klamerus ML, Vijan S, et al. Case management for patients with poorly controlled diabetes: a randomized controlled trial. Am J Med. 2004;116:732–9.
22. Choe HM, Mitrovich S, Dubay D, Hayward RA, Krein SL, Vijan S. Proactive case management of high risk patients with type 2 diabetes mellitus by a clinical pharmacist: a randomized controlled trial. Am J Manag Care. 2005;11:253–60.
23. Ishani A, Greer N, Taylor BC, Kubes L, Cole P, Atwood M, Clothier B, Ercan-Fang N. Effect of nurse case management compared with usual care on controlling cardiovascular risk factors in patients with diabetes: a randomized controlled trial. Diabetes Care. 2011;34(8):1689–94.
24. Sadur CN, Moline N, Costa M, et al. Diabetes management in a health maintenance organization: efficacy of care management using cluster visits. Diabetes Care. 1999;22:2011–7.
25. Peterson KA, Radosevich DM, O'Connor PJ, Nyman JA, Prineas RJ, Smith SA, Arneson TJ, Corbett VA, Weinhandl JC, Lange CJ, Hannan PJ. Improving diabetes care in practice: findings from the TRANSLATE trial. Diabetes Care. 2008;31(12):2238–43.
26. Polonsky WH, Earles J, Smith S, et al. Integrating medical management with diabetes self-management training: a randomized control trial of the diabetes outpatient intensive treatment program. Diabetes Care. 2003;26:3048–53.
27. Fleming B, Silver A, Ocepek-Welikson K, Keller D. The relationship between organizational systems and clinical quality in diabetes care. Am J Manag Care. 2004;10(12):934–44.
28. Solberg LI, Asche SE, Pawlson LG, Scholle SH, Shih SC. Practice systems are associated with high-quality care for diabetes. Am J Manag Care. 2008;14(2):85–92.
29. Nutting PA, Crabtree BF, Miller WL, Stange KC, Stewart E, Jaén C. Transforming physician practices to patient-centered medical homes: lessons from the national demonstration project. Health Aff (Millwood). 2011;30:439–45.
30. American College of Physicians. The advanced medical home: a patient-centered, physician-guided model of health care. Philadelphia: American College of Physicians; 2005. Position Paper. [cited 2015 Jun 16]. Available from: https://www.acponline.org/advocacy/current_policy_papers/assets/adv_med.pdf.
31. American Academy of Family Physicians (AAFP), American Academy of Pediatrics (AAP), American College of Physicians (ACP), American Osteopathic Association (AOA). Joint principles of the patient-centered medical home. 2007. [Cited 2015 Jun 16]. Available from: http://www.aafp.org/dam/AAFP/documents/practice_management/pcmh/initiatives/PCMHJoint.pdf
32. Wagner EH. The role of patient care teams in chronic disease management. BMJ. 2000;320:569–72.
33. Wagner EH, Sandhu N, Coleman K, Phillips KE, Sugarman JR. Improving care coordination in primary care. Med Care. 2014;52:S33–8.
34. Bojadzievski T, Gabbay RA. Patient-centered medical home and diabetes. Diabetes Care. 2011;34(4):1047–53.
35. National Committee on Quality Assurance. Patient-Centered Medical Home. [Cited 2015 Jun 16]. Available from: http://www.ncqa.org/Programs/Recognition/Practices/PatientCenteredMedicalHomePCMH/NewVersionofPCMH.aspx
36. Agency for Healthcare Research and Quality (AHRQ). Defining the PCMH. [cited 2015 Jun 22]. Available from: https://pcmh.ahrq.gov/page/defining-pcmh
37. Stange KC, Nutting PA, Miller WL, Jaén CR, Crabtree BF, Flocke SA, Gill JM. Defining and measuring the patient-centered medical home. J Gen Intern Med. 2010;25:601–12.
38. National Committee for Quality Assurance (NCQA) Care Coordination Standards. McColl Institute 2011. [Cited 2015 Jun 16]. Available from: http://www.improvingchroniccare.org/downloads/1_ncqa_care_coordination_process_measures.pdf
39. Daniel DM, Wagner EH, Coleman K, et al. Assessing progress toward becoming a patient-centered medical home: an assessment tool for practice transformation. Health Serv Res. 2013;48:1879–97.
40. Jortberg BT, Miller BF, Gabbay RA, Sparling K, Dickinson WP. Patient-centered medical home: how it affects psychosocial outcomes for diabetes. Curr Diabet Rep. 2012;12(6):721–8.
41. Paulus RA, Davis K, Steele GD. Continuous innovation in health care: implications of the Geisinger experience. Health Aff (Millwood). 2008;27:1235–45.

42. Friedberg MW, Rosenthal MB, Werner RM, Volpp KG, Schneider EC. Effects of a medical home and shared savings intervention on quality and utilization of care. JAMA Intern Med. 2015;175(8):1362–8.
43. McCarthy D, Mueller K, Tillmann I. HealthPartners: consumer-focused mission and collaborative approach support ambitious performance improvement agenda. New York: The Commonwealth Fund Publication; 2009. p. 1250. [Cited 2015 Jun 16]. Available from: http://www.commonwealthfund.org/~/media/files/publications/case-study/2009/jun/1250_mccarthy_healthpartners_case_study_61_for-pf.pdf.
44. Steiner BD, Denham AC, Ashkin E, Newton WP, Wroth T, Dobson Jr LA. Community care of North Carolina: improving care through community health networks. Ann Fam Med. 2008;6:361–7.
45. Colorado PCMH Multi-Payer. Multi-state pilot: a year in review. [cited 2015 Jun 16]. Available from: https://www.pcpcc.org/webinar/cmd-colorado-pcmh-multi-payer-multi-state-pilot-year-review
46. Alidina S, Schneider EC, Singer SJ, Rosenthal MB. Structural capabilities in small and medium-sized patient-centered medical homes. Am J Manag Care. 2014;20(7):e265–77.
47. Reid RJ, Coleman K, Johnson EA, Fishman PA, Hsu C, Soman MP, et al. The group health medical home at year two: cost savings, higher patient satisfaction, and less burnout for providers. Health Aff (Millwood). 2010;29(5):835–43.
48. Jaén CR, Ferrer RL, Miller WL, Palmer RF, Wood R, Davila M, et al. Patient outcomes at 26 months in the patient-centered medical home national demonstration project. Ann Fam Med. 2010;8(1 Suppl):S57–67. S92.
49. Miller BF, Kessler R, Peek CJ, Kallenberg GA. A national research agenda for research in collaborative care: papers from the collaborative care research network research development conference. AHRQ Publication No. 11-0067. 2011. [Cited 2015 Jun 16]. Available from: http://www.ahrq.gov/research/collaborativecare/
50. Jaber LA, Halapy H, Fernet M, Tummalapalli S, Diwakaran H. Evaluation of a pharmaceutical care model on diabetes management. Ann Pharmacother. 1996;30:238–43.
51. Johnson KA, Chen S, Cheng IN, Lou M, Gregerson P, Blieden C, et al. The impact of clinical pharmacy services integrated into medical homes on diabetes-related clinical outcomes. Ann Pharmacother. 2010;44:1877–86.
52. Choe HM, Bernstein SJ, Mueller BA, Walker PC, Stevenson JG, Standiford CJ. Pharmacist leads primary care team to improve diabetes care. Am J Health Syst Pharm. 2009;66(7):622–4.
53. Bodenheimer T, Willard-Grace R, Ghorob A. Expanding the roles of medical assistants: who does what in primary care? JAMA Intern Med. 2014;174:1025–6.
54. Bennett HD, Coleman EA, Parry C, Bodenheimer T, Chen EH. Health coaching for patients with chronic illness. Fam Pract Manag. 2010;17:24–9.
55. Ghorob A. Health coaching: teaching patients how to fish. Fam Pract Manag. 2013;20(3):40–2.
56. Naik AD, Palmer N, Petersen NJ, Street RL, Rao R, Suarez-Almazor M, Haider P. Comparative effectiveness of goal setting in diabetes mellitus group clinics. Arch Intern Med. 2011;171(5):453–9.
57. Willard-Grace R, Thom DH, Hessler D, Bodenheimer T, Chen EH. Health coaching to improve control of diabetes, hypertension and hyperlipidemia for low-income patients: a randomized controlled trial. Ann Fam Med. 2015;28(1):38–45.
58. Heisler M, Vijan S, Makki F, Piette JD. Diabetes control with reciprocal peer support versus nurse care management: a randomized trial. Ann Intern Med. 2010;153(8):507–15.
59. Thom DH, Ghorob A, Hessler D, De Vore D, Chen EH, Bodenheimer T. Peer health coaching improves glycemic in low-income patients with diabetes: results of a randomized controlled trial. Ann Fam Med. 2013;11:137–44.
60. Spencer MS, Rosland AM, Kieffer EC, Sinco BR, Valerio M, Palmisano G, et al. Effectiveness of a community health worker intervention among African- American and Latino adults with type 2 diabetes. Am J Public Health. 2011;101:2253–60.
61. Philis-Tsimikas A, Fortmann A, Lleva-Ocana L, Walker C, Gallo LC. Peer-led diabetes education programs in high-risk Mexican Americans improve glycemic control compared with standard approaches: a Project Dulce promotora randomized trial. Diabetes Care. 2011;34(9):1926–31.
62. Philis-Tsimikas A, Walker C, Rivard L, et al. Improvement in diabetes care of underinsured patients enrolled in Project Dulce. Diabetes Care. 2004;27:110–5.
63. California Health Workforce Alliance (CHWA), Taking Innovation to scale: community health workers, promoters, and the triple aim. A statewide assessment of the roles and contributions of California's community health workers. Preliminary findings, observations, and recommendations. Public Health Institute/California Health Workforce Alliance 2013. [cited 2015 Jun 16]. Available from: www.calhealthworkforce.org
64. Coventry P, Lovell K, Dickens C, Bower P, Chew-Graham C, McElvenny D, Hann M, Cherrington A, Garrett C, Gibbons CJ, Baguley C, Roughley K, Adeyemi I, Reeves D, Waheed W, Gask L. Integrated primary care for patients with mental and physical multimorbidity: cluster randomised controlled trial of collaborative care for patients with depression comorbid with diabetes or cardiovascular disease. BMJ. 2015;350:h638.

65. Katon W, Russo J, Lin EH, Schmittdiel J, Ciechanowski P, Ludman E, Peterson D, Young B, Von Korff M. Cost-effectiveness of a multicondition collaborative care intervention: a randomized controlled trial. Arch Gen Psychiatry. 2012;69(5):506–14.
66. Knowles SE, Chew-Graham C, Adeyemi I, Coupe N, Coventry PA. Managing depression in people with multimorbidity: a qualitative evaluation of an integrated collaborative care model. BMC Fam Pract. 2015;16(1):32.
67. Barello S, Graffigna G, Vegni E. Patient engagement as an emerging challenge for healthcare services: mapping the literature. Nurs Res Pract. 2012;2012:905934.
68. Graffigna G, Barello S, Libreri C, Bosio CA. How to engage type-2 diabetic patients in their own health management: implications for clinical practice. BMC Public Health. 2014;14:648.
69. Carman KL, Dardess P, Mauer M, et al. Patient and family engagement: a framework for understanding the elements and developing interventions and policies. Health Aff. 2013;32:223–31.
70. Hibbard JH, Greene J. What the evidence shows about patient activation: better health outcomes and care experiences; fewer data on costs. Health Aff (Millwood). 2013;32(2):207–14.
71. Hibbard JH, Stockard J, Mahoney ER, Tusler M. Development of the patient activation measure (PAM): conceptualizing and measuring activation in patients and consumers. Health Serv Res. 2004;39(4 Pt 1):1005–26.
72. Greene J, Hibbard JH, Sacks R, Overton V, Parrotta CD. When patient activation levels change, health outcomes and costs change, too. Health Aff (Millwood). 2015;34(3):431–7.
73. Bolen SD, Chandar A, Falck-Ytter C, Tyler C, Perzynski AT, Gertz AM, Sage P, Lewis S, Cobabe M, Ye Y, Menegay M, Windish DM. Effectiveness and safety of patient activation interventions for adults with type 2 diabetes: systematic review, meta-analysis, and meta-regression. J Gen Intern Med. 2014;29(8):1166–76.
74. Makoul G, Clayman ML. An integrative model of shared decision making in medical encounters. Patient Educ Couns. 2006;60:301–12.
75. Elwyn G, Frosch D, Thomson R, Joseph-Williams N, Lloyd A, Kinnersley P, Cording E, Tomson D, Dodd C, Rollnick S, Edwards A, Barry M. Shared decision making: a model for clinical practice. J Gen Intern Med. 2012;27:1361–7.
76. Elwyn G, Hutchings H, Edwards A, Rapport F, Wensing M, Cheung W, et al. The OPTION scale: measuring the extent that clinicians involve patients in decision-making tasks. Health Expect. 2005;8:34–40.
77. Dy SM. Instruments for evaluating shared medical decision making: a structured literature review. Med Care Res Rev. 2007;64:623–49.
78. Loh A, Simon D, Wills CE, Kriston L, Niebling W, Harter M. The effects of a shared decision-making intervention in primary care of depression: a cluster-randomized controlled trial. Pat Educ Counsel. 2007;67:324–32.
79. Elwyn G, Edwards A, Hood K, Robling M, Atwell C, Russell I, Wensing M, Grol R, Study Steering Group. Achieving involvement: process outcomes from a cluster randomized trial of shared decision making skill development and use of risk communication aids in general practice. Fam Pract. 2004;21(4):337–46.
80. Legare F, Stacey D, Pouliot S. Interprofessionalism and shared decision-making in primary care: a stepwise approach towards a new model. J Interprofess Care. 2011;25:18–25.
81. Bodenheimer T, Ghorob A, Willard-Grace R, Grumbach K. The 10 building blocks of high-performing primary care. Ann Fam Med. 2014;12:166–71.
82. Willard R, Bodenheimer T. The building blocks of high-performing primary care: lessons from the field. California HealthCare Foundation April 2012. [Cited 2015 Jun 16]. Available from: http://www.chcf.org/publications/2012/04/building-blocks-primary-care
83. Ghorob A, Bodenheimer T. Sharing the care to improve access to primary care. N Engl J Med. 2012;366(21):1955–7.
84. Balkhi AM, Reid AM, Westen SC, Olsen B, Janicke DM, Geffken GR. Telehealth interventions to reduce management complications in type 1 diabetes. World J Diabetes. 2015;6:371–9.
85. Marcolino MS, Maia JX, Alkmim MB, Boersma E, Ribeiro AL. Telemedicine application in the care of diabetes patients: systematic review and meta-analysis. PLoS ONE. 2013;8(11):e79246.
86. Piette JD, Weinberger M, McPhee SJ, Mah CA, Kraemer FB, Crapo LM. Do automated calls with nurse follow-up improve self-care and glycemic control among vulnerable patients with diabetes? Am J Med. 2000;108(1):20–7.
87. Schillinger D, Hammer H, Wang F, Palacios J, McLean I, Tang A, Youmans S, Handley M. Seeing in 3-D: examining the reach of diabetes self-management support strategies in a public health care system. Health Educ Behav. 2008;35(5):664–82.
88. Schillinger D, Handley M, Wang F, Hammer H. Effects of self-management support on structure, process, and outcomes among vulnerable patients with diabetes: a three-arm practical clinical trial. Diabetes Care. 2009;32(4):559–66.
89. Ratanawongsa N, Handley MA, Sarkar U, Quan J, Pfeifer K, Soria C, Schillinger D. Diabetes health information technology innovation to improve quality of life for health plan members in urban safety net. J Ambul Care Manag. 2014;37(2):127–37.

90. Chen AH, Kushel MB, Grumbach K, Yee Jr HF. Practice profile. A safety-net system gains efficiencies through "eReferrals" to specialists. Health Aff (Millwood). 2010;29:969–71.
91. Chen AH, Murphy EJ, Yee Jr HF. eReferral – a new model for integrated care. New Engl J Med. 2013;368:2450–3.
92. Straus SG, Chen AH, Yee Jr H, Kushel MB, Bell DS. Implementation of an electronic referral system for outpatient specialty care. AMIA Annu Symp Proc. 2011;2011:1337–46.
93. Scheibe MM, Imboden JB, Schmajuk G, Margaretten M, Graf JD, Chen AH, Yelin EH, Yazdany J. Efficiency gains for rheumatology consultation using a novel electronic referral system in a safety net health setting. Arthritis Care Res (Hoboken). 2015;67(8):1158–63.
94. Sewell JL, Day LW, Tuot DS, Alvarez R, Yu A, Chen AH. A brief, low-cost intervention improves the quality of ambulatory gastroenterology consultation notes. Am J Med. 2013;126(8):732–8.
95. Pereira K, Phillips B, Johnson C, Vorderstrasse A. Internet delivered diabetes self-management education: a review. Diabetes Technol Ther. 2015;17(1):55–63.
96. McIlhenny CV, Guzic BL, Knee DR, Wendekier CM, Demuth BR, Roberts JB. Using technology to deliver healthcare education to rural patients. Rural Remote Health. 2011;11:1798.
97. Avdal EU, Kizilci S, Demirel N. The effects of web-based diabetes education on diabetes care results: a randomized control study. Comput Inform Nurs. 2011;29(2 Suppl):Tc29–34.
98. Lorig K, Ritter PL, Laurent DD, Plant K, Green M, Jernigan VB, Case S. Online diabetes self-management program: a randomized study. Diabetes Care. 2010;33:1275–81.
99. Kim CJ, Kang DH. Utility of a web-based intervention for individuals with type 2 diabetes: the impact on physical activity levels and glycemic control. Comput Inform Nurs. 2006;24:337–45.
100. Noh JH, Cho YJ, Nam HW, Kim JH, Kim DJ, Yoo HS, Kwon YW, Woo MH, Cho JW, Hong MH, Yoo JH, Gu MJ, Kim SA, An KE, Jang SM, Kim EK, Yoo HJ. Web-based comprehensive information system for self-management of diabetes mellitus. Diabetes Technol Ther. 2010;12:333–7.
101. Song M, Choe MA, Kim KS, Yi MS, Lee I, Kim J, Lee M, Cho YM, Shim YS. An evaluation of web-based education as an alternative to group lectures for diabetes self-management. Nurs Health Sci. 2009;11:277–84.
102. Glasgow RE, Kurz D, King D, Dickman JM, Faber AJ, Halterman E, Woolley T, Toobert DJ, Strycker LA, Estabrooks PA, Osuna D, Ritzwoller D. Twelve-month outcomes of an Internet-based diabetes self-management support program. Patient Educ Couns. 2012;87:81–92.
103. Ralston JD, Hirsch IB, Hoath J, Mullen M, Cheadle A, Goldberg HI. Web-based collaborative care for type 2 diabetes: a pilot randomized trial. Diabetes Care. 2009;32(2):234–9.
104. McMahon GT, Gomes HE, Hohne SH, Hu TM-J, Levine BA, Conlon PR. Web-based care management in patients with poorly controlled diabetes mellitus. Diabetes Care. 2005;28(7):1624–9.
105. Bond GE, Burr RL, Wolf FM, Feldt K. The effects of a web-based intervention on psychosocial well-being among adults aged 60 and older with diabetes: a randomized trial. Diabetes Educ. 2010;36(3):446–5.
106. Azar M, Gabbay R. Web-based management of diabetes through glucose uploads: has the time come for telemedicine? Diabetes Res Clin Pract. 2009;83(1):9–17.
107. McMahon GT, Fonda SJ, Gomes HE, Alexis G, Conlin PR. A randomized comparison of online- and telephone-based care management with internet training alone in adult patients with poorly controlled type 2 diabetes. Diabetes Technol Ther. 2012;14(11):1060–7.
108. Liang X, Wang Q, Yang X, Cao J, Chen J, Mo X, Huang J, Wang L, Gu D. Effect of mobile phone intervention for diabetes on glycaemic control: a meta-analysis. Diabet Med. 2011;28(4):455–63.
109. Bell AM, Fonda SJ, Walker MS, Schmidt V, Vigersky RA. Mobile phone-based video messages for diabetes self-care support. J Diabetes Sci Technol. 2012;6(2):310–9.
110. Salber P, Niksch A. Digital health tools for diabetes. J Ambul Care Manag. 2015;38(2):196–9.
111. Quinn CC, Clough SS, Minor JM, Lender D, Okafor MC, Gruber-Baldini. A WellDoc mobile diabetes management randomized controlled trial: change in clinical and behavioral outcomes and patient and physician satisfaction. Diabetes Technol Ther. 2008;10(3):160–8.
112. Quinn CC, Gruber-Baldini AL, Shardell M, Weed K, Clough SS, Peeples M, Terrin M, Bronich-all L, Barr E, Lender D. Mobile diabetes intervention study: testing a personalized treatment/behavioral communication intervention for blood glucose control. Contemp Clin Trials. 2009;30(4):334–4.
113. Quinn CC, Shardell MD, Terrin ML, Barr EA, Ballew SH, Gruber-Baldini AL. Cluster-randomized trial of a mobile phone personalized behavioral intervention for blood glucose control. Diabetes Care. 2011;34(9):1934–42.
114. Nundy S, Dick JJ, Chou CH, Nocon RS, Chin MH, Peek ME. Mobile phone diabetes project led to improved glycemic control and net savings for Chicago plan participants. Health Aff (Millwood). 2014;33(2):265–72.
115. Clarke RM, Tseng CH, Brook RH, Brown AF. Tool used to assess how well community health centers function as medical homes may be flawed. Health Aff (Millwood). 2012;31(3):627–35.

116. Bray P, Cummings DM, Morrissey S, Thompson D, Holbert D, Wilson K, Lukosius E, Tanenberg R. Improved outcomes in diabetes care for rural African Americans. Ann Fam Med. 2013;11(2):145–50.
117. Moore K, Jiang L, Manson SM, Beals J, Henderson W, Pratte K, Acton KJ, Roubideaux Y. Case management to reduce cardiovascular disease risk in American Indians and Alaska Natives with diabetes: results from the Special Diabetes Program for Indians Healthy Heart Demonstration Project. Am J Public Health. 2014;104(11):e158–64.
118. Shea S, Weinstock RS, Starren J, Teresi J, Palmas W, Field L, et al. A randomized trial comparing telemedicine case management with usual care in older, ethnicity diverse, medically underserved patients with diabetes mellitus. J Am Med Inform Assoc. 2006;13:40–51.
119. Shane-McWhorter L, Lenert L, Petersen M, Woolsey S, McAdam-Marx C, Coursey JM, Whittaker TC, Hyer C, LaMarche D, Carroll P, Chuy L. The Utah remote monitoring project: improving health care one patient at a time. Diabetes Technol Ther. 2014;16(10):653–60.
120. Rogers EA, Hessler D, Dube K, Willard-Grace R, Gupta R, Bodenheimer T, Grumbach K. The panel management questionnaire: a tool to measure panel management capability. Perm J. 2015;19(2):4–9.
121. Edwards ST, Landon BE. Medicare's chronic care management payment – payment reform for primary care. N Engl J Med. 2014;371:2049–51.
122. Bindman AB. Nudging medical practice change one regulation at a time. JAMA. 2015;313:1197–8.
123. Gilmer TP, Philis-Tsimikas A, Walker C. Outcomes of Project Dulce: a culturally specific diabetes management program. Ann Pharmacother. 2005;39(5):817–22.
124. Gilmer TP, Roze S, Valentine WJ, et al. Cost-effectiveness of diabetes case management for low-income populations. Health Serv Res. 2007;42(5):1943–59.
125. Brown 3rd HS, Wilson KJ, Pagan JA, Arcari CM, Martinez M, Smith K, Reininger B. Cost-effectiveness analysis of a community health worker intervention for low-income Hispanic adults with diabetes. Prev Chronic Dis. 2012;9:E140.
126. Brownson CA, Hoerger TJ, Fisher EB, Kilpatrick KE. Cost-effectiveness of diabetes self-management programs in community primary care settings. Diabetes Educ. 2009;35(5):761–9.
127. Piette JD, Heisler M, Wagner TH. Cost-related medication underuse among chronically ill adults: the treatments people forgo, how often, and who is at risk. Am J Public Health. 2004;94(10):1782–7.
128. Hoerger TJ. Using costs in cost-effectiveness models for chronic diseases: lessons from diabetes. Med Care. 2009;47(7 Suppl 1):S21–7.

4 A Primary Health-Care System Approach to Improving Quality of Care and Outcomes in People with Diabetes: The University of Pittsburgh Medical Center Experience

Janice C. Zgibor, Francis X. Solano Jr., and Linda Siminerio

Introduction

Although substantial evidence exists demonstrating the efficacy of interventions for controlling risk factors for diabetes complications [1–6], dissemination into community practice is not widespread, for example, only 18 % of people with diabetes in the USA are achieving goals for HbA1c, blood pressure, and cholesterol (the ABCs) [7]. Since the majority of ambulatory care visits for diabetes take place in primary care, this environment provides an opportunity for significant improvement in diabetes outcomes on a population basis [8]. However, relying on a system that places the burden solely on primary care providers (PCPs) to reach evidence-based targets [9] for risk factor control may not be ideal. Traditional approaches used to enhance the quality of diabetes care including continuing medical education, self-study through medical literature or online courses, may improve knowledge short-term but do little to actually change quality of patient care [10, 11]. Primary care providers need innovative strategies to support the current demands for high quality care with limited resources. To achieve this, it is important to broaden our perspective to include models of care that may improve quality using more nontraditional approaches.

As early as 2000, the University of Pittsburgh Medical Center (UPMC) began adopting the elements of the Chronic Care model (CCM) [12–15] to enhance the quality of diabetes care using risk stratification, provider incentives, integration of care managers, travelling diabetes educators, population management, and collaboration with a health insurer. Many initiatives were undertaken and successful outcomes were achieved. This chapter highlights these initiatives and describes the detail that led to large-scale change in patient outcomes, diabetes care delivery, and population management.

J.C. Zgibor (✉)
Department of Epidemiology and Biostatistics, College of Public Health, University of South Florida, Tampa, FL, USA
e-mail: jzgibor@health.usf.edu

F.X. Solano Jr.
Community Medicine Inc, University of Pittsburgh Medical Center, Pittsburgh, PA, USA

Physician Services Division, University of Pittsburgh Medical Center, Pittsburgh, PA, USA

Division of General Internal Medicine, School of Medicine, University of Pittsburgh, Pittsburgh, PA, USA
e-mail: solanofx@upmc.edu

L. Siminerio
Division of Endocrinology, School of Medicine, University of Pittsburgh, Pittsburgh, PA, USA
e-mail: simineriol@upmc.edu

D. Simmons et al. (eds.), *Integrated Diabetes Care*, DOI 10.1007/978-3-319-13389-8_4

While several models of care are reported in the literature, the CCM was chosen to provide the framework to enhance diabetes care at the UPMC. The CCM posits that quality care is delivered using a comprehensive patient-centred approach that rewards outcomes not just processes of care. Previous research conducted on the effectiveness of the CCM demonstrated improvement in these parameters in a variety of primary health-care settings [16]. The elements of the CCM are reviewed in detail in Chap. 3. UPMC chose to implement the CCM to move towards strategies for the redesign of primary care, to improve processes and outcomes in people with diabetes. All elements of the CCM (health system, community, decision support, clinical information systems, self-management, and delivery system design) [12–15] were implemented in UPMC primary care practices over the 15-year timeframe described here.

Population Served

The University of Pittsburgh Medical Center (UPMC), established in 1990, is a global non-profit organization with more than 62,000 employees, 5500 affiliated physicians and 20 hospitals. There are more than 500 clinical locations that include doctors' offices in the Physicians Service Division and Community Medicine, Inc., (CMI) which has 150 primary care locations and 330 primary care providers. UPMC primarily serves a diverse population in western Pennsylvania [17] and provides care for more than 55,000 people with diabetes. There are approximately 600 primary care providers in UPMC. Primary care providers at UMPC and for this chapter include general practice, family practice and internal medicine physicians.

The University of Pittsburgh Medical Center also has an insurance division with more than three million members. UPMC Health Plan is the second largest health insurer in western Pennsylvania (PA) and serves Medicare, Medicaid, special needs populations, and workers' compensation. The insurer also serves parts of Ohio, West Virginia and Maryland [18].

Provider-Based Strategies for Quality Improvement

In 2000, UPMC embarked on a system-wide quality improvement initiative in the CMI practices. The philosophy of the quality improvement (QI) programme was to improve quality of care while "keeping it simple." This initiative was called *Intervention Now*!! Presently it includes up to 360 primary care physicians and 45,000 of their patients with diabetes. The leadership of CMI (the President of CMI and Medical Director and his administrative team) used the CCM framework for the initiative.

To launch the initiative, CMI leadership established evidence-based clinical goals. To disseminate these goals, the Medical Director of CMI met with primary care practices and presented results from recent studies, treatment goals, and strategies for improvement. There was no system-wide electronic health record (EHR) at the time, therefore data were entered onto flow sheets at the patient and practice levels. Physicians received information about local Diabetes Self-Management Education (DSME) programmes and were encouraged to refer patients to these programmes for education. Given the geographic distance of some of the CMI practices from the UPMC hub in Pittsburgh, PA, the Medical Director delivered the programme via teleconference. Initial targets for improvement were to intensify treatment in those with an HbA1c >9 %, statin use in those over the age of 40 at high risk for a cardiovascular event regardless of LDLc level, blood pressure control in those with a blood pressure >140/90 mmHg, ACE or ARB use for renal protection and aspirin use in those at high risk for a coronary heart disease event. The pilot phase of the initiative occurred in 2000 and included 148 volunteer providers. Average HbA1c was 7.6 % while 34 % of patients with diabetes had an HbA1c <7 %. By 2003, the initiative was adopted by 198 providers and approximately 25,000 of their patients. A reduction in average HbA1c to 6.9 % across all patients was reported with 61 % of patients achieving an HbA1c <7 %. Late adopters usually had worse glycaemic control, so this was unlikely to be due to "dilution" by the influx of patients with better glucose control. Eighty-three percent of practices lowered their patient's average HbA1c during the year of the intervention. There were practical limitations to this tracking method including accuracy, incomplete capture of patients and their HbA1c, and the potential for reporting bias. In order to facilitate more efficient data collection for HbA1c, the primary laboratory in the local area connected with the UMPC data network so that periodic data dumps could be extracted. This facilitated a more comprehensive data capture that was less prone to bias. The laboratory data were sent to physicians in an anonymized report on a quarterly basis. The Medical Director was then able to share anonymized data with the providers, which provided a means for them to examine their own data and compare their practice results to their peers. Physicians were ranked on their progress towards established goals. Improvements continued throughout CMI in all 198 primary care practices and a report from 2008 showed that 75 % of HbA1c tests were <7 %, an absolute improvement of 41 % from the beginning of the initiative. Since the proportion of patients with an HbA1c below goal had dra matically improved overtime, initiatives to control LDLc and blood pressure were started as the next phase in the quality improvement initiatives.

The Legacy of Implementation

Following the initial pilot work, several demonstration projects were simultaneously initiated to examine the most effective and globally acceptable means for implementation and adoption of the CCM. The demonstration projects implemented all elements of the CCM to varying degrees. Self-management is considered to be a core tenet of the CCM, thus at the foundation of these interventions was attention to diabetes self-management education and support (DSME/DSMS). This next section describes the role of DSME/DSMS within the context of quality improvement strategies and implementation of the CCM.

Patient-Centred Strategies-Diabetes Self-Management Education

The person living with diabetes is expected to make a multitude of daily self-management decisions and perform complex care activities. DSME/DSMS provides the foundation to help people with diabetes navigate these decisions and activities [19, 20]. DSME is the process of facilitating the knowledge, skill and ability necessary for diabetes self-care. DSMS refers to the support that is required for implementing and sustaining behaviours needed for self-management over the long term [21]. While different members of the health-care team and community can contribute to this process, initial DSME should be provided by a health professional while ongoing support can be provided by personnel within a practice and a variety of community-based resources. DSME/DSMS interventions are designed to: be culturally relevant, address patient's health beliefs, current knowledge, limitations, emotional concerns, family support, financial status, medical history, health literacy, and other factors that influence each person's ability to meet the challenges of self-management [21, 22].

DSME/DSMS are now considered to be a cornerstone of care, and have repeatedly been shown to improve diabetes-related outcomes [23–27]. In addition to significant improvements in HbA1c [20, 28–31], DSME is reported to have a positive impact on other clinical, behavioural and psychosocial aspects of diabetes [32, 33] and reduce the onset and/or advancement of diabetes complications [26] improve quality of life [34, 35], improve lifestyle behaviours [36], enhance self-efficacy and empowerment [37], increase healthy coping [38], and decrease the presence of diabetes-related distress [39] and depression [40]. DSME/DSMS has also been shown to be cost-effective by reducing hospital admissions and readmissions [41, 42] as well as estimated lifetime health-care costs related to a lower risk for complications [43].

While these improvements clearly reaffirm the importance of DSME, participation in DSME is low and educator services are underutilized [43–45]. It is the position of the American Diabetes

Association (ADA), Institute of Medicine and National Committee for Quality Assurance that all individuals with diabetes receive DSME/DSMS at diagnosis and as needed thereafter [9, 22, 46]. Despite these recommendations, recently released data show that only 6.8 % insured, newly diagnosed US adults with diabetes [45], and only 4 % of Medicare participants participated in DSME [43]. It has been suggested that the traditional way in which DSME is prescribed and delivered may be problematic [44]. Currently in the US, a physician must refer patients to DSME. In a national survey examining access, physicians reported that they want patients to receive DSME but find referral procedures difficult. Other challenges reported include a poor understanding of the need for and effectiveness of DSME. In addition, DSME/DSMS has historically been provided through didactic, formal programmes despite efforts underway to present diabetes content in a more dynamic and patient-focused approach. Survey authors concluded that efforts are needed to increase referral by physicians, follow-up by patients, and make DSME available in forms that make it attractive to patients and physicians [44].

Stepped Approach to Integrating DSME in Practice

We chose DSME/DSMS as the foundation of our implementation of the CCM for several reasons. First, the patient is responsible for the majority of their self-care outside of the physician office. DSME provides the skills necessary to do this self-management using a patient-centred approach. Second, primary care providers do not have the time to facilitate behaviour change strategies and ongoing support. Evidence demonstrates that this is a strength of DSME/DSMS. Third, diabetes educators are skilled clinicians with the expertise necessary to make therapeutic recommendations for treatment intensification. Finally, their role in US primary care is cost-effective. In this next section we describe our demonstration projects and the evolution of DSME/DSMS in primary care as it stands today.

Demonstration Projects

Phase 1: Exploring Referral and Participation Practices

In 2000, our research team began exploring DSME services when UPMC physicians reported a lack of access to diabetes education as a major barrier to quality care despite the fact that UPMC had supported hospital-based DSME programmes. The results of a needs assessment revealed that only three of the 19 DSME programmes were recognized by the ADA. This recognition ensures quality DSME services are delivered and enables programmes to bill for their services. UPMC applied for and received recognition for all programmes in November 2000 [47].

Phase 2: Addressing Access to DSME (2001–2003)

We explored improving access to DSME by implementing a care model shown to improve processes of care within primary care practices and patient outcomes. Again, the CCM provided the organizational approach with particular attention paid to team care and self-management [12–15]. A cluster randomized trial was implemented to examine the implementation of the CCM in an underserved, urban community [16]. Eleven primary care practices, along with their patients with either type 1 or type 2 diabetes (although the majority had type 2), were randomized to three groups: (1) CCM intervention where a diabetes educator provided DSME in the practice, (2) provider education where a series of problem-based cases were presented to physicians, and (3) usual care. On average, the CCM group showed a significant decline in HbA1c (0.6 %, $p=0.008$), while the other groups did not. The CCM group also showed improvement in patient knowledge ($p=0.07$) and empowerment ($p=0.02$).

Access to diabetes education in the rural areas was particularly problematic. To begin to explore these challenges, a study was conducted using the CCM was as a framework to test access to DSME in a rural area. A review of the practice population revealed that 95 % of patients with type 2 diabetes had significant cardiovascular disease risk factors; however, only 7 % had received relevant services like Medical Nutrition Therapy and none had received DSME. After integrating diabetes educator service into the practice, providers' adherence to the ADA Standards of Care significantly improved, diabetes educator utilization increased, and patients who received DSME had significant improvements in knowledge [48] and mean HbA1c from baseline to study end (7.2% vs. 6.5%, p=0.007). Results suggest that implementing a model that establishes a diabetes educator within the primary care setting is effective in improving process, clinical and behavioural outcomes [28].

In another study in a rural area, 295 patients with type 2 diabetes were identified within primary care practices, 162 (65%) reported they had never received DSME. Despite efforts by diabetes educators to improve awareness of local education services by primary care providers, 123 (76%) of the 162 patients had never received a referral. Those patients who received a referral had a higher number of risk factors and comorbid conditions than those who did not. Eighty-three percent of the patients, who received a referral from the primary care provider, however, had already participated in DSME. Studies suggest that physician recommendations are central to a patient's decision and physician referral has been positively associated with patient participation in health services. Our findings reflected this and affirmed the need to develop processes to improve physician referrals and receipt of DSME [30].

Efforts to explore our community's needs continued by examining our progress towards meeting the diabetes objectives in Healthy People 2010 goals (increase receipt of diabetes education for adults) [49] and potential challenges that still needed to be addressed in primary care [50]. UPMC primary care providers reported several barriers to outpatient DSME services that are consistent with other reports [44, 51]. Providers found the referral process difficult, expressed fears that patients are told to do things that they do not agree with, and that they may lose patients to specialists following DSME. In addition, providers and diabetes educators reported using different Electronic Health Record systems (EHR), thus eliminating opportunities for tracking patient DSME participation and direct communication between the provider and diabetes educators to address this significant challenge. A point of service education model was examined in four UPMC practices to address these issues [52]. A nurse diabetes educator offered DSME in the office on designated "diabetes days." The diabetes educator made therapy recommendations to the primary care provider based on patient assessments, trained staff on new therapies and served as a practice resource. The providers and the diabetes educator reported many advantages with the intervention that included increased communication on management plans and diabetes educators' involvement in medication initiation and adjustments. Patients reported more confidence in provider communication on treatment plans and satisfaction with ease of diabetes educator's access for inquiries [52]. These results again affirmed the role of diabetes educators delivering services in the primary care practices.

Our findings were encouraging; however, administrators challenged us to demonstrate how this could be supported and the benefits of DSME sustained? Attempts to answer these questions were made in a systematic way again using the CCM as a framework. DSME visits were tracked by reimbursement "G" codes in the UPMC database and compared between education delivered in primary care and hospital programmes. A two to threefold increase in the proportion of patients receiving DSME when delivered in primary care (24.7% versus hospital-based 8.3%, P<0.0001) was reported. In addition, diabetes educators were able to demonstrate their ability to generate revenue. At programme initiation, diabetes education services were a loss leader to the health system. In contrast, at conclusion, diabetes educators were covering costs through reimbursement [53]. The intent was not to suggest that DSME is a large revenue source or that hospital programmes will all be replaced by primary care, but rather that opportunities exist to expand this cost-neutral service and should be explored.

Phase 3: Examining Self-Management Support: An Expanded Role for Diabetes Educators? (2011–2012)

While arguments could be made for the financial benefits of diabetes educators in the short and long-term, evidence for sustained clinical effectiveness was still needed. There was also an additional need to explore ongoing DSMS, which was necessary to sustain improved outcomes following DSME [54]. In a comparative effectiveness research study DSME/DSMS was examined in three geographically/socioeconomically diverse primary care practice communities [53]. All type 2 patient-participants first received DSME from a diabetes educator over the course of 6 weeks. Participants were then randomized to receive 6 months of DSMS delivered by supervised "supporter" (peer, practice staff, or the diabetes educators). This supporter was trained and supervised by the diabetes educator. DSMS groups were compared to determine which support agent helped participants to maintain/ improve clinical and behavioural outcomes. Patients experienced a significant reduction in HbA1c values (0.9 %, p=0.0001) and significant improvements in empowerment [49], self-care [55] and distress scores [39] following DSME in the primary care practices. Although those in the diabetes educator group best sustained improved HbA1c, all groups maintained glycaemic improvements regardless of supporter. Study findings reaffirmed that DSME provided by diabetes educators in primary care is effective, DSMS supported by various agents trained and supervised by diabetes educators is feasible and has potential to be sustained.

Phase 4: Maximizing the Role of the Diabetes Educators in Primary Care (2012–2014)

The next phase in our demonstration projects moved towards the diabetes educators maximizing their expertise in both the behavioural and clinical aspects of diabetes care. Since our efforts to integrate diabetes educators into primary care were successful, it was logical to enhance the role of the diabetes educator in the practice setting. We implemented the Redesigning Effectiveness for Treatment in Diabetes Study (REMEDIES 4D) [56] to assess the differences in A1C, blood pressure, and LDLc levels (ABC) in participants to whom a diabetes educator intensified diabetes management by following the standardized, preapproved protocols compared with those who received usual care. This was a cluster randomized trial that took place in community-based primary care practices in Southwestern Pennsylvania among 240 type 2 diabetes participants who had at least one of the ABC levels above the ADA-recommended goals. At the end of the 1-year intervention, there was a significant difference in HbA1c between the intervention and usual care groups. The HbA1c in the intervention group decreased from 8.8 % to 7.3 %, while the HbA1c in the usual care group increased slightly from 8.2 % to 8.3 % (p=0.001). There was no significant difference between groups for LDLc or systolic blood pressure. Findings suggested that CDEs following standardized protocols is a feasible strategy and can effectively intensify treatment and improve glycaemic control.

In an effort to organize a system-wide approach to integrate and expand the role of the diabetes educator in primary care, we developed the "Glucose to Goal." programme. "Glucose to Goal" is a novel diabetes educator-driven, population-based management programme for patients with diabetes. The purpose of this project was to assess the feasibility of "Glucose to Goal," offered within the constructs of the ADA-recognized DSME programme within the UPMC network, and evaluate its impact on patient glycaemia. Three diabetes educators were introduced into primary care practices in their respective urban, suburban, and rural communities. Through the primary care EHR, diabetes educators proactively identified patients, reviewed lists with providers for diabetes educator referral, arranged diabetes educator visits and worked collaboratively with providers on treatment plans. HbA1c values were collected 1–3 months prior to DSME (baseline, HbA1c) to establish patient glycaemic control pre-DSME. Patients were categorized by HbA1c: ≤7 %, >7 % to 9 %, and >9 %. These values were compared to HbA1c levels at 3–6 and 9–12 months post DSME. HbA1c values were available in the EHR for 78 % of 143 patients (61.3 years, 51 % male) who met with a diabetes educator during the study period.

Average HbA1c values during the study period are shown in Fig. 4.1. For patients with baseline HbA1c ≤7 % (n=32), HbA1c levels

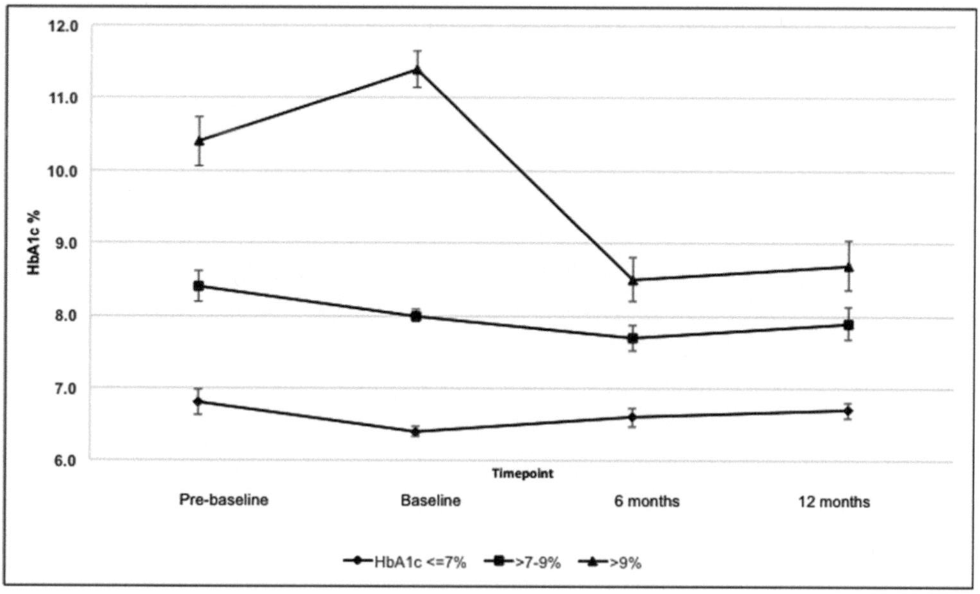

Fig. 4.1 HbA1c over time in UPMC Glucose to Goal programme

were maintained over time. For patients with baseline HbA1c >7–9 % (n=41), HbA1c was significantly reduced initially,, but trended upward at 12 months. For patients with baseline HbA1c >9 % (n=39), HbA1c was significantly reduced between prediabetes education visit and 6 months post- diabetes education visit(s) (−1.9; $p<0.001$) and this reduction was sustained at 12 months post-diabetes educator visit(s) (−1.7; $p<0.001$). Findings demonstrate the feasibility of this diabetes education-led primary care approach and confirm its benefits in all patients with type 2 diabetes, particularly for those at higher risk [57]. This study also reaffirms the need for ongoing patient support by diabetes educators in order to maintain glycaemic improvements over time.

In summary, the findings from our demonstration projects reflect challenges with referrals, the importance of referrals on patient participation, and the benefit the diabetes educator can have on patient outcomes in the primary care setting. Additionally, maximizing the role of diabetes educators to facilitate therapeutic management is feasible and effective. Our work provides the evidence for elevating the role of diabetes educators in primary care and assuring their place as a vital member of the health-care team.

Assessing Barriers to Practice Transformation

During the implementation of the demonstration projects, the CCM was gaining widespread attention; however, adoption of the elements of the CCM was not universal within our health system. It seemed that the early adopters were on board, while challenges remained for others. From March through October 2009, we sought to explore and enumerate the barriers to adopting the Model. Our research team partnered with diabetes educators in rural areas of western Pennsylvania to organize and participate in a qualitative study to gain insights into adoption of the CCM by primary care practices. These areas are shown on the map in the darker shaded areas (Fig. 4.2).

Our target geography was challenged by resources and lacked the infrastructure and support provided by a large health system as they were outside of the UPMC network. The rationale for exploring the barriers in resource poor areas was to identify methods for adopting the CCM from the most challenged areas that could be applied across a variety of primary care settings.

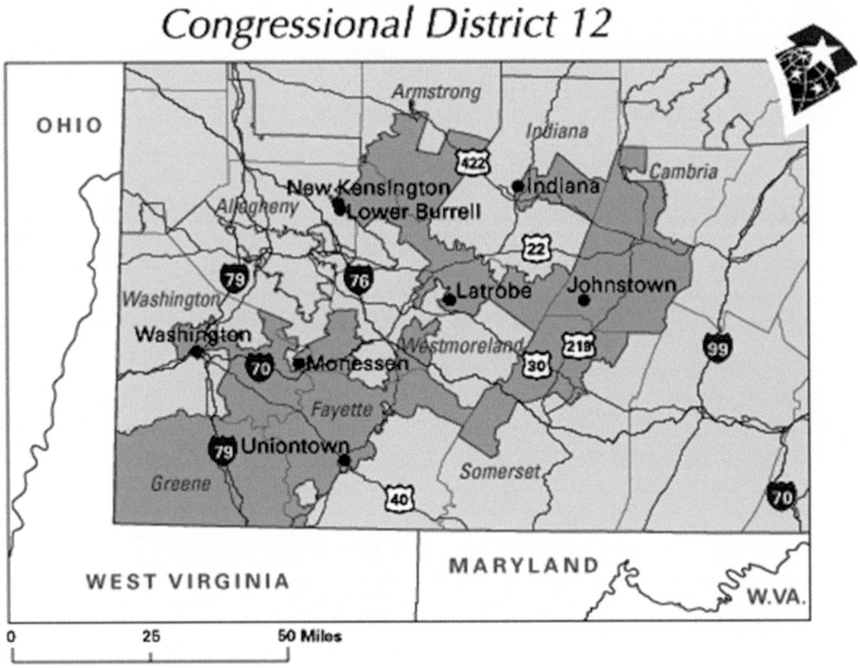

Fig. 4.2 Map of rural Southwestern Pennsylvania. The shaded area represents the general location of rural primary care practices

Following identification of 13 practices by the local diabetes educator, a trained qualitative interviewer conducted discussion groups in these practices. Groups ranged in size from three to five and included physicians, office managers, Licensed Practical Nurses (LPN) and medical assistants. A total of 49 health-care providers and office staff participated across the 13 practices. The format for the discussion group included brief introductions (10 min), the purpose of the discussion group (5 min), the CCM conceptual framework (20–30 min), discussion by the group (30–60 min), feedback and findings from the researchers (15 min), and question and answer (as needed). During the discussion, participants were asked to identify at least three elements of the CCM that could be implemented in their practice within the next month, 6-months and the next year. They were also asked prioritize implementation of the elements and enumerate the methods they would use to implement these elements. Researchers asked them to identify possible barriers to implementation. Problem-solving strategies were discussed and action steps for implementation were outlined. Following the discussion, the elements of the CCM that were of interest to the primary care providers in a particular practice were rolled out into that practice. Details of the themes identified in the discussion groups are summarized in Table 4.1. The most common element of the CCM identified by the practices for immediate implementation was DSMS/Delivery System Design or easier access to a diabetes educator. Providers believed that access to diabetes educators was essential to enhancing patient self-management and behaviour change. Practices also identified the need for resources to implement the Decision Support element of the CCM by having posters available as reminders to patients (e.g., foot care), flow sheets to track patient data, and easier access to current practice guidelines. The elements identified for long-term implementation were support from the Health System and Community. The element of least interest to the practices was Clinical Information Systems given financial barriers and lack of time or interest (EHRs were not in widespread use at this time).

Table 4.1 Themes identified by primary care practices during focus groups about the chronic care model

Element of the CCM	Themes identified
Health system	One staff person takes on numerous and sometimes disparate responsibilities
	The length of the visit was not long enough to address all patient needs
	Hosting other providers like CDEs was not feasible due to space limitations
	Lack of knowledge on reimbursement for services provided in the office
Community	Issues of territory or boundaries prohibited collaboration
	Patients were often unaware of opportunities to promote healthy lifestyles like group walks
	Community initiatives should not be one-time things, but rather they should aim for consistent, continuous efforts to offer education and raise awareness
	Existing community events could partner to offer wellness activities
Decision support	No quick way to examine longitudinal patterns in clinical outcomes
	Lack of knowledge about guidelines for diabetes care
Self-management	Lack of reimbursement for diabetes education activities
	Patient acknowledging that they need to manage their diabetes
	Dispel myths about diabetes
Delivery system design	Have a diabetes educator in the practice so that patients could see them at the time of their visits
	Group appointments
	Lack of administrative support for change
Clinical information systems	Interoperability of computers-hospitals had different computer systems leading to confusion and frustration
	No electronic health record

The research team provided assistance for implementation of the elements of the CCM prioritized by the primary care practices. Assistance was facilitated by the deployment of practice coaches. These coaches were nurses and mid-level providers with experience in diabetes education and quality improvement processes. These individuals worked with the research staff and met with the office managers, providers and office staff as needed. Their expertise allowed diabetes educators in rural sites to rely on those who had significant experience in troubleshooting quality improvement strategies. Having this expertise available to practices as issues arose was also important for addressing barriers in real time. Some of the topics with which the coaches were asked to assist included: methods for incorporating diabetes education into the practice, team-based diabetes care, requirements for ADA Recognition, National Committee for Quality Assurance (NCQA) certification, and billing and reimbursement for diabetes education services. The researchers also offered resources to the practices that included diabetes flow sheets, one-page informational sheets for diabetes self-management, time and location of local DSME/DSMS programmes, and educational materials for patients.

Perceived Patient Psychosocial Barriers

Throughout the discussions it became clear that staff and providers perceived that there were characteristics within the patient population that contributed to challenges in meeting expectations for self-management and clinical management of diabetes.

Most participants from the practices contended that patients did not know enough about diabetes to manage it properly. They recognized that some of this may be due to the failure of insurance companies to reimburse for diabetes education, but they also indicated that some of the limited knowledge is due to patients "not listening to what they are told by their doctor." Some participants admitted that, upon diagnosis, patients are inundated with too much information to digest it all at once. There were also misconceptions about diabetes noted during the discussions. For example, staff noted that patients think that "because their mother has diabetes, they know how to manage it." These and other local attitudes hampered the success of educational initiatives. The staff and providers also recognized that their patient populations are for the most part poor, which affects the kind of food that they can buy and their access to transportation and insurance coverage.

Summary of Findings

Providers and staff have characteristics that may impact how they care for patients with diabetes. Two important characteristics to consider are their attitudes towards change in the practice and their tendency to blame patients for their inability to take action and adhere to recommended treatment regimens. The former is seen in remarks like "my patients would never take to group appointments"; the latter is reflected in statements such as "they won't comply with their medication schedule." On the other hand, many of the providers and staff are quite committed to helping their patients better manage their diabetes and to providing the best care that they can.

A common barrier identified from the focus groups is that engaging the administration at the Health System level early on and obtaining the support from them was crucial for success of a sustainable programme. Administrative inertia would need to be overcome in order to establish a business model for sustainability of DSME services.

Driving Change into the Future

The Patient-Centered Medical Home (PCMH)

As described in this chapter, the PCMH model is grounded in the concepts of the CCM [13–16]. In this model, "practices seek to improve the quality, effectiveness, and efficiency of the care they deliver while responding to each patient's unique needs and preferences" [58]. The UPMC Health Plan initiated a PCMH pilot. Ten practices with 162 primary care physicians serving 23,930 Health Plan members participated in the pilot programme through 2010. The UPMC Health Plan provided six practice-based nurse care managers for the ten practices. Care managers received comprehensive training on diabetes and related co-morbidities from two diabetes educators. Three of the practice-based nurse care managers focused on helping patient members with one or more chronic conditions. Risk-stratification was used to identify high-risk patients. The care managers expanded their focus to address prevention, self-management of chronic conditions, reduction of clinical gaps in care (e.g., laboratory testing, eye exams), unplanned care, and use of duplicative services [59].

Practices provided office space, integration of the care manager into their work flow, and access to the EHR for scheduling and documentation. At the end of the pilot period, the ten PCMH practices were compared with the remainder of the practices in the primary care network. Overall, the practices participating in the PCMH pilot achieved significantly lower costs and reduced hospital readmissions. While emergency room (ER) visits and hospital admissions increased in both groups, the increase was proportionately lower in the PCMH practices (Fig. 4.3). When Healthcare Effectiveness Data and Information Set (HEDIS) indicators were compared, the PCMH sites outperformed the other sites on all measures between 2008 and 2010 (HbA1c tests: +6.6 % vs +3.4 %, eye exam: +23.2 vs 7.1 %, LDLc screen: +9.7 % vs +2.9 %, nephropathy monitoring: +6.8 % vs +4.8 %), although results were not statistically significantly different (Table 4.2). The return on investment was 160 % [56]. Those participating in the pilot also received support for completing the National Committee for Quality Assurance's (NCQA) application. Currently, some of the practices are NCQA designated PCMH; however, many of the elements of the PCMH are present throughout the UPMC primary care network.

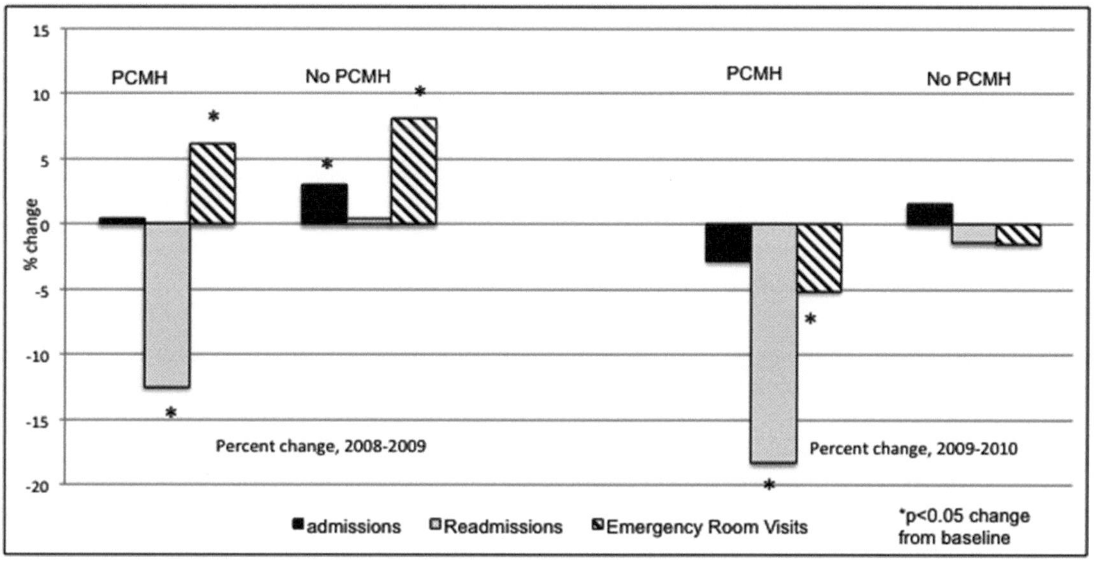

Fig. 4.3 Change in Hospital service use per 1000 members of UPMC Health Plan's Primary Care Network, 2008–2010. PCMH= patient centered medical home

Table 4.2 Change in performance on HEDIS measures in UMPC Health Plan Primary Care Network 2008–2010

	PCMH		No PCMH	
	2008	2010	2008	2010
HbA1c tests (%)	84.1	90.7	82.7	86.1
Eye exams (%)	60.6	83.8	50.6	57.7
LDLc screening (%)	80.3	90.0	80.6	83.5
Nephropathy monitoring (%)	82.6	89.4	75.4	80.2
PCMH= Patient-Centered Medical Home				

Data from Rosenberg et al. [59]

Meaningful Use

Meaningful Use (MU), a programme administered by the Center for Medicare and Medicaid Services (CMS), is designed to improve quality, safety, efficiency, and reduce health disparities. It also proposes to engage patients and their families, improve care coordination, population and public health while maintaining patient privacy. The ultimate goal of MU is to improve clinical outcomes, increase transparency and efficiency, empower individuals, and provide more robust research data on health systems [60]. The MU programme was also designed to incentivize physicians to implement an electronic record. MU is being rolled out in three stages at UPMC. Stage 1 (2011–2012): data capture and sharing; Stage 2 (2014): advance clinical processes (2016): improved outcomes. CMS provides incentive payments as MU parameters are adopted. Approximately $44,000 is available per eligible provider. Hospitals may receive $2 million or more. Currently, UPMC is in Stage 2 of MU, though UPMC has put several ongoing initiatives in place to meet the all of the parameters of MU. These included, but are not limited to, initiatives addressing quality of care, finance, and information technology. The primary barrier to implementation continues to be resources including funds, personnel, and support for rollout. While this barrier exists, UPMC has managed to overcome these barriers and roll out the required elements.

Infrastructure

UPMC continues to move forward with initiatives to improve the quality of care and outcomes in people with diabetes. Over the course of 15 years of integrating care, the EpicCare medical record system [61] was implemented in all CMI practices. This system has core metrics for quality of care. These metrics are directly tied to incentives for the providers and the health system. The physicians need to successfully obtain all of the metrics in order to receive the incentives. This EHR has a tool called "Healthy Planet" which is a population-based tool for disease management. To facilitate population management, there are currently patient registries for asthma, diabetes, preventive care and hypertension. Registries for cardiovascular, renal, and liver disease are in development.

CMI is also in the process of establishing "PODS" to drive population management. These pods are determined geographically and serve approximately 25,000 patients. These Pods provide support to the primary care providers through care management teams. These teams consist of an advanced practice nurse, a behavioural specialist, and CDEs. This team works together with the primary care provider to address chronic conditions. Their focus is to decrease variability in care, improve quality and give the physician more time to focus on complex patients. There are currently 5 Pods with the eventual goal of 20 Pods throughout the UPMC health system.

In summary, diabetes care and integration of nontraditional approaches to deliver that care have evolved over a 15-year periods at UPMC. There continues to be enthusiasm, support, and dedication to improving the care and outcomes for people with diabetes using cutting edge strategies. There also continues to be challenges at the patient, provider and system levels; however, innovative approaches are continually implemented to meet the needs of the rapidly growing population of people with diabetes in a dynamic health-care environment.

References

1. Hansson L, Zanchetti A, Carruthers SG, Dahlof B, Elmfeldt D, Julius S, et al. Effects of intensive blood-pressure lowering and low dose aspirin in patients with hypertension: principal results of the Hypertension Optimal Treatment (HOT) randomised trial. Lancet. 1998;351:1755–62.
2. LIPID Study Group. Long-term effectiveness and safety of pravastatin in 9014 patients with coronary heart disease and average cholesterol concentrations: the LIPID trial. 2002.
3. The ALLHAT Officers and Coordinators for the ALLHAT Collaborative Research Group. Major outcomes in moderately hypercholesterolemic, hypertensive patients randomized to pravastatin vs usual care: the antihypertensive and lipid-lowering treatment to prevent heart attack trial. JAMA. 2002;288(23):2998–3007.
4. Ridker PM, Rifai N, Pfeffer MA, Sacks FM, Moye LA, Goldman S, et al. Inflammation, pravastatin, and the risk of coronary events after myocardial infarction in patients with average cholesterol levels. Cholesterol and Recurrent Events (CARE) investigators. Circulation. 1998;98(9):839–44.
5. UK Prospective Diabetes Study Group. Tight blood pressure control and risk of macrovascular and microvascular complications in type 2 diabetes: UKPDS 38. BMJ. 1998;317:703–13.
6. Intensive blood-glucose control with sulphonylureas or insulin compared with conventional treatment and risk of complications in patients with type 2 diabetes (UKPDS 33). The Lancet. 1998;352(9131):837–53.
7. Stark Casagrande S, Fradkin JE, Saydah SH, Rust KF, Cowie CC. The prevalence of meeting A1C, blood pressure, and LDL goals among people with diabetes, 1988–2010. Diabetes Care. 2013;36(8):2271–9.
8. Janes GR. Ambulatory medical care for diabetes. In: Group NDD, editor. Diabetes in America. Bethesda: National Institutes of Health; 1995. p. 541–52.
9. American Diabetes Association. Standards of medical care in diabetes, 2015. Diabetes Care. 2015;38 Suppl 1:S5–87.
10. Bloom BS. Effects of continuing medical education on improving physician clinical care and patient health: a review of systematic reviews – effects of continuing medical education on improving physician clinical care and patient health_0.pdf [Internet]. [cited 2016 Apr 19]. Available from: https://aetcnec.ucsf.edu/sites/aetcnec.ucsf.edu/files/Effects%20of%20continuing%20medical%20education%20on%20improving%20physician%20clinical%20care%20and%20patient%20health_0.pdf
11. VanNieuwenborg L, Goossens M, De Lepeleire J, Schoenmakers B. Continuing medical education for general practitioners: a practice format. Postgrad Med J. 2016;92(1086):217–22.
12. Wagner EH, Austin BT, Korff MV. Improving outcomes in chronic illness. Manag Care Q. 1996;4(2):12–25.
13. Wagner EH, Austin BT, Korff MV. Organizing care for patients with chronic illness. Mill Bank Q. 1996;74(4):511–44.
14. Wagner EH, Bennett SM, Austin BT, Greene SM, Schaefer JK, Vonkorff M. Finding common ground: patient-centeredness and evidence-based chronic illness care. J Altern Complement Med. 2005;11(supplement 1):s7–15.

15. Wagner EH, Glasgow RE, Davis C, Bonomi AE, Provost L, McCulloch D, et al. Quality improvement in chronic illness care: a collaborative approach. Jt Comm J Qual Improv. 2001;27(2):63–80.
16. Piatt GA, Orchard TJ, Emerson S, Simmons D, Songer TJ, Brooks MM, et al. Translating the chronic care model into the community: results from a randomized controlled trial of a multifaceted diabetes care intervention. Diabetes Care. 2006;29(4):811–7.
17. University of Pittsburgh Medical Center. UPMC Facts and Figures [Internet]. 2015. Available from: http://www.upmc.com/about/facts/numbers/Pages/default.aspx
18. University of Pittsburgh Medical Center Health Plan. UPMC health plan: our company [Internet]. 2014. Available from: http://www.upmchealthplan.com/about/who-we-are/about-our-company.aspx
19. Brown SA. Studies of educational interventions and outcomes in diabetic adults: a meta-analysis revisited. Patient Educ Couns. 1990;16(3):189–215.
20. Norris SL, Lau J, Smith SJ, Schmid CH, Engelgau MM. Self-management education for adults with type 2 diabetes: a meta-analysis of the effect on glycemic control. Diabetes Care. 2002;25(7):1159–71.
21. Haas L, Maryniuk M, Beck J, Cox CE, Duker P, Edwards L, et al. National standards for diabetes self-management education and support. Diabetes Care. 2013;36(Supplement_1):S100–8.
22. Powers MA, Bardsley J, Cypress M, Duker P, Funnell MM, Hess Fischl A, et al. Diabetes self-management education and support in type 2 diabetes: a joint position statement of the American Diabetes Association, the American Association of Diabetes Educators, and the Academy of Nutrition and Dietetics. Diabetes Care. 2015;38(7):1372–82.
23. Brunisholz K, Briot P, Hamilton S, Joy E, Lomax M, Barton N, et al. Diabetes self-management education improves quality of care and clinical outcomes determined by a diabetes bundle measure. J Multidiscip Healthc. 2014;533.
24. Weaver RG, Hemmelgarn BR, Rabi DM, Sargious PM, Edwards AL, Manns BJ, et al. Association between participation in a brief diabetes education programme and glycaemic control in adults with newly diagnosed diabetes. Diabet Med. 2014;31(12):1610–4.
25. Steinsbekk A, Rygg L, Lisulo M, Rise MB, Fretheim A. Group based diabetes self-management education compared to routine treatment for people with type 2 diabetes mellitus. A systematic review with meta-analysis. BMC Health Serv Res. 2012;12(1):213.
26. Fan L, Sidani S. Effectiveness of diabetes self-management education intervention elements: a meta-analysis. Can J Diabetes. 2009;33(1):18–26.
27. Ellis SE, Speroff T, Dittus RS, Brown A, Pichert JW, Elasy TA. Diabetes patient education: a meta-analysis and meta-regression. Patient Educ Couns. 2004;52(1):97–105.
28. Siminerio LM. Implementing the chronic care model for improvements in diabetes care and education in a rural primary care practice. Diabetes Educ. 2005;31(2):225–34.
29. Siminerio L, Ruppert K, Huber K, Toledo FGS. Telemedicine for Reach, Education, Access, and Treatment (TREAT): linking telemedicine with diabetes self-management education to improve care in rural communities. Diabetes Educ. 2014;40(6):797–805.
30. Ruppert K, Uhler A, Siminerio L. Examining patient risk factors, comorbid conditions, participation, and physician referrals to a rural diabetes self-management education program. Diabetes Educ. 2010;36(4):603–12.
31. Tshiananga JKT, Kocher S, Weber C, Erny-Albrecht K, Berndt K, Neeser K. The effect of nurse-led diabetes self-management education on glycosylated hemoglobin and cardiovascular risk factors: a meta-analysis. Diabetes Educ. 2012;38(1):108–23.
32. Welch G, Zagarins SE, Feinberg RG, Garb JL. Motivational interviewing delivered by diabetes educators: does it improve blood glucose control among poorly controlled type 2 diabetes patients? Diabetes Res Clin Pract. 2011;91(1):54–60.
33. Gary TL, Genkinger JM, Guallar E, Peyrot M, Brancati FL. Meta-analysis of randomized educational and behavioral interventions in type 2 diabetes. Diabetes Educ. 2003;29(3):488–501.
34. Cooke D, Bond R, Lawton J, Rankin D, Heller S, Clark M, et al. Structured type 1 diabetes education delivered within routine care: impact on glycemic control and diabetes-specific quality of life. Diabetes Care. 2013;36(2):270–2.
35. Cochran J, Conn VS. Meta-analysis of quality of life outcomes following diabetes self-management training. Diabetes Educ. 2008;34(5):815–23.
36. Toobert DJ, Glasgow RE, Strycker LA, Barrera M, Radcliffe JL, Wander RC, et al. Biologic and quality-of-life outcomes from the Mediterranean lifestyle program: a randomized clinical trial. Diabetes Care. 2003;26(8):2288–93.
37. Funnell MM, Anderson RM. Empowerment and self-management of diabetes. Clin Diabetes. 2004;22(3):123–7.
38. Thorpe CT, Fahey LE, Johnson H, Deshpande M, Thorpe JM, Fisher EB. Facilitating healthy coping in patients with diabetes: a systematic review. Diabetes Educ. 2013;39(1):33–52.
39. Fisher L, Hessler DM, Polonsky WH, Mullan J. When is diabetes distress clinically meaningful?: Establishing cut points for the diabetes distress scale. Diabetes Care. 2012;35(2):259–64.
40. de Groot M, Doyle T, Kushnick M, Shubrook J, Merrill J, Rabideau E, et al. Can lifestyle interventions do more than reduce diabetes risk? Treating depression in adults with type 2 diabetes with exercise and cognitive behavioral therapy. Curr Diabet Rep. 2012;12(2):157–66.
41. Healy SJ, Black D, Harris C, Lorenz A, Dungan KM. Inpatient diabetes education is associated with less frequent hospital readmission among patients

with poor glycemic control. Diabetes Care. 2013;36(10):2960–7.

42. Robbins JM, Thatcher GE, Webb DA, Valdmanis VG. Nutritionist visits, diabetes classes, and hospitalization rates and charges: the urban diabetes study. Diabetes Care. 2008;31(4):655–60.
43. Duncan I, Ahmed T, Li Q, Stetson B, Ruggiero L, Burton K, et al. Assessing the value of the diabetes educator. Diabetes Educ. 2011;37(5):638–57.
44. Peyrot M, Rubin RR, Funnell MM, Siminerio LM. Access to diabetes self-management education: results of National surveys of patients, educators, and physicians. Diabetes Educ. 2009;35(2):246–63.
45. Li R, Shrestha SS, Lipman R, Burrows NR, Kolb LE, Rutledge S, et al. Diabetes self-management education and training among privately insured persons with newly diagnosed diabetes – United States, 2011–2012. MMWR Morb Mortal Wkly Rep. 2014;63(46):1045–9.
46. American Medical Association (AMA) and the National Committee for Quality Assurance (NCQA) [Internet]. Adult diabetes: performance measures. AMA-convened physician consortium for performance Improvement; 014; Available from: http://www.ama-assn.org/apps/listserv/x-check/qmeasure.cgi?submit=PCPI
47. Siminerio L, Zgibor J, Solano FX. Implementing the chronic care model for improvements in diabetes practice and outcomes in primary care: the University of Pittsburgh Medical Center experience. Clin Diabetes. 2004;22(2):54–8.
48. Fitzgerald JT, Funnell MM, Hess GE, Barr PA, Anderson RM, Hiss RG, et al. The reliability and validity of a brief diabetes knowledge test. Diabetes Care. 1998;21(5):706–10.
49. U.S. Department of Health and Human Services. Healthy people 2010: understanding and improving health. 2nd ed. Washington, DC: U.S Government Printing Office; 2010.
50. Krall J, Gabbay R, Zickmund S, Hamm ME, Williams KR, Siminerio L. Current perspectives on psychological insulin resistance: primary care provider and patient views. Diabetes Technol Ther. 2015;17(4):268–74.
51. Siminerio LM, Ruppert K, Emerson S, Solano FX, Piatt GA. Delivering Diabetes Self-Management Education (DSME) in primary care: the Pittsburgh Regional Initiative for Diabetes Education (PRIDE). Dis Manag Health Outcomes. 2008;16(4):267–72.
52. Siminerio LM. Deploying the chronic care model to implement and sustain diabetes self-management training programs. Diabetes Educ. 2006;32(2):253–60.
53. Siminerio L, Ruppert KM, Gabbay RA. Who can provide diabetes self-management support in primary care? Findings from a randomized controlled trial. Diabetes Educ. 2013;39(5):705–13.
54. Anderson RM, Fitzgerald JT, Gruppen LD, Funnell MM, Oh MS. The diabetes empowerment scale-short form (DES-SF). Diabetes Care. 2003;26(5):1641–2.
55. Toobert DJ, Hampson SE, Glasgow RE. The summary of diabetes self-care activities measure: results from 7 studies and a revised scale. Diabetes Care. 2000;23(7):943–50.
56. Zgibor JC, Kuo S, Emerson S, Gittinger P, Solano FX, Tilves D, et al. Rationale, design, and implementation of a cluster randomized trial using certified diabetes educators to intensify treatment for glycemia, blood pressure and lipid control: REMEDIES 4D. Contemp Clin Trials. 2014;39(1):124–31.
57. Siminerio L. Improving glycemia in primary care: a model integrating diabetes education into practice. Boston: American Diabetes Association; 2015. 75th Scientific Sessions.
58. American Academy of Family Physicians. The patient centered medical home [Internet]. 2015. Available from: http://www.aafp.org/practice-management/transformation/pcmh.html
59. Rosenberg CN, Peele P, Keyser D, McAnallen S, Holder D. Results from a patient-centered medical home pilot at UPMC health plan hold lessons for broader adoption of the model. Health Aff (Millwood). 2012;31(11):2423–31.
60. US Department of Health & Human Services. EHR incentives & certification [Internet]. 2015. Available from: https://www.healthit.gov/providers-professionals/meaningful-use-definition-objectives
61. Epic [Internet]. [cited 2016 Apr 19]. Available from: https://www.epic.com/Software

5 Integrated Diabetes Care in Hong Kong: From Research to Practice to Policy

Roseanne O. Yeung, Junmei Yin, and Juliana C.N. Chan

Introduction

Hong Kong is a unique densely populated metropolitan city with heavy Western influences in a Chinese society. Given its colonial history, Western acculturation has been occurring in Hong Kong before most other areas in China, and so it provides a window into the potential future of the rest of China given its rapid economic and industrial development over the last century.

Over seven million people live in the 1104 km^2 city-state, and health care is provided by both the public and private sectors. The public health-care system is managed under the Hospital Authority (HA), a statutory body that provides acute hospital and ambulatory care services including 42 public hospitals and institutions, 47 Specialist Outpatient Clinics, and 73 General Outpatient Clinics. Most recent estimates suggest the adult prevalence of diabetes is 9.9 % 1.

This chapter discusses the evolution of diabetes care delivery at the Prince of Wales Hospital (PWH) and the Chinese University of Hong Kong (CUHK) into the current Joint Asia Diabetes Evaluation (JADE) programme, a multipronged quality improvement initiative. It also highlights the studies carried out at PWH and CUHK that have examined the data of Hong Kong citizens with diabetes, and how this information has and continues to influence diabetes care delivery to meet the local needs.

R.O. Yeung (✉)
Division of Endocrinology, Department of Medicine, University of Alberta, Edmonton, Alberta, Canada

Hong Kong Institute of Diabetes and Obesity, The Chinese University of Hong Kong, Hong Kong, China
e-mail: ryeung@ualberta.ca

J. Yin
Department of Medicine and Therapeutics, The Chinese University of Hong Kong, Hong Kong, China
e-mail: Suky605@163.com

J.C.N. Chan
Department of Medicine and Therapeutics, The Chinese University of Hong Kong, Hong Kong, China

Hong Kong Institute of Diabetes and Obesity, The Chinese University of Hong Kong, Hong Kong, China

International Diabetes Centre of Education, The Chinese University of Hong Kong, Prince of Wales Hospital, Satin, Hong Kong, China
e-mail: jchan@cuhk.edu.hk

D. Simmons et al. (eds.), *Integrated Diabetes Care*, DOI 10.1007/978-3-319-13389-8_5

Clinical Care: The CUHK-PWH Integrated Diabetes Care Programme

Adapting Lessons from Clinical Trials: Protocol-Driven Care as the Standard of Care

PWH is the public teaching hospital affiliated with the CUHK and serves more than 1.2 million people from all socio-economic backgrounds, and is governed by the HA. Hong Kong's public health-care system is heavily subsidized where 90 % of patients with chronic disease, including diabetes, receive care from the HA clinics and hospitals. All patients have access to medications, investigations, and professional consultations for a nominal fee (US$10 per clinic visit, US$1.5 per drug item each lasting 3–4 months). Since 1995, the HA has introduced a territory-wide Clinical Management System (CMS) which captures all critical clinical information including hospitalization, emergency room attendance, laboratory investigations, and drug dispensing information. Authorized personnel can retrieve patient data by using the Hong Kong Identity Card number, a unique identification number issued by the Hong Kong Government to all Hong Kong residents.

Led by CUHK clinician scientists and HA health-care professionals, the Diabetes and Endocrine Centre in PWH is a multidisciplinary centre that provides diabetes complication assessment, diabetes education and endocrine investigations to patients referred to PWH. It is also a training centre for medical doctors, nurses and other health-care professionals on diabetes management and education. It is dedicated to provide comprehensive multidisciplinary care to patients with diabetes through risk assessment and stratification, patient education and empowerment, periodic monitoring to prevent diabetes-related complications, and improving quality of life.

In 1989, the CUHK researchers carried out a 1-year randomized trial of enalapril versus nifedipine in 102 patients with type 2 diabetes and hypertension [2]. Both groups had improvements in blood pressure and albuminuria, so the study protocol was continued for another 4 years. During these 5 years, the study clinicians compared their experiences between usual care in the HA clinics to that within the clinical trial clinic. Usual care was poorly coordinated and fragmented, as the clinician could only spend an average of 8–12 min per patient and had little support to educate and reinforce the patient on lifestyle changes, treatment adherence and self-management. These patients were usually seen every 4–6 months by different generalists or specialists within a busy and crowded clinic setting. At each visit, blood pressure, fasting blood glucose and fructosamine were measured by clinic nurses. Annual assessments were recommended, but not dictated. By contrast, with the salary of a research nurse, the "clinical trial clinic" was set up in a 200 ft^2 room within the teaching block where patients were seen by doctors according to the protocol with visits every four months once stable. On average, each consultation lasted 15–20 min with predefined assessment for advancement of therapy, as needed. The research nurse served as a coordinator and liaison between the doctors and patients. Apart from performing clinical assessments (e.g. blood pressure, body weight, laboratory sample collection), the nurses also reinforced treatment plans and provided education and support which contributed towards a trusting relationship between patients and care team. Guided by the protocol, biochemical testing was more rigorous with measurement of glycated haemoglobin and lipid profile at least every 6 months and renal function including tests for albuminuria at least annually. Annual foot and retinal examination were also mandated in the trial clinic.

After 5 years, the follow-up study demonstrated the durability of these medications in blood pressure control with fewer clinical events, which motivated the team to explore the broader impact of this structured clinical setting on patient outcomes [3]. After 7 years of implementing the enalapril versus nifedipine protocol, a case-cohort study was undertaken to compare those in the trial versus those receiving usual care [4]. The latter patients were not eligible for the original trial due to lower blood pressure at the time (<160/90 mmHg). They were matched on a 1:1 basis with all those in the trial on age, sex, and duration of diabetes, among other clinical characteristics. At baseline, patients in the trial had higher prevalence of neuropathy and retinopathy. However, by the end of 7 years, the usual care group had higher blood pressures and fasting blood glucose than those in the trial group. More strikingly, 24.7 % of the usual care group died, compared to 8.8 % of those in the trial group with an adjusted relative risk of death of 0.21 (95 % CI 0.07, 0.65, P=0.006) in favour of the trial group. The team concluded that diabetes management by protocol-driven care improved survival and clinical outcomes in patients.

Standardization of Workflow

Given the large improvements seen with structured care in this setting, the CUHK-PWH team created a standardized and structured intake process based on the St. Vincent's Declaration Eurodiab Protocol in 1995 to improve care delivery [5]. Due to the shortage of manpower, nurses were trained to perform protocol-driven diabetes assessment and screening for common complications of diabetes. Changes were made to the workflow by creating two to three additional sessions at the Diabetes Centre where 20–25 patients would have comprehensive assessments (CA) carried out by one to two nurses and a few healthcare assistants in each session.

In detail, patients attended the Diabetes Centre for CA after fasting for at least 8 h. Trained nurses collected information on socio-economic status, medical history, family history, medication use and adherence, lifestyle, and self-care behaviours from the patients using structured preprinted forms. Significant medical history of co-morbidities was cross-checked with either the referring physician and/or the CMS. Lifestyle factors included smoking status, self-monitoring of blood glucose (SMBG) frequency, exercise frequency, and adherence to a balanced diet within the previous 3 months. Hypoglycaemia was assessed by asking patients if they had experienced hypoglycaemia during the previous 3 months.

Blood pressure and anthropometric measurement including body mass index (BMI) and waist circumference (WC) were taken using standardized procedures. Visual acuity and retinal photography were performed by trained nurses and later technicians, and reviewed by endocrinologists for typical features of diabetic retinopathy. Standardized monofilament and graduated tuning fork examinations were used to detect sensory neuropathy. Blood and urine samples were collected for fasting plasma glucose, HbA1c, lipid profile (total cholesterol, low density-lipoprotein cholesterol LDL-C, high density-lipoprotein cholesterol HDL-C and triglycerides), renal function and urinary albumin-to-creatinine ratio (ACR).

Big Data to Drive Improvements: The Hong Kong Diabetes Registry

Recognizing the importance of quality data in improving care, the Hong Kong Diabetes Registry (HKDR) was established in 1995 using the data from the structured assessments. Resources from both HA and CUHK were put towards meticulously prospectively collecting the data, and clerks were hired to enter and manage the data for quality assurance purposes. This rich clinical dataset has provided the means to examine clinical research questions in a timely and efficient manner. This registry has led to many dozens of publications which provide numerous descriptive analyses of the local diabetic population, which previously had not been well defined. This included the rarity of autoimmune diabetes even in the young population; low BMI with propensity for central obesity; secular changes of clinical outcomes, initially dominated by stroke and renal failure in the 1990s, coronary heart disease in the 2000, and more recently heart failure and cancer as survival continues to improve with better risk factor management and interventions. These epidemiological findings have subsequently been reported by many Asian investigators which have led to the acceptance by the scientific community regarding the "Asian phenotype," or better referred as a "phenotype in transition," characterized by early onset of disease with beta cell insufficiency, metabolic syndrome, and a propensity for renal disease and cancer 6. Given the paucity of randomized clinical trials in Asian populations, researchers have been able to replicate results from other parts of the world in order to validate questions in their own local population, in addition to examining novel research questions.

Given the volume of patients in the clinics, the team's earliest work from the HKDR prioritized the development of prediction models, to allow for more efficient, data-driven risk stratification of patients. After accruing data for a decade on over 7000 patients, the team established 5-year probabilities for major diabetes-related complications as defined by the International Code for Diseases retrieved from the CMS. These included end stage renal disease [7], stroke [8], coronary heart disease [9], heart failure [10], and mortality [11]. These risk equations have a 70–90 % sensitivity and specificity of predicting outcomes based on the parameters collected in the registry.

From Pilot Projects to Public Health Programmes in the Hospital Authority (HA)

Among the over 40 public hospitals run by HA, there are 17 public-funded diabetes centres coordinated by diabetologists and nurse educators that provide two to three weekly sessions of complication screening to all patients referred by the public hospitals and community-based clinics. The benefits of team-based periodic comprehensive assessments, disease management and peer support programmes, designed by specialists and coordinated by trained nurses, pharmacists and health-care assistants on clinical outcomes (death, cardiovascular-renal disease, hospitalizations) had been rigorously evaluated in peer-reviewed publications. These results were presented at hospital management conferences with mass media coverage to inform payers and the public. Along with efforts from other colleagues, these quality improvement programmes have contributed to the corporate strategy of the HA, which is the major health-care provider in Hong Kong, to develop career paths for nurse specialists and establishment of diabetes centres and pharmacist-led adherence clinics to provide assessment, education and integrated care programmes in major public hospitals in order to reduce the burden of chronic disease. These programmes were also timely in light of the development of the territory-wide CMS which enabled the HA to adapt the HKDR care protocol and develop standard templates for data collection for all diabetes centres. All centres use the same template for diabetes assessment, derived from the HKDR, which has now enrolled 350,000 patients with diabetes, accounting for 90 % of people diagnosed with diabetes in HK with a population of seven million and an estimated prevalence of 10 %, where only 50–70 % have been diagnosed. More recently, this diabetes complication screening service was extended to the publicly-funded community-based family clinics for risk stratification and triage purposes, and evaluation has shown a reduction of mortality (adjusted HR 0.363; 95 % CI, 0.308–0.428) using this programme [12]. However, due to the heavy service demands and resource constraints, there are still variations among different hospitals and clinics in delivering diabetes care despite the same Electronic Medical Record (EMR) templates. As a teaching hospital, the CUHK-PWH team continues to leverage the academic resources including research funding and postgraduate students to test pilot programmes and use research results to influence clinical practice. Here are a few examples of how research data can be used to change practice and influence policy.

Medication Adherence and Follow-Up

In 1998, the CUHK-PWH team carried out a 2-year randomized trial evaluating the impact of a pharmacist-led telephone counselling intervention to promote medication adherence on mortality in non-adherent patients prescribed at least five chronic medications attending the usual care specialist clinics [13]. As part of her MPhil thesis, a pharmacist identified eligible non-adherent patients based on a 20–30 min medication assessment interview, and defined adherence as taking 80–120 % of the prescribed daily medications. Adherence was assessed at screening, randomization, and after 2 years. The intervention consisted of a pharmacist making six to eight phone calls lasting 10–15 min per call to the patient between physician visits. The pharmacist clarified misconceptions of medications, asked about side effects, reinforced the importance of adherence, and provided basic counselling on self-care and lifestyle management. Patients were encouraged to report side effects, self-initiated changes in medication, and concerns to their attending doctors. The control group received no phone calls. After 2 years, 38 (17 %) patients had died in the control group compared to 25 (11 %) in the intervention group (adjusted relative risk: 0.59, 95 % CI 0.35–0.87, P=0.039). Notably, half of the patients who initially consented but defaulted on follow-up died within the 2-year period. These defaulters had similar clinical and demographic characteristics as the patients who were followed, except that their adherence scores were lower at baseline.

In another PhD project, the pharmacist candidate implemented a structured care programme in patients with types 2 diabetes and renal impairment and demonstrated the marked benefits in reducing cardiovascular disease and end stage renal disease after 2 years compared to usual care [14]. These results were replicated in a multicentre study where the use of a doctor-nurse team, guided by a protocol with predefined care processes and treatment targets (A1c <7 %, BP <130/80 mmHg, LDL-C <2.6 mmol/L, triglyceride <1.7 mmol/L, persistence of renin angiotensin system (RAS) inhibitors), increased the rate of attaining ≥3 targets by threefold (61 % versus 28 %). Patients who attained ≥3 targets was translated into relative risk reduction of 0.43 (95 % CI: 0.21–0.86) for end stage renal disease after 2 years [15]. These findings reinforced the importance of using protocols and frequent follow-up to treat to multiple targets and reinforce treatment adherence in these patients with silent disease, which have provided the rationale for the design of the JADE programme (see later section in this chapter).

Negative Emotions

The lifelong commitments to medication adherence and lifestyle modification make diabetes self-management both physically and emotionally taxing. The psychological burdens result from insulin injection, self-monitoring of blood glucose, dietary restriction, as well as fear of complications, which may significantly increase negative emotions in patients with diabetes. Depression, anxiety, and distress are prevalent mental afflictions found in patients with diabetes [16–19]. In a survey involving 189 patients with type 2 diabetes attending the PWH clinic, 20–50 % experienced diabetes-related distress using validated questionnaires. These symptoms of distress closely correlate with obesity and HbA1c [20]. Another study with a consecutive cohort of 586 outpatients with type 2 diabetes showed that the prevalence of depression was 18.3 % in Hong Kong Chinese patients with type 2 diabetes. Furthermore, depression was associated with poor glycaemic control and self-reported hypoglycaemia, in part due to poor adherence [21]. With the aid of the HKDR, the team conducted a prospective study involving 7835 patients with type 2 diabetes without cardiovascular disease (CVD) at baseline, and found that 153 patients were diagnosed with major depression by psychiatrists in public hospitals. After adjusting for conventional risk factors, depression was independently associated with a two to threefold increase in the risk of incident CVD [22].

Treatment Gaps in Young Onset Diabetes

As diabetes prevalence increases in younger populations and based on clinical observations regarding the poor outcomes in these subjects, the CUHK-PWH team used the registry to explore the impact of young-onset diabetes, a therapeutic challenge which has not been well defined. Using the HKDR, the team reported that one in five patients with type 2 diabetes were diagnosed before the age of 40. Compared to those with later onset of disease (≥40 years), patients with young-onset diabetes had worse metabolic control, under-prescription of life saving drugs such as statins and RAS inhibitors, with a higher cumulative event rate driven by longer disease duration [23]. These data also indicate that the rate of cardiovascular-renal complications in young type 2 diabetes patients have eclipsed those in type 1 diabetes, due to the amplifying effects of silent risk factors including obesity, hypertension, and dyslipidaemia [24]. The focus on preventing and delivering early preventive care has sparked the team to conduct community outreach programmes to engage tech-savvy younger people to assess and monitor their risk for diabetes using mobile phone applications (see section in this chapter on Yao Chung Kit Diabetes Assessment Centre for discussion of Community Outreach).

Genetic Risk

The establishment of the HKDR was accompanied by a biobank from consenting participants, and has allowed for novel genomic research (see section in this chapter on CUHK Diabetes: Genomics Research and Biobanking for further details). Areas of active research include discovery for genetic markers of diabetes and its complications including cancer. Apart from conducting linkage analysis using family-based cohorts recruited through the registry [25] and validating the first wave of genetic variants discovered in genome wide association studies in our Chinese population [26], the group has also used these resources to discover genetic variants associated with increased cancer risk [27], end stage renal disease [28], cardiovascular-renal disease [29–33], and young-onset diabetes [34–37], some of which have been validated in a recent meta-analysis [38].

Biochemical Markers

The registry contains many biochemical parameters linked to the development of complications, and have allowed exploration of a number of associations that are informing areas of future interventional research. Examples include:

- Critical importance of albuminuria and renal dysfunction as prognostic markers for cardiovascular-renal complications and their multiple determinants including metabolic syndrome [39]
- Association of HbA1c variability (mean standard deviation) with development of chronic kidney disease and cardiovascular disease independent of mean HbA1c and other confounders [40]
- Association of severe hypoglycaemia requiring hospitalization with increased mortality mainly due to cancer and chronic kidney disease [41]
- Association of cancer risk with (1) copresence of low triglycerides and low LDL-C and (2) copresence of high HDL-C and low LDL-C plus albuminuria, suggesting the importance of dysregulation of lipid metabolism in cancer development in type 2 diabetes [42]
- Patients with low C-peptide who received insulin had lower cardiovascular events and mortality than those on insulin with high C-peptide highlighting subphenotype-treatment interactions and the possible use of C-peptide to guide therapy [43]
- Both white blood cell count and haematocrit were independent predictors of mortality in type 2 diabetes which raise the hypothesis regarding the roles of inflammation and erythropoiesis in diabetes [44, 45]

These findings help to inform the pathophysiological understanding of this complex disease by better characterizing phenotypes, and providing the premise for formulating hypothesis for mechanistic and interventional studies with high clinical relevance.

Cancer and Diabetes

Diabetes has been associated with increased cancer risk, but the underlying mechanism is poorly understood. The linkage between the longitudinal clinical data within the HKDR and the cancer outcome data in the CMS has provided important observational findings to help elucidate these connections. Detailed pharmacoepidemiological analyses revealed attenuated cancer risk in patients treated with insulin and oral antidiabetic drugs compared with non-users of these drugs [46–48]. The team has further observed significant drug-subphenotype interactions with attenuated cancer risk in:

1. metformin users with low HDL-C
2. RAS inhibitor users with high WBC count
3. statin users with copresence of low LDL-C plus albuminuria or low triglyceride [49, 50].

These observations corroborate with experimental findings of possible consequences of hyperglycaemia on dysregulation of cholesterol metabolism as well as activation of RAS and adenosine 5′-monophosphate-activated protein kinase pathways, all of which may be implicated in cancer development. In support of these notions, the registry was used to confirm the additive effects of optimal glycaemic control and use of RAS inhibitors and statins on reduced cancer risk [51]. By combining the experimental and epidemiological observations, the CUHK-PWH diabetes team has formulated the hypothesis that early identification and optimization of multiple risk factors including early use of statins and RAS inhibitors may normalize the internal milieu to reduce cancer risk in type 2 diabetes, although large-scale, randomized clinical trials will be needed to confirm these hypothesis [52].

Diabetes and Chronic Hepatitis B Infection

Given the high prevalence of chronic hepatitis B infection in the region, the CUHK-PWH diabetes team was among the first to document the increased risk of renal and cardiovascular complications in people with chronic hepatitis B infection and diabetes compared to having diabetes alone [53, 54]. Furthermore, the rich dataset allowed the team to investigate the impact of treatment of risk factors in hepatitis B infected patients and found that the use of statins and insulin were associated with greatly reduced risk of development of hepatocellular carcinoma [55], providing the basis for designing clinical trials in this area.

The JADE Programme: Evolving Health Information Technology

In 2007, the Asia Diabetes Foundation (ADF) was founded as a non-profit research-promoting entity under the governance of the CUHK Foundation to transfer this large body of knowledge through technological enhancements to further improve the efficiency of care delivery and conduct of research. The ADF is a charitable organization dedicated to develop and validate innovative chronic disease management models with the aim to make quality care sustainable, affordable and accessible. The prime achievement of the ADF is the development of the JADE programme, a *state-of-the-art* web-based information technology that incorporate diabetes care protocols, validated risk engine, and clinical decision support tools to maximize the delivery of quality care and enable both health-care providers and patients to make informed decisions.

Supported by an educational grant, an endocrinologist was seconded for 2 years to develop the JADE programme, alongside a programming team and a project coordinator. The JADE programme began enrolling patients in 2007 as a quality improvement initiative to engage both physicians and patients. The JADE software consists of a web-based portal that uses technology to digitize risk stratification and protocol-driven care. The existing paper templates based on protocols recommended by international bodies were transformed into online forms, and the database was upgraded to a larger, more robust system. JADE assessment relies on a specified clinical workflow that integrates multiple care components to enable health-care providers to establish a diabetes registry with built in matrixes for documentation of key performance indexes. The key features of this web-based quality improvement programme include (Figs. 5.1 and 5.2):

1. Templates to guide standardized assessment workflow and data capture
2. Validated risk equations to estimate 5-year probability of major clinical events

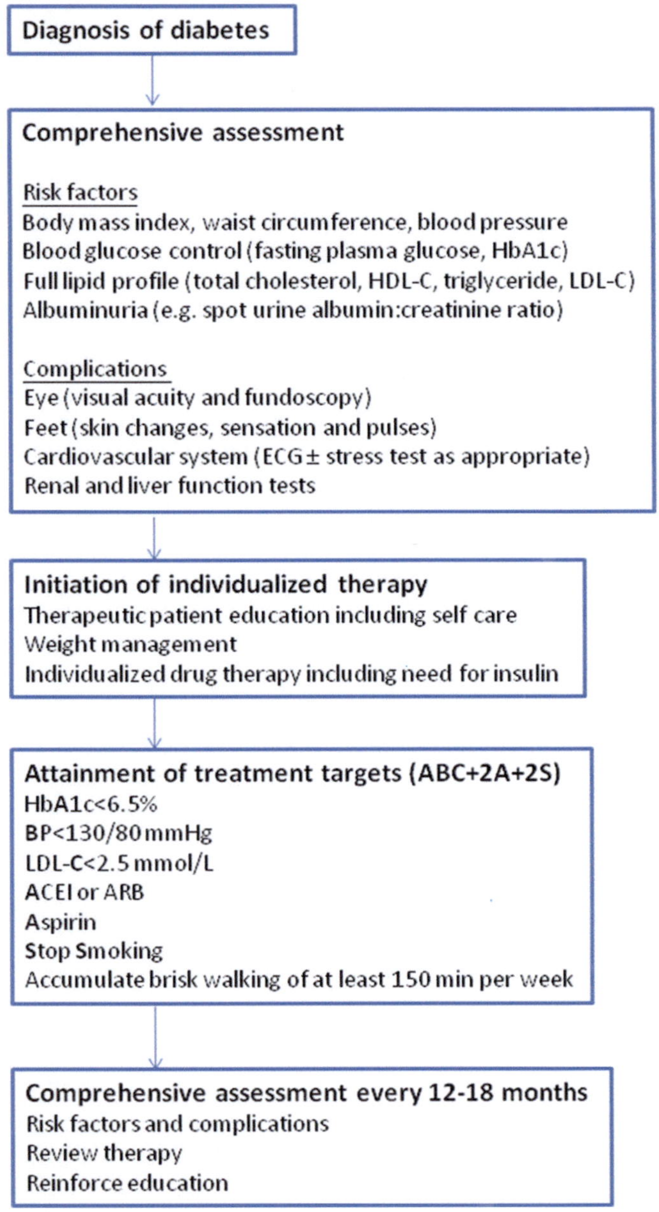

Fig. 5.1 Integrated diabetes care protocol recommended by the Plan of Action (2006–2010) for the Western Pacific Declaration on Diabetes (WPDD) (Adapted by the Joint Asia Diabetes Evaluation programme, designed by the Asia Diabetes Foundation (ADF). The protocol was based on Alberti et al. [74]; and Asian-Pacific Type 2 Diabetes Policy Group. Type 2 diabetes – practical targets and treatments. International Diabetes Institution and In Vivo Communications Asia Pte Co. Ltd., 2005)

3. Personalized reports with graphs and bar charts illustrating risk categories, current control of risk factors with easy communication of target values, notably A1c, blood pressure, LDL-C (ABC) and body weight
4. Individualized decision support for both doctors and patients, triggered by attained ABC targets and body weight, to empower self-management, reduce clinical inertia, and promote shared decision-making
5. Built in matrixes which displays the proportions of patients attaining various treatment targets and risk categories and their changes over time

These data are entered into a computer programme with predefined definitions of risk factors, complications and treatment targets to generate a one-page summary report which enable the physicians to efficiently identify gaps

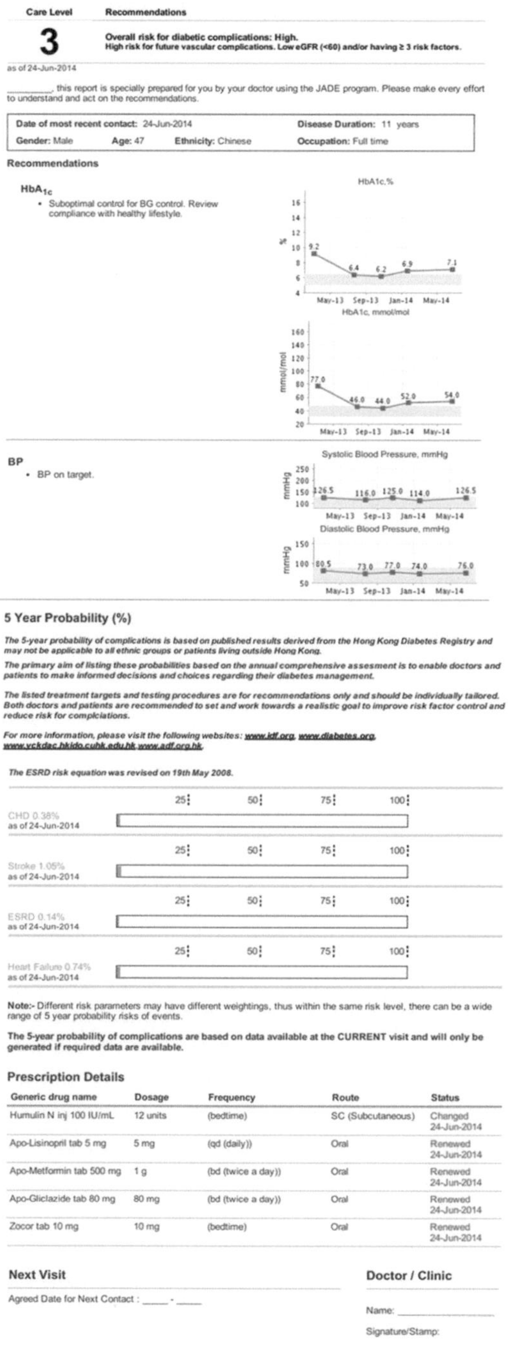

Care Level **Recommendations**

3 **Overall risk for diabetic complications: High.**
High risk for future vascular complications. Low eGFR (<60) and/or having ≥ 3 risk factors.

as of 24-Jun-2014

________, this report is specially prepared for you by your doctor using the JADE program. Please make every effort to understand and act on the recommendations.

Date of most recent contact: 24-Jun-2014			**Disease Duration:** 11 years
Gender: Male	**Age:** 47	**Ethnicity:** Chinese	**Occupation:** Full time

Recommendations

HbA1c

- Suboptimal control for BG control. Review compliance with healthy lifestyle.

BP

- BP on target.

5 Year Probability (%)

The 5-year probability of complications is based on published results derived from the Hong Kong Diabetes Registry and may not be applicable to all ethnic groups or patients living outside Hong Kong.

The primary aim of listing these probabilities based on the annual comprehensive assesment is to enable doctors and patients to make informed decisions and choices regarding their diabetes management.

The listed treatment targets and testing procedures are for recommendations only and should be individually tailored. Both doctors and patients are recommended to set and work towards a realistic goal to improve risk factor control and reduce risk for compliciations.

For more information, please visit the following websites: www.idf.org, www.diabetes.org, www.yckdac.hkido.cuhk.edu.hk, www.adf.org.hk.

The ESRD risk equation was revised on 19th May 2008.

CHD 0.38% as of 24-Jun-2014 (25 50 75 100)

Stroke 1.05% as of 24-Jun-2014 (25 50 75 100)

ESRD 0.14% as of 24-Jun-2014 (25 50 75 100)

Heart Failure 0.74% as of 24-Jun-2014 (25 50 75 100)

Note:- Different risk parameters may have different weightings, thus within the same risk level, there can be a wide range of 5 year probability risks of events.

The 5-year probability of complications are based on data available at the CURRENT visit and will only be generated if required data are available.

Prescription Details

Generic drug name	Dosage	Frequency	Route	Status
Humulin N inj 100 IU/mL	12 units	(bedtime)	SC (Subcutaneous)	Changed 24-Jun-2014
Apo-Lisinopril tab 5 mg	5 mg	(qd (daily))	Oral	Renewed 24-Jun-2014
Apo-Metformin tab 500 mg	1 g	(bd (twice a day))	Oral	Renewed 24-Jun-2014
Apo-Gliclazide tab 80 mg	80 mg	(bd (twice a day))	Oral	Renewed 24-Jun-2014
Zocor tab 10 mg	10 mg	(bedtime)	Oral	Renewed 24-Jun-2014

Next Visit

Agreed Date for Next Contact : ____ - ____

Doctor / Clinic

Name: ____________

Signature/Stamp:

Fig. 5.2 A sample of comprehensive assessment (CA) report for patient generated by the Joint Asia Diabetes Evaluation programme (Used with permission of Asia Diabetes Foundation, Hong Kong)

in treatment and make recommendations for each patient. Depending on the setting and workflow, these data collected by nurses or doctors, can be entered by clerical staff to be mailed to the referring physician and patient to promote shared decision-making. A prospective JADE research registry has been established through these periodic assessments.

Facilitating Knowledge Transfer and Clinical Decision-Making

The process of knowledge transfer in clinical medicine includes multiple steps and stakeholders, the simplest being:

(i) The patient conveys information to one or more health-care providers
(ii) The health-care provider(s) investigates with additional history, physical examination, or specialized investigations
(iii) The health-care provider(s) synthesizes the data to determine a potential diagnosis and treatment plan
(iv) The health-care provider(s) shares the potential diagnosis and treatment plan with the patient
(v) The patient and health-care provider(s) engage in shared decision-making to carry out plan

Each health-care system has its unique challenges of knowledge transfer and communication. Nevertheless, the challenges faced by the Hong Kong's public health-care system, modelled after the UK National Health System, are likely to be shared by many developing areas in Asia where universal health-care coverage for chronic disease like diabetes is becoming an urgent government priority. During the life journey of a person with diabetes, s/he will have multiple encounters with many health-care professionals including primary care physicians, specialists, nurses, other allied health professionals working in different settings including private and public as well as hospital and community clinics. Failed communication at any of these steps may result in the patient slipping through the cracks of the fragmented care continuum.

The CUHK-PWH team recognizes the challenges at each step and continues to make great efforts, based on feedback from users, to enhance the functionality of the JADE portal and design the JADE report to promote collaborative, multidisciplinary care, resulting in the creation of two JADE reports: one for the health-care provider, and one for the patient.

Communicating Between Professionals: JADE Health-Care Provider Reports

The JADE Health-Care Provider Report addresses the first three steps of the knowledge transfer process:

(i) The patient conveys information to one or more health-care providers,
(ii) The health-care provider(s) performs history taking, physical examination, or specialized investigations,
(iii) The health-care provider(s) synthesizes the data to create a problem list and treatment plan.

In addressing the first two steps, the team established the minimum data set required for collection using the template-guided process of information gathering between the patient and the health-care providers. By standardizing the type of information gathered and the format in which the information is conveyed, all team members can quickly and easily find and interpret information, decreasing the amount of searching through records.

Once the information is collected, the challenge lies in synthesizing the data for diagnostic and treatment purposes given the amount of medical knowledge required and the ever-expanding scientific literature. One of the biggest clinical obstacles is properly risk-stratifying patients to determine the appropriate level of intervention. The CUHK-PWH team capitalized on the local knowledge generated from the HKDR, and built a risk stratification engine in the JADE portal based on the published and internally validated risk equations for diabetes complications. A simple, practical clinical assessment consisting of four JADE risk categories was based on the learnings from the HKDR including the various risk equations (Fig. 5.3). These internally-validated risk categories respectively predict an annual all-event rate of 8 % (level 4, very high risk), 5 % (level 3, high risk), 3 % (level 2, moderate risk), 1 % (level 1, low risk). The CA report displays the patient's 5-year probabilities of clinical events (stroke, coronary heart disease, heart failure and ESRD) based on these validated risk equations.

Based on the risk category, a physician must then identify appropriate unmet gaps to prevent development or worsening of disease by controlling the four most modifiable risk factors (ABC and body weight). In order to help physicians identify evidence-based gaps and reduce clinical inertia, clinical decision support based on the International Diabetes Federation (IDF) clinical practice guidelines were integrated into the reports.

Communicating with the Patient: JADE Patient Reports

Multi-target clinical care focusing on glycaemic control, blood pressure, and lipids had been shown to reduce the development of diabetes-related complications and mortality in the landmark STENO-2 study [56]. The findings, based on data collected in a controlled randomized clinical trial setting, were subsequently confirmed in the HKDR which showed that attainment of ABC targets reduced events in a real-world setting [57]. To promote health literacy and empowerment, patients are informed about their ABC and body weight targets with decision support to help them achieve these goals.

The JADE patient report was created in order to complete steps 4 and 5 of the knowledge transfer process:

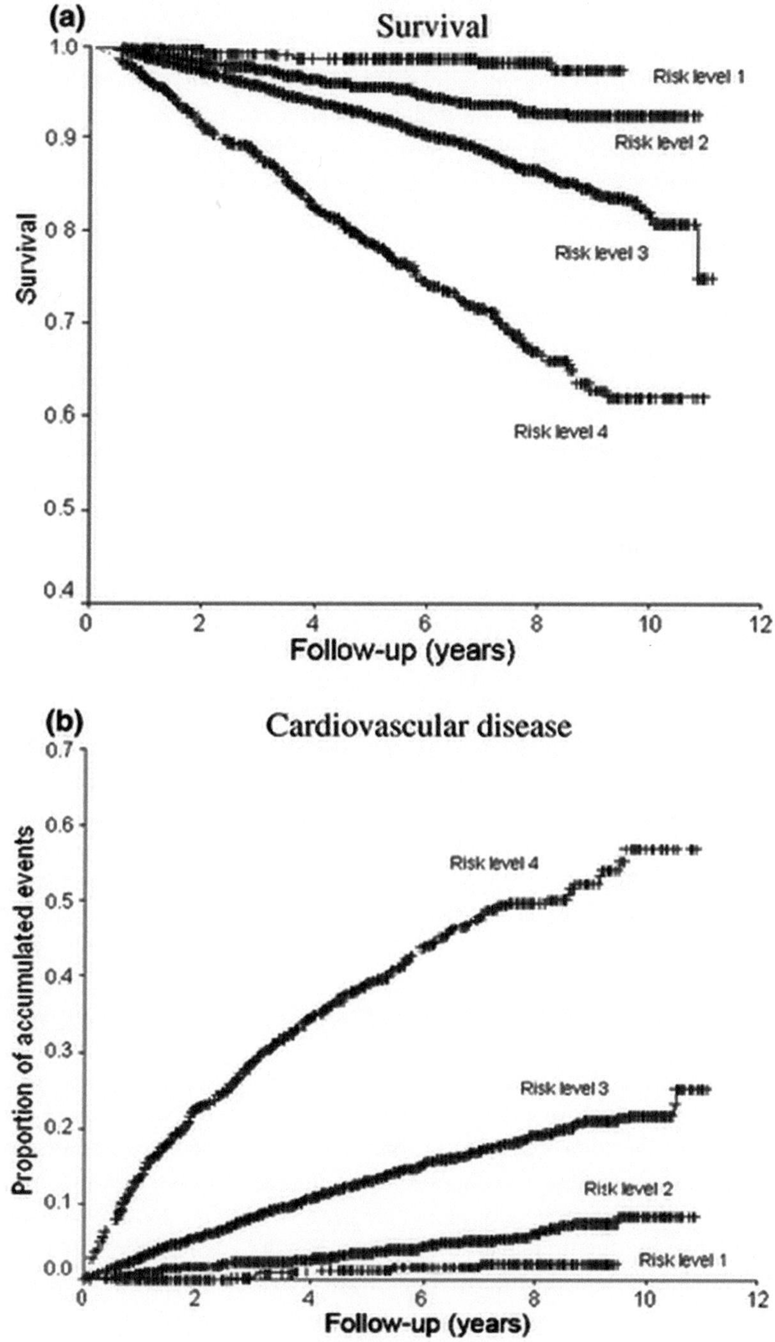

Fig. 5.3 (**a**, **b**) Kaplan–Meier analysis of survival and clinical event rates in 7534 Chinese type 2 diabetic patients categorized into different risk levels using the Risk Engine of the Joint Asia Diabetes Evaluation (JADE) programme. Log rank test: $P<0.001$ in both analyses. Risk level: level 1, low risk ($n=452$), level 2, moderate risk ($n=1468$), level 3, high risk ($n=4476$), level 4, very high risk ($n=1138$) (Reprinted with permission from Chan et al. [75])

(i) The health-care provider(s) shares the potential diagnosis and treatment plan with the patient
(ii) The patient and health-care provider engage in shared decision-making to carry out plan

The JADE report was designed to educate and empower the patient to self-manage with clear goal-directed feedback. After electronic entry of the data collected during the annual or biannual CA, the JADE portal generated a CA report for the patient (Fig. 5.2). This report shows the results of the assessments with emphasis on key modifiable risk factors including HbA1c, BP, LDL-C and body weight, and trend of these risk factors over time in a graphic representation. The ABC targets were set at HbA1c <7 %, BP <130/80 mmHg and LDL-C <2.6 mmol/L, based on the IDF recommendations [58]. The patient report also includes the risk stratification engine, and informs the patient of their 5-year probabilities of clinical events. The report also contains practical suggestions in layman terms to promote patient self-care and medication adherence in order to reach multiple treatment targets.

The JADE e-portal also has the functionality to generate follow-up (FU) reports to help track quality of diabetes care with decision support between CAs. As long as the key modifiable risk factors (HbA1c, BP, LDL-C and body weight) are assessed and entered into the portal, a personalized FU report displaying the patient's trends of ABC (HbA1c, BP, LDL-C) control and body weight with individualized reminders for self-care can be generated as a reinforcement tool to empower the patient. This FU report provides an important tool to track progress and promote ongoing dialogue between patients and healthcare professionals for shared decision-making.

Closing the Loop: Patient Education

Among the many challenges of patient self-management, lack of education and empowerment are the two most cited barriers [59]. Sufficient knowledge is unquestionably important in self-care, especially in people with low health literacy and limited access to diabetes education. Several systematic reviews showed that self-management education with comprehensive lifestyle interventions improved glycaemic and cardiovascular risk factor control [60–62]. In a meta-analysis, quality improvement measures targeted at patients, systems, and care providers all had positive impacts on metabolic control among patients with diabetes with patient education focusing on personalized goal-setting and action planning, having the largest effect size of 0.48 % reduction in mean HbA1c [63]. Moreover, patient empowerment, which motivates patients with diabetes to actively participate in decision-making regarding their self-care rather than simply comply with physician's instruction, is a further step to increase one's ability to think critically and act autonomously.

In order to efficiently empower patients, group classes were created to educate and reinforce patients on the basic of diabetes management. Patients are asked to return to the Diabetes Centre 6–8 weeks after their initial CA to collect their reports and attend a diabetes empowerment class led by diabetes nurse specialist. During this 2-h group session, the patients are informed of their assessment results and educated about self-management knowledge on diet, medication, physical activity, self-monitoring of blood glucose, and psychological health. They are also taught to interpret the JADE reports and emphasize the importance of attaining multiple treatment targets. The nurse uses both didactic and interactive approaches to teach and motivate the patients to be more engaged in self-management.

This care delivery model combining logistics, knowledge transfer, and information technology enables integrated and holistic care to patients with diabetes (Fig. 5.4). Starting with the primary care physician or other referring physician, a patient with diabetes is identified and referred for CA by the specialist team. A multidisciplinary team performs the CA and inputs the results into the JADE portal, generating the two personalized feedback reports as mentioned above. Patients are asked to return to PWH 4–6 weeks after the CA to attend a nurse-led empowerment class where they are educated about self-management knowledge and taught to interpret the JADE patient report. Patients follow up with their primary care physicians, who are empowered with the JADE professional report recommendations and arrange follow-up with the patients at appropriate time periods based on risk assessment (the majority being 3–4 months), where higher risk patients are booked in more frequently. Periodic specialist-reviewed CA are suggested every 12–24 months to help primary care physicians

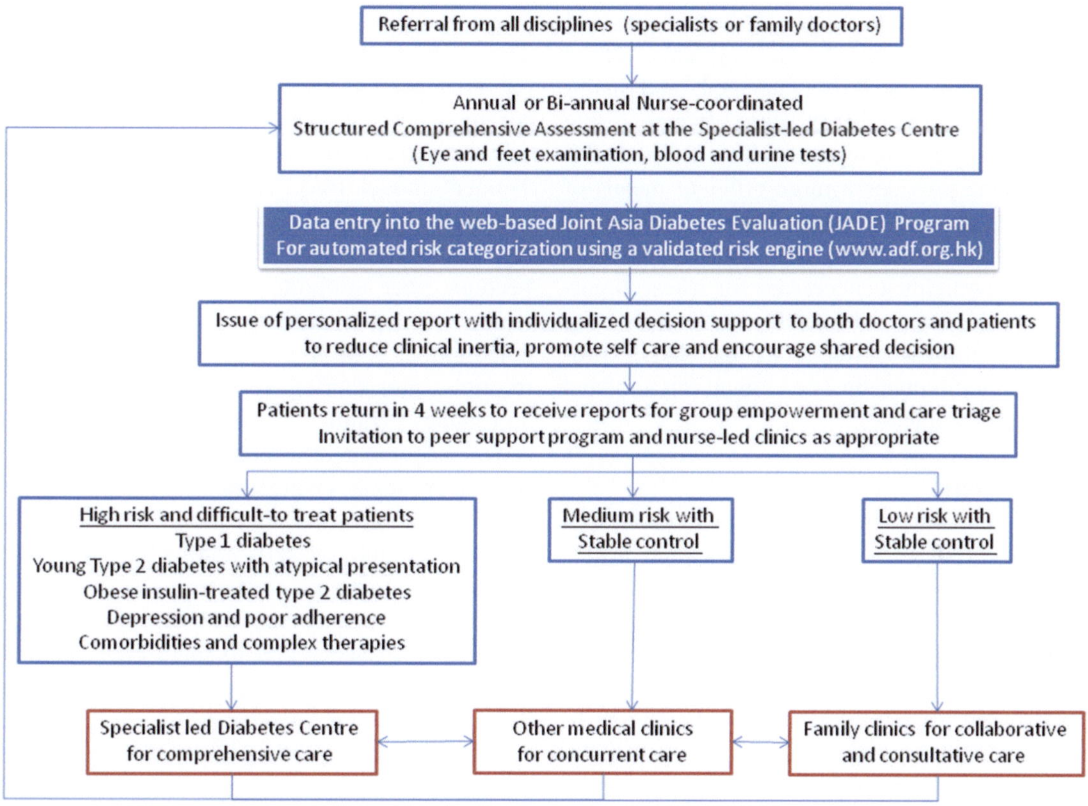

Fig. 5.4 Workflow of the multicomponent integrated diabetes care programme at the Chinese University of Hong Kong – Prince of Wales Hospital International Diabetes Federation Centre of Education, Hong Kong

and patients stay connected to the latest evidence-based treatments, clinical trial opportunities, and specialty programmes.

Innovation in JADE: More Efficient Data Infrastructure for Clinical Trials

Prospective cohort studies are always limited by bias, and evidence-based medicine requires planned, prospective evaluation of interventions to demonstrate efficacy. However, the costs of obtaining efficacy data in diabetes are growing exponentially as regulatory bodies demand data demonstrating superiority over existing treatments, long-term non-inferiority data in regards to cardiovascular outcomes, and cost-effectiveness [64, 65]. At present, many trials are funded by industry as major funding bodies continue to have budget cuts, leading many to question the validity of the data given the industry's inherent conflict of interest over profitability versus best patient care. As more medications come to market, there is a growing need for comparative effectiveness studies looking at medications within the same class and multiple medication class combinations, yet this research is difficult, time consuming, and often unpalatable to industry funding because of unclear benefits. And when evaluating cost-effectiveness, many of the existing studies are limited due to forced assumptions, since robust longitudinal clinical data are often unavailable [66]. Furthermore, few systems are in place for quality ongoing clinical surveillance once medications are approved.

Data Collection

Clinical trials are expensive because of the detail and depth of data required on each patient, which often require separate databases to be developed outside of the usual-care electronic medical records or paper-based chart systems. These databases must be built, managed, and maintained from scratch every time, often requiring double-entry of data by research staff. The JADE programme provides a more efficient means of collecting the key clinical variables in its comprehensive assessments, and allows researchers to add new fields as necessary for research purposes. This obviates the need for redundant entry into non-clinical systems, as the JADE programme is simultaneously a clinical care tool and prospective database.

Recruitment

The identification of patients for clinical trial recruitment starts with informing either healthcare professionals or patients of the trial inclusion criteria. Professionals must identify patients by relying on memory while sifting through paper charts, or using filtering capabilities if available in existing electronic medical records. A large number of trials fail because of inadequate recruitment [67]. The JADE programme has allowed for ready identification of eligible clinical trial participants because of its detailed clinical database.

Longitudinal Benefit

One of the greatest challenges in clinical trials is maintaining the contact between researchers and patients over many years. By pairing a study platform with clinical care, JADE facilitates long-term contact with the patient, as part of routine periodic follow-up. This also allows researchers to evaluate longer term outcomes than many previous trials, given the great expense in maintaining databases for the tracking of longitudinal outcomes.

Case Example of Enabling Research and Quality Improvement: PEARL Study

Clinicians on the CUHK-PWH team recognized the potential of empowering people with diabetes to help each other after seeing some of the positive interactions in the diabetes education class. These observations led to the development of the Peer support, Empowerment, And Remote communication Linked by information technology (PEARL) Study, based on a "Train-the-Trainer" model [68]. The team identified and invited friendly and knowledgeable patients with type 2 diabetes with an HbA1c less than 8 % to become peer supporters. A multidisciplinary team designed a curriculum of training, which consisted of four 8-h workshops incorporating tutorials, case sharing, reflections, role-playing, and games. Training focused on basic diabetes self-management information on diet, exercise, poor sleep, stress, changes in daily routines, body weight, medications, concurrent illnesses, and the importance of self-monitoring of blood glucose. Training was also provided regarding communication and empathic listening. Peer supporters were encouraged to share their positive experiences to assist their peers to manage diabetes on a day-to-day basis.

All patients undergoing comprehensive assessments were invited to join the study, and those who agreed were randomized to receive either peer support or usual care within the JADE programme where patients received periodic CA and quarterly FU reports through the mail. After 1 year, those managed by the JADE programme had significant improvement in risk factor control through reduced clinical inertia and improved self-care. Although patients who received additional peer support did not have further improvement in cardio-metabolic control, they had reduced hospitalization rates after one year of intervention. In a post hoc analysis, patients with significant negative emotions who had poor cardio-metabolic risk factor control such as hyperglycaemia, high BMI, and CKD, benefited most from peer support with hospitalization rate similar to those without negative emotions in whom peer support did not have effects on hospitalization. In these high risk patients with multiple risk factors and complications as well as negative emotions, peer support further improved psychological well-being and drug adherence. Furthermore, the peer supporters showed sustained glycaemic control, and improvements in self-care and health-related quality of life over 4 years of being involved with the programme [69].

Lessons learned from that trial have allowed for the development of the second iteration of the PEARL study, currently underway. In the second iteration, there has been the additional systematic evaluation of providing periodic personalized FU reports on metabolic control and hospitalization in patients with both type 1 and type 2 diabetes managed by the JADE programme. It includes almost all the patients referred to the PWH Diabetes Centre for annual CA from February 26 to December 1, 2013. A group of high-risk patients was offered peer support and randomized to receive two JADE FU reports by mail after their clinic visits. Patients not offered peer support were also randomized to receive two JADE FU reports. The primary outcome was change in HbA1c at month 12, as well as rate, frequency, and length of stay of hospitalization during the 12 months. The secondary outcomes include risk factor control, attainment of treatment targets, rate and frequency of emergency room visits, and changes in cognitive-psychosocial-behavioural parameters. The primary results show that patients who received additional FU reports had greater reduction in HbA1c compared to those under usual care, and patients with peer support had further improvements in psychosocial well-being, self-empowerment, and quality of life [70]. This programme forms the basis of another PhD thesis, which highlights the benefits of using an academic-health-care institution-foundation partnership to generate new knowledge and inform clinical practice, as advocated in the emerging field of improvement science [71].

The third iteration of the PEARL programme is in the planning stages. However, this serves as an example of an iterative quality improvement programme that has been greatly augmented by the JADE data collection platform, allowing for quality research at reduced cost given much of the data platform and clinical processes are already in place. In this programme, the team has been able to translate knowledge from the clinical efficacy setting of a randomized controlled trial, to adapting and implementing lessons learned into a clinical effectiveness setting, and adhering to principles of continuous quality improvement.

CUHK Diabetes Clinical Research Centre

Established since 1999, the CUHK Diabetes Clinical Research Centre has conducted nearly 100 phase two to four clinical trials of novel compounds and devices, to address unmet needs in diabetes, obesity, cardiovascular and renal diseases. Conducted trials included pharmaceutical-sponsored multicentre international studies and investigator-initiated studies. Apart from addressing the primary research questions, execution of clinical trials provide direct clinical benefits through education, intensified monitoring and structured care. Established principles of the research centre include:

(i) Protecting human rights
(ii) Ensuring that studies are conducted in accordance to Good Clinical Practice
(iii) Ensuring data quality and integrity for public dissemination
(iv) Adhering to Standards of Operation

Apart from fundraising to support other research programmes, the Diabetes Clinical Research Centre also serves as a training centre where fellows, nurses, health care, research and administrative personnel work in a collaborative and cohesive manner to gather and translate evidence to clinical practice through a bedside-to-bench-to-beside approach.

CUHK Diabetes: Genomics Research and Biobanking

Since 1994, the unit has embarked on an overarching strategy to combine epidemiology, applied genomics, clinical trials, and translational research with the ultimate goal to use clinical, biochemical, and genetic markers to identify high risk subjects for early intervention and prevention of complications. A biobank was established, containing multiple prospective case-control, family-based, adolescent/youth and mother-offspring cohorts. These interlinking research programmes which aim to discover markers to predict diabetes and its complications, have formed the basis of large scale epidemiological studies to examine the prevalence and natural history of childhood obesity, multiple forms of diabetes (e.g., young-onset diabetes, gestational diabetes), and possible interventions. This rich dataset has also facilitated global and region-wide research with the CUHK-PWH team being a key member in the Global Diabetes Consortium funded by the National Institute of Health in the United States and the Asian Genetic Epidemiology Network (AGEN) Consortium, which, for example, has enabled the discovery of new loci for type 2 diabetes in East Asians [72].

Building Professional Capacity: Hong Kong Institute of Diabetes and Obesity

The Hong Kong Institute of Diabetes and Obesity (HKIDO) is an education and research institute established under the CUHK in 2005, funded by donations, grants, contract research, to deliver training and education courses to health-care professional from both locally and in the Asia region, with the aim to strengthen professional capacity. In turn, proceeds from these conferences and courses have provided the much needed seed funding to sustain the continuous data analysis and genomic programme which are not inexpensive.

The key education programmes and conferences conducted include:

- Hong Kong Diabetes and Cardiovascular Risk Factors East-Meets-West Symposium held annually since 1999 http://www.hkido.cuhk.edu.hk/SymposiumsWorkshops/EMWSymposium2015/WelcomeMessage.aspx
- Diploma in Diabetes Management and Education since 2002
- Masters Course in Endocrinology, Diabetes and Metabolism since 2004 http://www.hkido.cuhk.edu.hk/Programmes/MScinEndocrinology,DiabetesandMetabolism/OverviewandObjectives.aspx
- Diploma in General Endocrinology and Metabolism since 2004
- Diabetes Preventing the Preventable Forum held annually since 2011 http://www.idfce-hk.org/dpp2015/

Yao Chung Kit Diabetes Assessment Centre

In 2007, the Yao Chung Kit (YCK) Diabetes Assessment Centre http://www.yckdac.hkido.cuhk.edu.hk/en/index.html was established through a generous donation from the Yao Yiu Sai Education and Charitable Memorial Fund to the CUHK to increase the accessibility, affordability and sustainability of this much needed risk stratification programme to benefit the growing population of patients with diabetes in the community. Given the dual private and public health-care systems in Hong Kong, the YCK Diabetes Assessment Centre offers an affordable private option for expedited care, as waiting lists for a CA at the HA Diabetes Centre can be up to a year or more. Services provided in YCK Diabetes Assessment Centre include comprehensive JADE-based diabetes CA and risk evaluation, with available 24 h ambulatory blood pressure monitoring and 24 h continuous glucose monitoring. Lifestyle-focused diabetes education classes are also provided, including exercise workshops, cooking classes, and diabetes conversation map workshops. Referrals can be made by physician or self-referral by the patient, allowing motivated patients readier access to services. By supporting private doctors in the community to provide a more holistic, quality-assured and affordable care, the YCK Diabetes Assessment Centre aims to provide an alternative option to patients who can afford a more personalized service to reduce the growing burden on the public system, while at the same time building a network of like-minded doctors and care professionals to improve diabetes care in the community.

Community Engagement: OPAL and RUBY

Supported by university and government grants, the YCK Diabetes Assessment Centre takes on an additional role of reaching out to the community to raise awareness and detect high risk subjects for early intervention. In the nurse-led Outreach Program to raise Awareness and Lifestyle Modification (OPAL), volunteers, peer supporters and health-care workers use simple tools and point of care tests to screen for prediabetes, diabetes and metabolic syndrome in workplaces and public spaces, often in partnership with interested employers and non-governmental organizations. Using various community and family-based cohorts, a validated risk equation for developing diabetes has been developed [73] and made into a web-based engine and mobile phone application, known as Risk Understanding By Yourself (RUBY). These technologies aim to engage website visitors and mobile-users to self-assess their risk of diabetes with recommendations including periodic monitoring and connection to health-care providers if they are at risk (http://rubyapp.adf.org.hk/#).

Beyond Hong Kong: Experience to Date

Though started in Hong Kong, the vision of the JADE programme is to create a virtual environment to enable sharing of best practices and empower informed decisions and self-management in people with diabetes across Asia. This platform, with multiple languages, has now been adopted by more than 300 sites in ten other Asian countries/regions: China, India, Indonesia, Malaysia, Philippines, South Korea, Singapore, Taiwan, Thailand, and Vietnam. This has enabled regional collaborations with cross-national comparisons and gap identification.

As an example, the prevalence of diabetes is increasing in young adults across Asia, but little is known about the metabolic control or burden of diabetes in this population. Data were extracted from 245 sites for cross sectional evaluation, and comparisons were made between those with young-onset diabetes (diagnosis before age 40) and late-onset diabetes (diagnosis at age 40 or older) [16]. Of the 41,029 patients with data available, 18 % had young-onset diabetes. The young-onset group had longer disease duration than those with late-onset diabetes (10 versus 5 years), with worse glycaemic control (mean HbA1c 8.32 % [SD 2.03] vs 7.69 % [1.82]; $p<0.001$). Despite their worse risk profiles, these young onset patients were also less likely to receive statins for documented dyslipidaemia, and less likely to be on antihypertensive medications for documented hypertension. These prospectively collected data, using the same protocol, provide a reasonable estimate of real-world practices. By identifying the variation in practice across settings, clinicians, policy makers, and public health experts are better equipped to examine the system and population differences to account for these differing gaps. Adoption of broad interventions or secular changes, such as the introduction of new practice guidelines, can be evaluated using more detailed clinical data, on a much larger population level, and used to guide future interventions, which can be continuously tracked in a quality improvement cycle. The clinical decision algorithms and reporting tools embedded in the JADE programme provide a means to disseminate the latest knowledge and provide a closed-loop approach to knowledge translation from the findings directly obtained from the included population.

JADE: Future Considerations

As technology advances, the JADE programme will endeavour to keep up with the demands of improving user interface and user experience for diabetes care delivery. Increasingly, the private and public sectors are recognizing the potential of using technology to deliver self-reported and self-tracked data for chronic disease management, with ever-expanding mobile applications and medical devices. Our team hopes to build interoperability between web-based JADE programme and mobile devices which measure objective physical

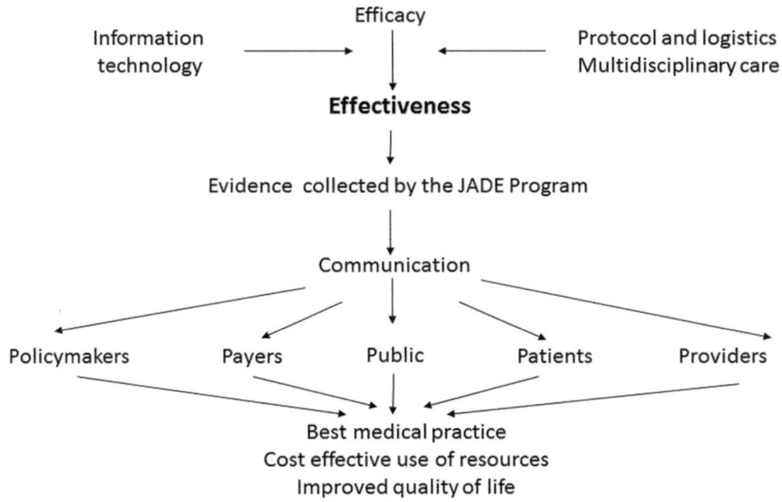

Fig. 5.5 The JADE programme advocates to use logistics, information technology and team-based care to change practice and influence policy through ongoing collaborative research efforts (Reprinted with permission from Chan et al. [76])

data (e.g., glucometers, insulin pumps, blood pressure) to enable even better risk assessment and monitoring to improve clinical decision-making. A focus on longitudinally capturing self-reported data such as quality of life and patient satisfaction through convenient technological methods will also allow for better clinical care and more accurate health economic evaluation.

JADE Summary

Since 1989, the CUHK-PWH diabetes team has amassed considerable knowledge, from the microscopic world of molecular biology to the macroscopic realm of clinical epidemiology and translational medicine. With a strong focus on local needs, the CUHK-PWH team has been able to identify and develop approaches to overcome many of the barriers of chronic disease management through the use of structured workflow, information technology, team-based care, and rigorous evaluation (Fig. 5.5). The team recognizes the importance of facilitating communication of the evidence at all levels, from patients to care providers to policy makers. The JADE programme serves as an important prototype to demonstrate how collection of registry data can enhance care, identify gaps, and improve outcomes, while all in the spectre of usual clinical practice. This serves as a hopeful example to promote international collaborative research efforts, focused on providing more holistic, personalized, evidence-based care.

References

1. Information Services Department, Hong Kong SAR Government. Feb 2016. Available from: http://www.gov.hk/en/about/abouthk/factsheets/docs/public_health.pdf
2. Chan JC, Cockram CS, Nicholls MG, Cheung CK, Swaminathan R. Comparison of enalapril and nifedipine in treating non-insulin dependent diabetes associated with hypertension: one year analysis. BMJ. 1992;305(6860):981–5.
3. Chan JC, Ko GT, Leung DH, Cheung RC, Cheung MY, So WY, et al. Long-term effects of angiotensin-converting enzyme inhibition and metabolic control in hypertensive type 2 diabetic patients. Kidney Int. 2000;57(2):590–600.
4. So WY, Tong PCY, Ko GTC, Leung WYS, Chow C-C, Yeung VTF, et al. Effects of protocol-driven care versus usual outpatient clinic care on survival rates in patients with type 2 diabetes. Am J Manag Care. 2003;9(9):606–15.
5. Piwernetz K, Home PD, Snorgaard O, Antsiferov M, Staehr-Johansen K, Krans M. Monitoring the targets of the St Vincent Declaration and the implementation of quality management in diabetes care: the DIABCARE initiative. The DIABCARE Monitoring Group of the St Vincent Declaration Steering Committee. Diabet Med. 1993;10(4):371–7.
6. Chan JCN, Malik V, Jia W, Kadowaki T, Yajnik CS, Yoon K-H, et al. Diabetes in Asia: epidemiology, risk factors, and pathophysiology. JAMA. 2009;301(20):2129–40.

7. Yang X, So W, Kong A, Clarke P, Ho C, Lam C, et al. End-stage renal disease risk equations for Hong Kong Chinese patients with type 2 diabetes: Hong Kong Diabetes Registry. Diabetologia. 2006;49(10):2299–308.
8. Yang X, So W-Y, Kong APS, Ho C-S, Lam CWK, Stevens RJ, et al. Development and validation of stroke risk equation for Hong Kong Chinese patients with type 2 diabetes: the Hong Kong Diabetes Registry. Diabetes Care. 2007;30(1):65–70.
9. Yang X, Ma RC, So W-Y, Ko GT, Kong AP, Lam CW, et al. Impacts of chronic kidney disease and albuminuria on associations between coronary heart disease and its traditional risk factors in type 2 diabetic patients – the Hong Kong Diabetes Registry. Cardiovasc Diabetol. 2007;6:37.
10. Yang X, Ma R, So W-Y, Kong A, Ko GT, Ho C-S, et al. Development and validation of a risk score for hospitalization for heart failure in patients with type 2 diabetes mellitus. Cardiovasc Diabetol. 2008;7(1):9.
11. Yang X, So WY, Tong PCY, Ma RCW, Kong APS, Lam CWK, et al. Development and validation of an all-cause mortality risk score in type 2 diabetes. Arch Intern Med. 2008;168(5):451–7.
12. Jiao F, Fung CSC, Wan YF, McGhee SM, Wong CKH, Dai D, et al. Long-term effects of the multidisciplinary risk assessment and management program for patients with diabetes mellitus (RAMP-DM): a population-based cohort study. Cardiovasc Diabetol. 2015;14:105.
13. Wu JYF, Leung WYS, Chang S, Lee B, Zee B, Tong PCY, et al. Effectiveness of telephone counselling by a pharmacist in reducing mortality in patients receiving polypharmacy: randomised controlled trial. BMJ. 2006;333(7567):522.
14. Leung WYS, So W-Y, Tong PCY, Chan NN, Chan JCN. Effects of structured care by a pharmacist-diabetes specialist team in patients with type 2 diabetic nephropathy. Am J Med. 2005;118(12):1414.
15. Chan JC, So W-Y, Yeung C-Y, Ko GT, Lau I-T, Tsang M-W, et al. Effects of structured versus usual care on renal endpoint in type 2 diabetes: the SURE study: a randomized multicenter translational study. Diabetes Care. 2009;32(6):977–82.
16. Das-Munshi J, Stewart R, Ismail K, Bebbington PE, Jenkins R, Prince MJ. Diabetes, common mental disorders, and disability: findings from the UK National Psychiatric Morbidity Survey. Psychosom Med. Jan;69(6):543–50.
17. Anderson RJ, Freedland KE, Clouse RE, Lustman PJ. The prevalence of comorbid depression in adults with diabetes: a meta-analysis. Diabetes Care. 2001;24(6):1069–78.
18. Grigsby AB, Anderson RJ, Freedland KE, Clouse RE, Lustman PJ. Prevalence of anxiety in adults with diabetes: a systematic review. J Psychosom Res. 2002;53(6):1053–60.
19. Golden SH. A review of the evidence for a neuroendocrine link between stress, depression and diabetes mellitus. Curr Diabetes Rev. 2007;3(4):252–9.
20. Ting RZW, Nan H, Yu MWM, Kong APS, Ma RCW, Wong RYM, et al. Diabetes-related distress and physical and psychological health in Chinese type 2 diabetic patients. Diabetes Care. 2011;34(5):1094–6.
21. Zhang Y, Ting R, Lam M, Lam J, Nan H, Yeung R, et al. Measuring depressive symptoms using the Patient Health Questionnaire-9 in Hong Kong Chinese subjects with type 2 diabetes. J Affect Disord. 2013;151(2):660–6. Elsevier.
22. Ting RZW, Lau ESH, Ozaki R, Lau WWY, Kong APS, Luk AOY, et al. High risk for cardiovascular disease in Chinese type 2 diabetic patients with major depression – a 7-year prospective analysis of the Hong Kong Diabetes Registry. J Affect Disord. 2013;149(1–3):129–35.
23. Chan JC, Lau ES, Luk AO, Cheung KK, Kong AP, Yu LW, et al. Premature mortality and co-morbidities in young-onset diabetes – a 7 year prospective analysis. Am J Med. 2014;127(7):616–24.
24. Luk AOY, Lau ESH, So WY, Ma RCW, Kong APS, Ozaki R, et al. Prospective study on the incidences of cardiovascular-renal complications in Chinese patients with young-onset type 1 and type 2 diabetes. Diabetes Care. 2014;37(1):149–57.
25. Ng MCY, So W-Y, Cox NJ, Lam VKL, Cockram CS, Critchley JAJH, et al. Genome-wide scan for type 2 diabetes loci in Hong Kong Chinese and confirmation of a susceptibility locus on chromosome 1q21-q25. Diabetes. 2004;53(6):1609–13.
26. Ng MCY, Park KS, Oh B, Tam CHT, Cho YM, Shin HD, et al. Implication of genetic variants near TCF7L2, SLC30A8, HHEX, CDKAL1, CDKN2A/B, IGF2BP2, and FTO in type 2 diabetes and obesity in 6,719 Asians. Diabetes. 2008;57(8):2226–33.
27. Ma RCW, So WY, Tam CHT, Luk AO, Ho JSK, Wang Y, et al. Genetic variants for type 2 diabetes and new-onset cancer in Chinese with type 2 diabetes. Diabetes Res Clin Pract. 2014;103(2):328–37.
28. Ma RCW, Tam CHT, Wang Y, Luk AO, Hu C, Yang X, et al. Genetic variants of the protein kinase C-beta 1 gene and development of end-stage renal disease in patients with type 2 diabetes. JAMA. 2010;304(8):881–9.
29. Wang Y, Luk AOY, Ma RCW, So W-Y, Tam CHT, Ng MCY, et al. Predictive role of multilocus genetic polymorphisms in cardiovascular disease and inflammation-related genes on chronic kidney disease in type 2 diabetes – an 8-year prospective cohort analysis of 1163 patients. Nephrol Dial Transplant. 2012;27(1):190–6.
30. Ho JSK, Germer S, Tam CHT, So W-Y, Martin M, Ma RCW, et al. Association of the PPARG Pro12Ala polymorphism with type 2 diabetes and incident coronary heart disease in a Hong Kong Chinese population. Diabetes Res Clin Pract. 2012;97(3):483–91.
31. So W-Y, Wang Y, Ng MCY, Yang X, Ma RCW, Lam V, et al. Aldose reductase genotypes and cardiorenal complications: an 8-year prospective analysis of 1,074 type 2 diabetic patients. Diabetes Care. 2008;31(11):2148–53.

32. Wang Y, Ng MCY, Lee S-C, So W-Y, Tong PCY, Cockram CS, et al. Phenotypic heterogeneity and associations of two aldose reductase gene polymorphisms with nephropathy and retinopathy in type 2 diabetes. Diabetes Care. 2003;26(8):2410–5.
33. Baum L, Ng MCY, So W-Y, Lam VKL, Wang Y, Poon E, et al. Effect of hepatic lipase -514C->T polymorphism and its interactions with apolipoprotein C3–482C->T and apolipoprotein E exon 4 polymorphisms on the risk of nephropathy in Chinese type 2 diabetic patients. Diabetes Care. 2005;28(7):1704–9.
34. Ma RCW, Lee HM, Lam VKL, Tam CHT, Ho JSK, Zhao H-L, et al. Familial young-onset diabetes, prediabetes and cardiovascular disease are associated with genetic variants of DACH1 in Chinese. PLoS ONE. 2014;9(1):e84770.
35. Lam VKL, Ma RCW, Lee HM, Hu C, Park KS, Furuta H, et al. Genetic associations of type 2 diabetes with islet amyloid polypeptide processing and degrading pathways in Asian populations. PLoS ONE. 2013;8(6):e62378.
36. Ma RCW, Hu C, Tam CH, Zhang R, Kwan P, Leung TF, et al. Genome-wide association study in a Chinese population identifies a susceptibility locus for type 2 diabetes at 7q32 near PAX4. Diabetologia. 2013;56(6):1291–305.
37. Ng MCY, Lam VKL, Tam CHT, Chan AWH, So W-Y, Ma RCW, et al. Association of the POU class 2 homeobox 1 gene (POU2F1) with susceptibility to type 2 diabetes in Chinese populations. Diabet Med. 2010;27(12):1443–9.
38. Mooyaart AL, Valk EJJ, van Es LA, Bruijn JA, de Heer E, Freedman BI, et al. Genetic associations in diabetic nephropathy: a meta-analysis. Diabetologia. 2011;54(3):544–53.
39. So WY, Kong APS, Ma RCW, Ozaki R, Szeto CC, Chan NN, et al. Glomerular filtration rate, cardiorenal end points, and all-cause mortality in type 2 diabetic patients. Diabetes Care. 2006;29(9):2046–52.
40. Luk AOY, So W-Y, Ma RCW, Kong APS, Ozaki R, Ng VSW, et al. Metabolic syndrome predicts new onset of chronic kidney disease in 5,829 patients with type 2 diabetes: a 5-year prospective analysis of the Hong Kong Diabetes Registry. Diabetes Care. 2008;31(12):2357–61.
41. Kong APS, Yang X, Luk A, Ma RCW, So WY, Ozaki R, et al. Severe hypoglycemia identifies vulnerable patients with type 2 diabetes at risk for premature death and all-site cancer: the Hong Kong Diabetes Registry. Diabetes Care. 2014;37(4):1024–31.
42. Yang X, So WY, Ma RCW, Kong APS, Lee HM, Xu G, et al. Synergistic effects of low LDL cholesterol with other factors for the risk of cancer in type 2 diabetes: the Hong Kong Diabetes Registry. Acta Diabetol. 2012;49 Suppl 1:S185–93.
43. Ko GT, So WY, Tong PC, Chan WB, Yang X, Ma RC, et al. Effect of interactions between C peptide levels and insulin treatment on clinical outcomes among patients with type 2 diabetes mellitus. CMAJ. 2009;180(9):919–26.
44. So W, Yang X, Ma R, Kong A, Lam C, Ho C, et al. Risk factors in V-shaped risk associations with all-cause mortality in type 2 diabetes—The Hong Kong Diabetes Registry. Diabetes Metab Res Rev. 2008;24(3):238–46.
45. Tong PCY, Kong APS, So W-Y, Ng MHL, Yang X, Ng MCY, et al. Hematocrit, independent of chronic kidney disease, predicts adverse cardiovascular outcomes in Chinese patients with type 2 diabetes. Diabetes Care. 2006;29(11):2439–44.
46. Yang X, So WY, Ma RCW, Yu LWY, Ko GTC, Kong APS, et al. Use of sulphonylurea and cancer in type 2 diabetes-the Hong Kong Diabetes Registry. Diabetes Res Clin Pract. 2010;90(3):343–51.
47. Yang X, So W-Y, Ma RCW, Yu LWL, Kong APS, Lee HM, et al. Use of thiazolidinedione and cancer risk in type 2 diabetes: the Hong Kong Diabetes Registry. Diabetes Res Clin Pract. 2012;97(1):e13–7.
48. Yang X, Ko GTC, So WY, Ma RCW, Yu LWL, Kong APS, et al. Associations of hyperglycemia and insulin usage with the risk of cancer in type 2 diabetes: the Hong Kong Diabetes Registry. Diabetes. 2010;59(5):1254–60.
49. Yang X, Ma RCW, So WY, Ko GTC, Kong APS, Zhao H, et al. White blood cell count and renin-angiotensin system inhibitors for the risk of cancer in type 2 diabetes. Diabetes Res Clin Pract. 2010;87(1):117–25.
50. Yang X, So W-Y, Ma RCW, Ko GTC, Kong APS, Wang Q, et al. Predicting values of lipids and white blood cell count for all-site cancer in type 2 diabetes. Endocrinol Relat Cancer. 2008;15(2):597–607.
51. Kong APS, Yang X, So W-Y, Luk A, Ma RCW, Ozaki R, et al. Additive effects of blood glucose lowering drugs, statins and renin-angiotensin system blockers on all-site cancer risk in patients with type 2 diabetes. BMC Med. 2014;12:76.
52. Yang X, So W-Y, Ma RCW, Kong APS, Xu G, Chan JCN. Diabetes and cancer: the mechanistic implications of epidemiological analyses from the Hong Kong Diabetes Registry. Diabetes Metab Res Rev. 2012;28(5):379–87.
53. Cheng AYS, Kong APS, Wong VWS, So WY, Chan HLY, Ho CS, et al. Chronic hepatitis B viral infection independently predicts renal outcome in type 2 diabetic patients. Diabetologia. 2006;49(8):1777–84.
54. Lo MKW, Lee K-F, Chan NN, Leung WYS, Ko GTC, Chan W-B, et al. Effects of gender, Helicobacter pylori and hepatitis B virus serology status on cardiovascular and renal complications in Chinese type 2 diabetic patients with overt nephropathy. Diabetes Obes Metab. 2004;6(3):223–30.
55. Yang X, Wang Y, Luk AOY, So WY, Ma RCW, Kong APS, et al. Enhancers and attenuators of risk associations of chronic hepatitis B virus infection with hepatocellular carcinoma in type 2 diabetes. Endocrinol Relat Cancer. 2013;20(2):161–71.
56. Gaede P, Vedel P, Larsen N, Jensen GV, Parving HH, Pedersen O. Multifactorial intervention and cardiovascular disease in patients with type 2 diabetes. N Engl J Med. 2003;30;348(5):383–93.

57. Kong APS, Yang X, Ko GTC, So W-Y, Chan W-B, Ma RCW, et al. Effects of treatment targets on subsequent cardiovascular events in Chinese patients with type 2 diabetes. Diabetes Care. 2007;30(4):953–9.
58. International Diabetes Federation. Global guideline for type 2 diabetes: recommendations for standard, comprehensive, and minimal care. Diabet Med. 2006;23(6):579–93.
59. Ahola AJ, Groop P-H. Barriers to self-management of diabetes. Diabet Med. 2013;30(4):413–20.
60. Loveman E, Cave C, Green C, Royle P, Dunn N, Waugh N. The clinical and cost-effectiveness of patient education models for diabetes: a systematic review and economic evaluation. Health Technol Assess. 2003;7(22):iii. 1–190.
61. Loveman E, Frampton GK, Clegg AJ. The clinical effectiveness of diabetes education models for type 2 diabetes: a systematic review. Health Technol Assess. 2008;12(9):1–116. iii.
62. Jarvis J, Skinner TC, Carey ME, Davies MJ. How can structured self-management patient education improve outcomes in people with type 2 diabetes? Diabetes Obes Metab. 2010;12(1):12–9.
63. Tricco AC, Ivers NM, Grimshaw JM, Moher D, Turner L, Galipeau J, et al. Effectiveness of quality improvement strategies on the management of diabetes: a systematic review and meta-analysis. Lancet. 2012;379(9833):2252–61. Elsevier Ltd.
64. U.S. Department of Health and Human Services Food and Drug Administration Center for Drug Evaluation and Research (CDER). Guidance for Industry Diabetes Mellitus–evaluating cardiovascular risk in new antidiabetic therapies to treat type 2 diabetes Internet; 2008 cited 2015 May 17. Available from: http://www.fda.gov/downloads/drugs/guidancecomplianceregulatoryinformation/guidances/ucm071627.pdf
65. Avorn J. The $2.6 billion pill – methodologic and policy considerations. N Engl J Med. 2015;372(20):1877–9.
66. Hay J, Jackson J. Panel 2: methodological issues in conducting pharmacoeconomic evaluations – modeling studies. Value Health. 1999;2(2):78–81.
67. McDonald AM, Treweek S, Shakur H, Free C, Knight R, Speed C, et al. Using a business model approach and marketing techniques for recruitment to clinical trials. Trials. 2011;12(1):74.
68. Chan JCN, Sui Y, Oldenburg B, Zhang Y, Chung HHY, Goggins W, et al. Effects of telephone-based peer support in patients with type 2 diabetes mellitus receiving integrated care. JAMA Intern Med. 2014;174(6):972–81.
69. Yin JM, Wong R, Au S, Chung HY, Lau M, Lin L, Tsang CC, Lau KP, Ozaki R, So WY, Ko G, Luk A, Yeung R, Chan JC, Yin JM, Wong R, Au S, Chung HY, Lau M, Lin L, Tsang CC, Lau KP, Ozaki R, So WY, Ko G, Luk A, Yeung RCJ. Effects of being a peer supporter on diabetes management in people with type 2 diabetes. Ann Fam Med. 2015;13 Suppl 1:S42–9.
70. Yin J. A quality improvement project evaluating the effect of personalized feedback report and Peer support in patients with diabetes in Hong Kong. PhD dissertation. The Chinese University of Hong Kong. 2015. ProQuest LLC.
71. Marshall M, Pronovost P, Dixon-Woods M. Promotion of improvement as a science. Lancet. 2013;381(9864):419–21.
72. Cho YS, Chen C-H, Hu C, Long J, Ong RTH, Sim X, et al. Meta-analysis of genome-wide association studies identifies eight new loci for type 2 diabetes in east Asians. Nat Genet. 2012;44(1):67–72.
73. Ko G, So W, Tong P, Ma R, Kong A, Ozaki R, et al. A simple risk score to identify Southern Chinese at high risk for diabetes. Diabet Med. 2010;27(6):644–9.
74. Alberti KG, Zimmet P, Shaw J. International Diabetes Federation: a consensus on type 2 diabetes prevention. Diabet Med. 2007;24:451–63.
75. Chan J, So W, Ko G, Tong P, Yang X, Ma R, et al. The Joint Asia Diabetes Evaluation (JADE) Program: a web-based program to translate evidence to clinical practice in Type 2 diabetes. Diabet Med. 2009;26(7):693–9.
76. Chan JCN, Ozaki R, Luk A, Kong APS, Ma RCW, Chow FCC, et al. Delivery of integrated diabetes care using logistics and information technology – the Joint Asia Diabetes Evaluation (JADE) program. Diabetes Res Clin Pract. 2014;106(Suppl):S295–304.

Approaches to Integrated Diabetes Care: A South African Approach

6

Larry A. Distiller and Michael A.J. Brown

Part I: Background to the South African Health Care System

South Africa has an estimated population of 54 million people [1]. The Department of Health holds overall responsibility for healthcare, with a specific responsibility for the public sector. Because of high levels of poverty and unemployment, the bulk of the burden of healthcare is borne by the state, with 84 % of the population receiving some portion of their healthcare from the public (Government) sector. Sixty-eight percent of the population does not use any private care at all, and a further 16 % of the population rely on the public sector for hospital care, but use the private sector for primary care, paying out of their own pockets. Despite this burden, Government spending on healthcare comprises less than half of total health expenditure. In 2013, the remaining 16 % of the population (8.64 million people) paid for private health insurance cover (often with a monthly contribution from their employers), from 87 Registered Medical Insurance companies or Medical Schemes (down from 93 schemes in 2012, as schemes are battling to maintain the legislated monetary reserves and amalgamate or fold). The private sector generally supplies excellent care, but faces constant media and opportunistic political accusations of profiteering off the health burden of South Africa.

Healthcare disparities are worsened by the fact that around 70 % of all doctors and most specialists only work in the private sector; the remaining 30 % serve the public sector [2, 3].

A health intelligence report [4] on the future of healthcare in Africa [4], considers South Africa "by many health measures," as "the most advanced of the Sub-Saharan nations," with the biggest and most well developed, high-quality, private health insurance sector, and the largest and best-trained health workforce in Africa. It is also formulating a universal national health insurance (NHI) system, one of the first and most ambitious on the continent, in attempt to bring healthcare equality to all. However, the same report indicates that South Africa also experiences many healthcare problems facing other African countries, including high rates of maternal, infant and child mortality, chronic conditions including diabetes, hypertension and obesity, injuries and violence, and communicable diseases like HIV and tuberculosis. Additionally, many health services underperform on service delivery, with a background of poor management, deteriorating infrastructure, and underfunding. This has increased healthcare inequality. The private-sector health insurance system is seen as both an asset and a potential obstacle to implementing an NHI system [4]. Based on many patient reports, treatment of patients with diabetes

L.A. Distiller (✉) • M.A.J. Brown
Centre for Diabetes and Endocrinology (Pty) Ltd, Johannesburg, South Africa
e-mail: LarryD@CDEDiabetes.co.za; MichaelB@CDEDiabetes.co.za

D. Simmons et al. (eds.), *Integrated Diabetes Care*, DOI 10.1007/978-3-319-13389-8_6

in the public health sector is also under-resourced and underfunded. Some Academic Hospital diabetes clinics endeavour to provide full care, but overall, these clinics are understaffed and overextended by large patient numbers. While they do offer comprehensive diabetes education, and eye and foot screening, circumstances limit their reach and fragment their care. For example, patients verbalize that they often choose not to lose their place in 6–8 h pharmacy queues, thereby missing potentially useful consultations with dieticians and other diabetes team members.

Part II: The Growing Burden of Diabetes

Diabetes imposes a massive economic burden on all healthcare systems, accounting for 11 % of total global healthcare expenditure on adults in 2013. In the next 20 years, the "developing world" is expected to be affected most by the diabetes pandemic, with 77 % of people with diabetes living in low- and middle-income countries. Africa is, and will be, particularly hard-hit with 76 % of deaths due to diabetes occurring in people under 60 years of age, the highest continental proportion of people with diabetes being undiagnosed (62.5 %) and the largest predicted continental increase in prevalence (109.1 % by 2035) [5].

With the spreading diabetes pandemic and the advent of newer, more expensive drugs to treat the condition, it can be anticipated that costs of diabetes care over the coming decades will increase incrementally. While the exact prevalence of diabetes in South Africa is unknown, the 2014 International Diabetes Federation (IDF) estimated prevalence of diabetes for South Africa was 8.39 % [6], which suggests a possible total of up to 4,530,000 patients with diabetes, 737,000 in the private healthcare sector, and a further 3,800,000 in the public sector.

Worldwide funders, whether they are governments, National Health Services, or private Health Insurance companies, are desperately looking for a way to reduce costs without reducing quality of care. A number of commonly used interventions have proved to be cost-effective [7]. These include:

- the use of angiotensin-converting-enzyme inhibitors (ACE inhibitors (ACE-I)) for intensive blood pressure control
- ACE-I or angiotensin receptor blockers (ARB) for renal disease
- comprehensive foot care
- intensive risk-factor control
- intensive insulin therapy for type 1 diabetes
- life-style modification and
- screening for and early treatment of retinopathy.

While these are all important components of long-term care, the economic consequences of such treatment protocols can be overwhelming for any healthcare funder. Consequently, many funders, be they Private or Government, resort to developing Managed Care Programmes to contain costs while trying to provide quality, affordable care to their patients.

Part III: Managed Care Programmes in South Africa

Regulation 8 of the Medical Schemes Act of 1998 [8] requires South African Medical Schemes to pay in full for the costs of diagnosis, treatment and care of 270 medical conditions and 25 common chronic conditions, including diabetes mellitus. These "Prescribed Minimum Benefits" (PMB) are a set of defined benefits to ensure that all medical scheme members have access to certain minimum health services, regardless of the option they have chosen. "Treatment protocols" which provide guidelines for appropriate treatment for each of the chronic PMB conditions have been published in the Government Gazette.

To contain the costs of providing such cover, while ensuring good quality treatment, certain measures have been taken to ensure that schemes can cover those members who need it, without putting the scheme at financial risk. Accordingly schemes are entitled to contract with "designated service providers" (specified groups of hospitals, clinics, doctors, retail pharmacies, etc.) to provide treatment for PMB conditions. However, this fact must be stated in the scheme rules and patients must be informed about where and how they can get medication and treatment from that provider. Patients who do not abide by the rules about which providers to use, may face having to pay all or part of the costs of their treatment themselves.

Often, designated service providers institute managed care programmes to standardize and control care rendered in a safe and cost-effective manner. However, many of these programmes concentrate on *cost-savings* rather than *patient service utilization* and *improved clinical outcomes*. These programmes fall into several categories:

- Programmes driven by *drug formularies*, which may exclude or restrict some more expensive and newer pharmaceutical agents. In many instances, this also extends to restricting (in patients with type 1 diabetes) or disallowing entirely (in type 2 patients) testing strips for home glucose monitoring. However, overall, the costs of medication, including insulin, accounts for just 7 % of all healthcare costs related to diabetes [9].
- Programmes that *restrict the frequency of patient visits* to doctors and that *restrict access to specialist care*. The number of visits to other healthcare providers such as dietitians, podiatrists and ophthalmologists are also limited as a "cost-cutting" exercise. Not surprisingly, these funders do not even acknowledge the need for, or the role of, the Diabetes Nurse Educator and do not fund education sessions. This passes PMB muster because the "Treatment Protocols" [10, 11] focus on attainment of glycaemic targets, using mainly an algorithmic pharmacological approach, and Council for Medical Scheme PMB guidance [12] only specifies:
  - "Consultations with your treating provider (GP or specialist – if authorized by your scheme)
  - Lifestyle modification interventions such as dietary and disease education."

  The type of provider is unspecified and thus the essential role of the Diabetes Nurse Educator in diabetes care [13] is ignored.
- Programmes that *restrict the number of laboratory investigations* that can be performed annually. A typical limit of services in seen in Fig. 6.1, as per a form sent to patients who are on this particular funders "Management Programme."
- Programmes that make use of *telephonic case manager contact* from time to time to "check how patients are doing."

While these approaches may save some costs in the short-term, Managed Care Programmes which do not address patient outcomes nor reduce long term complications, ignore the fact that that the majority of the costs for treating diabetes, even in the medium term, are due to the treatment of acute and chronic complications and for inpatient hospital care [14]. Additionally, it is well established that poor long-term clinical outcomes increase the cost burden of managing the patient with diabetes by up to 250 %. Outpatient care provided in clinics or doctor's offices, accounts for less than one-quarter of the costs of accruing to a cohort of patients with diabetes [15]. Despite this, a recent study of 11 different funders in South Africa [16] showed that utilization of necessary outpatient services to monitor diabetes control and screen for potential complications is grossly inadequate. On average, only 48.37 % of patients have an HbA1c measured annually, 35.08 % have their lipids monitored, 31.55 % are tested for microalbuminuria, 20.79 % see an ophthalmologist annually and 2.39 % see a podiatrist (Fig. 6.2).

Clearly, if the economic costs of diabetes are to be contained, any approach needs to incorporate a managed care initiative that will promote

Tariff Code	Description	Number of Services
000192	GP - Consultation/Visit: long duration	2
000192	Specialist Consultation/Visit: long duration (Physician)	1
000192	Specialist Consultation/Visit: long duration (Ophthalmologist)	1
001232	ECG Without Effort	1
003003	Fundus contact lens or 90D lens examination	1
003009	Basic capital equipment used in Specialist rooms	1
003014	Test:Tonometry	1
004025	Blood Test: Cholesterol HDL/LDL/Trig	1
004032	Blood Test: Creatinine level	1
004050	Blood Test: Glocose Strip Test	2
004064	Blood Test: Haemoglobin A1C measurement	2
004113	Blood Test: Potassium level	1
004114	Blood Test: Sodium level	1
004151	Blood Test: Urea level	1
004188	Urine Test: Dipstick	2
068302	Podiatrist Consultation 11 - 20 minutes	1
084205	Dietician Consultation	1

Fig. 6.1 A typical diabetes managed care programme as promoted by a medical funder

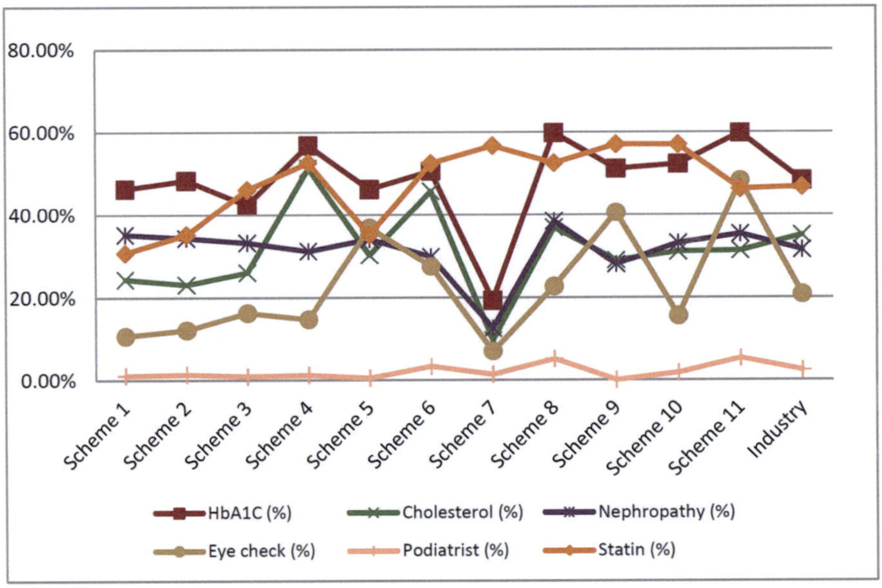

Fig. 6.2 Patient utilization of services across 11 medical aid schemes (funders) in South Africa (Used with permission from HQA [16])

better care and control of diabetes and other co-morbidities, reduce both acute and all-cause hospitalization rates, and be proactive in promoting patient health rather than reactively treating complications and problems as they arise. Most importantly, none of this will be implementable unless the system of care is designed around the *patient's perspective* of their diabetes and the needed care, the so-called "*integrated care*" of diabetes [17].

Part IV: The CDE "Diabetes Management Programme" (DMP): Past to Present

With the intensive care results and the other care insights provided by the Diabetes Control and Complications Trial (DCCT) [18], fresh in our minds, the "Centre for Diabetes and Endocrinology" was initially established as a single "Centre of Excellence" in 1994. It was staffed by two endocrinologists, two nurse educators, a registered dietician, a podiatrist, a clinical psychologist, a pharmacist and a biokineticist and effectively provided a "one-stop shop" for our patients. With all services in one place, and a well-managed appointment system, patients experienced minimal waiting and optimal consultation times. They could continue with their lives with minimal disruption. This was in stark contrast to the prevailing situation – diabetes care resources available to South Africans were generally grossly inadequate. Additionally, medical aid schemes did not appropriately fund private sector diabetes care and the resultant outcomes were generally suboptimal. We had a vision to create an all-encompassing and comprehensive diabetes treatment and management Centre, which allowed us to implement correct and appropriate diabetes care principles. However, within a very short time after opening our Centre, we faced bankruptcy as the salaries of the allied health professionals and the costs our ancillary services could only be funded from the consultation fees of the two founding medical practitioners.

We had to make a plan to survive. With our current crisis being the muse of innovation, we approached a medical aid scheme with our care offering and a simple but compelling financial equation. We knew that we could manage the monthly treatment costs of a person with diabetes for "X." We also knew that with the current hospital-centric diabetes management approaches of the time, the medical funders were paying a higher figure "Z." Could we not agree to meet somewhere in-between at a mutually agreed monthly, per patient capitation fee, "Y'? With a contractually bound promise of community-based, holistic care that prevented unnecessary hospitalization (with the Centre being responsible for the costs thereof if we failed to prevent this), our diabetes care team would receive fair professional remuneration for proactive diabetes management. The medical aid scheme would receive state-of-the art care (and improved outcomes) for their members with diabetes *and* the ability to budget for their reduced diabetes risk. This was groundbreaking thinking at that time; the concept of managed healthcare and the idea of ring-fencing, capitating and managing a condition like diabetes was alien in South Africa. In 1995, in a great leap of faith, and possibly with a glimpse into the future, this medical aid scheme contracted the services of the CDE. In the first month of operations, the CDE had 13 patients under management.

We recognized that to provide good diabetes care across South Africa, more than one "Centre of Excellence" would be required. This was also needed to meet the expectations of our first funder, which had members across South Africa. As a result, we established a founding preferred provider network of 14 CDE Centres within months. At the helm at each of these initial "Centres of Excellence," was either an Endocrinologist or a specialist Diabetologist.

Over the past 20 years, the Centre for Diabetes and Endocrinology has expanded from these 14 Centres, to a national network offering the services of 31 Endocrinologists/Diabetologists, 48 Specialist Physicians (Internists), 165 "Centres of Excellence" run by trained and dedicated General Practitioners and Family Physicians, and 610 contracted primary care doctors (Fig. 6.3). This network effectively offers primary, secondary and tertiary levels of expertise and care nationally in the private sector.

In tandem with the growth of the CDE Provider Network, the number of patients under our management has risen steadily – At the end of May 2015, our national network of 220 Centres (some Centres have more than one CDE-accredited doctor) were responsible for the care of 20,569 patients. Two thousand eight hundred ninety one (14.1 %) had type 1 diabetes and 17,678 (85.9 %), type 2 diabetes. Of the people with type 2 diabetes, 50.4 % (8903) were on oral

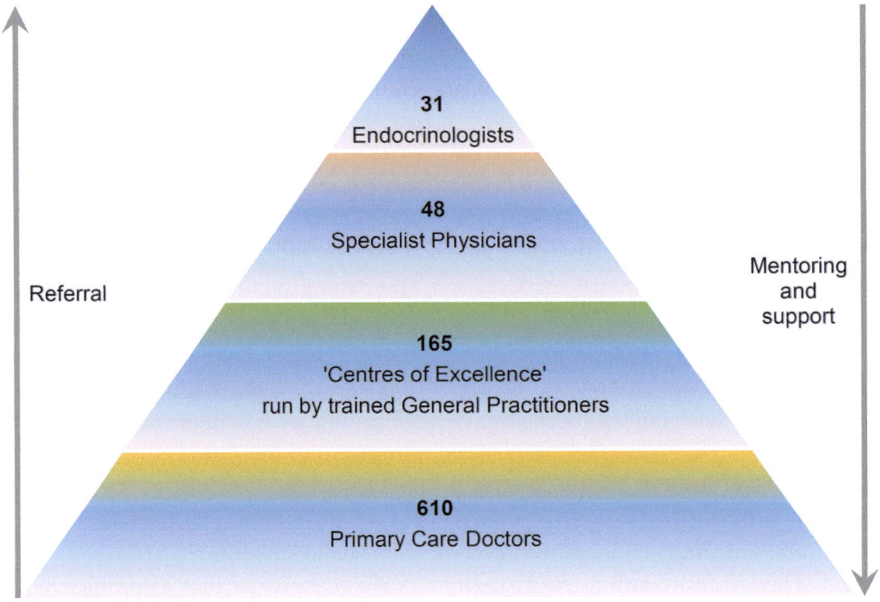

Fig. 6.3 The CDE network pyramid

glucose-lowering agents alone and 49.6 % (8775) required insulin therapy, with or without the addition of oral agents.

Persons with diabetes covered by the medical schemes and contracted to receive care via the CDE DMP encompass all of the multiple ethnic groups found in South Africa and much of the socioeconomic spectrum from blue-collar workers to company directors. We are keen to expand our best practice care to all South Africans with diabetes.

In response to the needs of funders who cannot afford the CDE traditional "Comprehensive Care Plan," from 2015 the CDE has introduced a "Standard Care Plan," which has a capitation fee more palatable to funders with tight financial margins, albeit with reduced "benefits." Within this new model, payment responsibility for medicines and some services falls away from the ambit of the capitation fee. Our Centres are, however, expected to refer to the core members of the diabetes team as usual, and maintain the highest possible standard of care, even though they will not be paying for all aspects directly. With this approach, we hope to enable access to improved diabetes care to many people for whom this was previously not possible. The clinical outcomes of this approach have yet to be ascertained. In this chapter, we discuss the CDE "Comprehensive Care Plan."

Part V: Structure and Principles of the CDE DMP and Diabetes Care Network

The contracted servicing doctor (Centre) receives a set monthly capitation fee, in advance, for caring for patients contracted to receive their diabetes care from that Centre. A two-tier fee structure exists, with a lower fee being paid for patients on oral glucose-lowering agents alone and a higher fee for those requiring insulin, irrespective of whether the insulin-requiring patient has type 1 or type 2 diabetes. The fee is negotiated annually based on the anticipated costs of providing all guaranteed services, plus a fair margin for the Centre taking the risk for those patients who require more intensive management, the cost of acute diabetes related hospital admissions, inflation and the choice of more expensive treatment modalities for selected patients. Centres are paid according to the number of patients they have contracted to service. Funds must be utilized to provide all services, including clinical care, supply of all diabetes medication and accessories (including meters and testing materials for self-monitoring of blood glucose), and specified laboratory investigations (The annual measurement of lipids, renal function, and microalbuminuria is part of the guaranteed services, and careful monitoring of blood pressure is expected at every visit). Should it be found necessary, the Medical Scheme funds treatment for co-morbid conditions outside of the monthly capitation fee. We guarantee all medical schemes that contract the CDE Network an absolute minimum level of servicing for their patients as stated in the CDE "Minimum Care Guidelines" (Table 6.1). However, subjects often receive additional services in excess of these Guidelines, depending on their individual clinical circumstances.

Each Centre of Excellence is required to have on staff, in addition to the responsible doctor, a trained Diabetes Nurse Educator (DNE) to act as the primary team contact for their DMP members and to facilitate the process of patient empowerment and self-management. Each Centre must also contract with or employ both a dietitian and a podiatrist to provide the guaranteed services to the patients. For diabetes-related emergencies, every Centre must provide a direct 24-h emergency telephone number ("Hotline").

Via this novel diabetes-care model, CDE Centres are empowered to decide on medication for the optimal treatment of their patients with diabetes – no formulary restrictions are imposed. Since each Centre must pay for the medication and insulin from the set capitation fee, the treating doctor is responsible for deciding which treatment regimen is the most cost- and quality-effective for each patient. Thus, the onus falls on the individual Centre to absorb the costs of prescribing more expensive treatment modalities should they be deemed clinically advantageous. Our Centres are generally happy to do this, because they are clearly taught that the CDE DMP has an in-built level of cross subsidization (like medical aid schemes) where any available funds remaining from patients on less-expensive regimens "cover" the "deficit" accrued by patients on more expensive regimens.

Table 6.1 "Minimum Care Guidelines" as contractually agreed to between CDE diabetes centres and contracted funders

Service	Minimum frequency
Consultations:	
Doctor	2×annually
Nurse educator	2×annually
Dietitian (nutritional guidance)	1×annually
Podiatrist (foot care)	1×annually (screening)
Ophthalmologist (eye care)	1×annually (screening)
Exercise physiologist (Biokineticist)	If required
Clinical psychologist	If required
Laboratory tests to monitor diabetes:	
HbA1c	6-monthly
Lipogram	1×annually
Renal function, microalbuminuria	1×annually
24/7/365 "Hotline" for emergencies and advice	
All diabetes medications and monitoring equipment	
Insulin's and tablets	As prescribed
Blood glucose metres and test strips	As prescribed
Glucagon hypo kit	All patients on insulin therapy – replaced on use⁄expiry
Ketone test strips	All patients with type 1 diabetes – replaced on use⁄expiry
Insulin pens/syringes, needles, lancets	As prescribed
Risk assumption for hospitalization costs for acute diabetes emergencies	

Furthermore, each contracted Centre is directly responsible for all additional costs incurred should a person with diabetes under that Centre's care be admitted to hospital for a "diabetes emergency" (defined as a primary admission diagnosis of hypoglycaemia, hyperglycaemia, hyperosmolar non-ketotic coma (HONK) or diabetic ketoacidosis (DKA)). This is based on the experience that admissions for such acute metabolic events are largely avoidable in patients who have received adequate diabetes education and who are sufficiently self-empowered and have the opportunity to call their Centre via the contractually mandated 24-h emergency Hotline should they develop any acute problems. Again, our Centres are happy to assume this risk (once they have a financially viable minimum of 20 capitated patients under their care), because the contracted doctors soon learn that with good care, they have the power to avoid these events. This voluntary risk assumption for the costs of hospitalization is a powerful guarantee to our funding partners that the CDE and its Provider Network will do the job they have contracted to do. The DMP, however, does not cover the treatment cost of any chronic complication or the treatment of other co-morbidities or risk factors, and the hospital admission costs for diabetes complications or non-diabetes-related illness. Our contracts with Funders clearly state these exclusions, as the funding risk for these events would exceed the capacity of the DMP budget, which is clearly based on the *daily management costs of diabetes.*

Part VI: The CDE DMP: Outcomes

Note: Since people tend to change medical schemes from time to time, with membership of the DMP depending on whether their current medical scheme was contracted to the DMP or not, long term follow-up for all patients is not always possible.

Glycaemic Control

A sustained reduction in HbA1c of approximately 1.5 % in subjects with both type 1 and type 2 diabetes has been achieved (Fig. 6.4) [19].

Although the HbA1c assays were not standardized across the country, each patient had his or her HbA1c performed at the same laboratory longitudinally, so that the starting HbA1c for each patient effectively acted as its own control. Reasons for the sustained improvement might relate to the high compliance rate ensured by the CDE Programme as well as responsiveness to person-centred advice on lifestyle modification needed and an aggressive "treat-to-target" approach taught to and adopted by the CDE Centres. While a mean HbA1c for type 1 patients of 7.7 % (±1.2 % SD, Median 7.6 %) after 5 years is not at the recommended target of 7 %, it approaches the 7.6 % suggested by the VISS (Vascular diabetic complications In Southeast Sweden) study to be the cut-off for the prevention of proliferative retinopathy and macroalbuminuria [20]. It is significantly better than the mean HbA1c seen at many diabetes clinics, which may be in excess of 8 % [21, 22]. The mean HbA1c of 7.4 % (±1.36 % SD, median 7.1 %) achieved in our type 2 patients, is considerably better than that seen in many surveys in people with type 2 diabetes including the United Kingdom Prospective Diabetes Study (UKPDS) 10-year follow-up data (mean HbA1c of both the intensive and the conventional therapy groups evened out at about 8 %) [23].

Hospital Admissions

Hospital admission remains the top healthcare cost in the private healthcare sector in South Africa, accounting for 39.1 % of the total paid out by Medical Schemes in the 2013 financial year [3]. Specifically for diabetes, the all cause hospital admission rate for patients with diabetes is threefold higher than that seen in the nondiabetic population [24]. Additionally, a study of the Economic Costs of Diabetes in the U.S. in 2012 [25] showed that for people with diabetes, hospital inpatient care accounted for 43 % of the total medical cost of diabetes. Therefore, any programme that can result in even a slight reduction in the number of acute diabetes-related admissions has the potential of substantial cost savings in any healthcare system.

In this context, we have seen a significant overall reduction in all acute diabetes-related hospital admissions for patients on the CDE DMP. Our previously reported hospital admission rates [19] for patients requiring admission for acute metabolic decompensation (where the entire hospital bill was paid by their treating CDE doctor) were 6 admissions per 1000 patient-years for type 1 and 1 admission per 1000 patient-years for type 2 subjects. This was achieved with no patient mortality resulting from acute metabolic

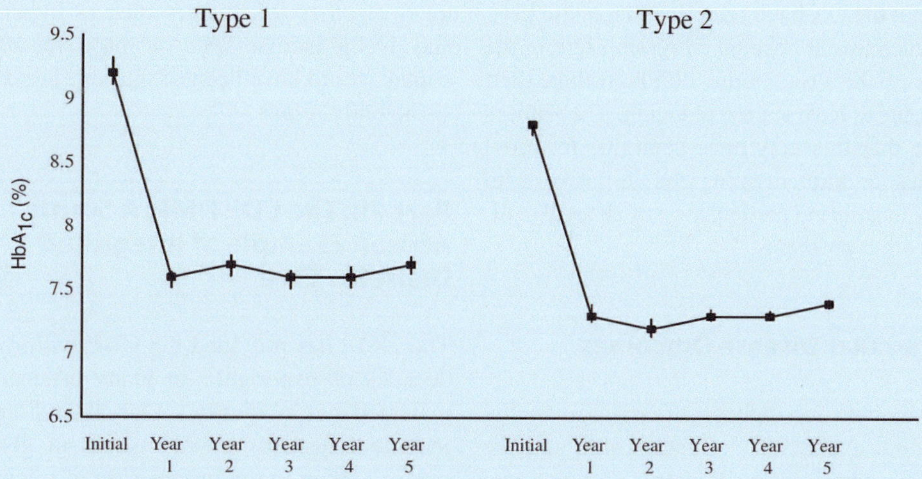

		Initial	1 year	2 years	3 years	4 years	5 years
Type 1	Mean ±SD (%)	9.2±2.1	7.6±1.8	7.7±1.8	7.6±1.3	7.6±1.3	7.7±1.2
	Median (%)	8.9	7.4	7.5	7.4	7.5	7.5
	95% confidence limits	9.11-9.32	7.52-7.64	7.61-7.77	7.51-7.65	7.52-7.68	7.63-7.76
Type 2	Mean ±SD	8.8±1.95	7.3±1.55	7.2±1.62	7.3±1.42	7.3±1.41	7.4±1.36
	Median	8.6	7.1	7.0	7.0	7.2	7.1
	95% confidence limits	8.72-8.81	7.26-7.39	7.14-7.28	7.27-7.35	7.28-7.34	7.37-7.43

Fig. 6.4 Five-year follow-up of 2726 type 1 and 14,317 type 2 patients with diabetes who were part of the CDE Diabetes Management Programme for more than 5 years (Used with permission from Distiller et al. [19])

causes (hypoglycaemia, hyperglycaemia or DKA). We have had no admissions for the crisis of HONK in over 10 years, a condition that is still prevalent in many academic hospital settings [26]. Hospital admission rates for these conditions in this group of patients prior to joining the DMP were not obtainable, nor are there any published figures for hospital admissions for acute diabetes-related causes available in South Africa. The CDE DMP cohort also showed a 40 % overall reduction in hospital admission rates and a 20 % reduction in length of hospital stay for hospital admission diagnoses related directly or indirectly to the diabetes (acute or chronic complications). All-cause hospital admission rates were reduced from 210 admissions per 1000 patient-years for the first year on the DMP to <100 admissions per 1000 patient years in subsequent years. This reduction was sustained for the full 5 years of the study [19].

Since mortality rates were not taken into account, it could be argued that those patients with major illness or extensive arterial disease when joining the DMP could have died subsequently, leaving those in better health and with less reason for hospital admission on the Programme over subsequent years. However, the phenomenon of managed, better-controlled persons with diabetes requiring hospital admission less often than unmanaged and uncontrolled subjects is well-described. One managed care approach in Pennsylvania (USA) [27] was associated with a major reduction in the total number of admissions per patient per year, down from 0.16 to 0.12 over a 2-year period. They also documented less inpatient days and fewer emergency room visits. Another integrated diabetes disease management programme across five States in the USA also reported a 22 % reduction in hospital admission rates [28] and several other studies have confirmed this [29, 30]. Attempts at an Integrated Care Initiative in the UK have been less successful [31], with an increase in hospital admission rate in the first year of the Programme, although thereafter, costs appear to have started reducing. The authors speculate that this may have been due to initial difficulties in implementing the initiative with difficulty in assuring participation of all local staff, amongst other problems.

Microvascular Disease Outcomes

Prevalence data for diabetic microvascular disease are not available for South Africa and are difficult to source internationally. The National Health and Nutrition Examination Survey (NHANES) 1999–2004 survey reported chronic kidney disease to be present in 27.8 % and eye disease in 18.9 % of people with diabetes in the USA [32]. Microalbuminuria was present in 20–40 % of patients with diabetes [33]. The Wisconsin Epidemiologic Study of Diabetic Retinopathy (WESDR) reported some retinopathy in nearly all persons who had had type 1 diabetes for 20 years [34] and in nearly 80 % of those who had had type 2 diabetes for the same duration [35]. Up to 21 % of newly diagnosed type 2 patients have some degree of retinopathy at time of diagnosis [36]. A series of patients who were assessed for retinopathy at the time of joining the CDE DMP, showed a prevalence of 35.2 % for the type 1 patients (background retinopathy 26 % and referable retinopathy 9.2 %) and 20.5 % in the type 2 diabetes (14.1 % background retinopathy and 6.4 % referable retinopathy) [37]. This was in line with the internationally reported figures. In individuals who were on the CDE DMP for over 5 years, the prevalence of retinopathy was 28 % for the type 1 patients and 26.6 % for the type 2 patients [19]. The incidence of nephropathy (15.8 % in patients with type 1 and 22.6 % in patients with type 2 diabetes) was clearly lower than might have been expected for a mean duration of diabetes of 15.2 years in the type 1 group and 9.3 years for the type 2 subjects. This is probably attributable to the improved levels of glycaemic control, but also to better overall patient care and attention to and aggressive treatment of other risk factors such as hypertension and dyslipidaemia. Data on macrovascular outcomes would have been of interest, but were not sufficiently robust.

Part VII: The CDE DMP: A South African Example of Integrated Diabetes Care

The DMP has provided the CDE with over two decades of experience in many aspects of the managed care of diabetes. Our clinical outcomes include long-term improvements in glycaemic control, delay in the progression of microvascular complications and reductions in hospital admissions for both acute metabolic emergencies and all other causes.

The cost savings and resulting improvements in quality of life for the patients served are self-evident. Although no formal quality of life assessments have been performed, we have, however, been recognized for excellence in managed healthcare, by being awarded eight PMR.africa Managed Healthcare Awards since 2002 (the majority being "Diamond Arrow" Awards (ranked 1st overall and rated at least 4, 10 out of 5, 00 – equivalent to outstanding). The PMR.africa Awards are designed to recognize and enhance excellence in a range of industries and to set a benchmark in each sector. These externally and independently adjudicated awards are the culmination of a research process by PMR.africa, whereby companies and institutions are rated based on respondents' perceptions with a strong focus on evaluating and measuring customer service and customer satisfaction. Importantly, a company, department, institution and individual cannot "enter" the research process, but must always be nominated and rated by the respondents. In the case of managed care companies, excellence is rated by input from a random, national sample of 100 respondents (Chairmen and Principal Officers of listed/large companies as well as Fund Managers, Trustees, Medical Advisors/Directors and Assessors representing Medical Aid Schemes and Administrators).

Table 6.2 Differences between the CDE diabetes management programme and "usual" disease management programmes for diabetes

"Usual" programmes	CDE Diabetes Management Programme
Maximum visits per year laid down	Minimum visits guaranteed. Maximum unlimited
Drug formularies	Drugs used depends only on doctor's judgement
Success measured by cost savings	Success measured by outcomes, not cost-savings
Clinical outcomes largely ignored	Clinical outcomes are key performance indicators to justify DMP existence
No transfer of risk	Risk of acute hospital admission costs transferred to provider
Task orientated	Person-centred

Important inherent differences exist between the CDE DMP and more conventional Managed Care programmes for diabetes (Table 6.2). However, we believe that our focus on and attention to the provision of integrated diabetes care, since our inception, has been one of the main reasons for our many successes.

A Definition of Integrated Diabetes Care

Diabetes UK (2014) [17] offers the following definition: "Integrated care is about designing a system that focuses on the *patient's perspective of care*. The delivery of integrated care is facilitated by integration of the processes, methods and tools, which enable patients to move between services according to need. Integrated diabetes care means vertical integration between primary, community and specialist care. This is distinct from the wider agenda of horizontally integrated health and social care."

Important Patient/Provider Principles of Integrated Diabetes Care

This definition tells us that the delivery of diabetes services must be designed around the *patient's perspective of care* and the needs that accrue as a result. Diabetes mellitus is a complex, chronic, physical/psychosocial/spiritual condition that affects every part of the human experience. This gives rise to a number of challenges that we have experienced over the years, which make the understanding of the patient perspective even more important [38, 39] Healthcare professionals (and people with diabetes) often need experience and specialized training and knowledge to achieve this mutual understanding. The resultant care principles from these insights are role-modelled in all that we do and are included in all our healthcare-provider training courses. Once we understand these challenges and care principles, insight into the patient perspective and process of care becomes easier for all involved:

- *Chronicity*: People with diabetes battle to accept the life-long nature of their condition – in the mind of the patient, the traditional expectation of "cure" is insufficiently replaced by the concept of a lifetime of "control" of lifestyle, blood glucose, blood pressure, serum cholesterol and body weight. Chronicity is not only a major task for the patient to deal with, but also for the *caregiver* who needs to assume a *new professional identity as a chronic care specialist*. "Treatment" of a chronic condition with a physical domain bias using an "acute-care" approach will inevitably lead to imbalance, "non-compliance" and failure to control. This can be a large spiritual, psychosocial and financial burden.
- *Change*: Diabetes is a life-changing condition. One cannot hope to facilitate the process of change (a major developmental task in diabetes) and adjust to a condition that must be mainly self-managed and that requires life-long care and control, if one cannot identify with and manage this process oneself. This applies equally to patients and their caregivers. Change, however, is not an on-off switch, but often a long and stop-start-relapse process requiring a high degree of reflection, self-awareness, and the testing of the validity of our own attitudes, values and beliefs about something (in this case diabetes). It is these

"internal" drives that determine our eventual behaviour and what our patients/clients experience as a result.

- *One size does not fit all*: One practitioner does not have the necessary knowledge and skills to treat all the different effects of diabetes. Team-facilitated management was shown in the Diabetes Control and Complications Trial (DCCT) to be a vital element in the control of type 1 diabetes by "Intensive Therapy" [40]. In addition to the doctor, input from the diabetes educator, dietitian, podiatrist, ophthalmologist, pharmacist, biokineticist and psychologist (amongst others), is necessary at different times to maximize insight, care and quality of life. The critical role of the diabetes nurse educator is reinforced by the CDE experience over the years that every CDE Centre that has won one of our eight Annual Clinical Excellence Awards, designed to recognize outstanding patient care in various categories, has had as its coordinator, an outstanding diabetes nurse educator.
- *Self-care* is vital and is a major challenge for Health Professionals to facilitate when they and their patients are used to conventional (acute) care approaches. The focus is on the *prevention of ill health* and *not* its treatment.
- *Continuity*: Care must be organized around a person who has a life full of events, both good and bad. The aim is to build up a coherent picture of their needs and their health status over time. Ideally, the same caregivers should facilitate this care at each visit to engender trust and to improve the continuity of thought, process and action.
- *Congruence in care*: everyone in the Health Team should not only be giving the same information, but should also have the same insightful approach (based on a set of commonly shared and communicated values attitudes and beliefs) towards diabetes management. The person with diabetes will be reassured by the agreement and harmony they see and be more confident (a feeling of "self-efficacy") to practise what they have been taught.
- *Concordance* (or agreement within the Team, including the patient): A person with diabetes has to balance the demands of life, diabetes and diabetes management with the emotional, spiritual, structural, financial, and social resources available to them. Everybody must understand and accept the degree of tension that is being experienced and of the ability of the person with diabetes to cope with it. This will help to ensure an open, trusting care process and achieve maximum adherence to therapy.
- *Communication*: Good communication is a prerequisite to concordance – patient and diabetes team must be open and truthful at all times and most importantly must *listen* to each other.
- *Conceptions* of diabetes: previous experiences of diabetes treatment successes and failures result in a set of values, attitudes and beliefs, which guide future feelings and behaviours towards diabetes. We must assess these and factor them into any treatment plan.

Important Structural Principles of Integrated Diabetes Care

For the person with diabetes to self-manage their condition, they need the support of a diabetes team that provides care responsive to their needs from diagnosis to the management of chronic complications of diabetes. Diabetes UK lists the following five "key enablers of integration" [17]:

1. Integrated Information Technology Systems
2. Aligned finances and responsibility
3. Care planning
4. Clinical engagement and leadership
5. Robust clinical governance

How Does the CDE DMP Approach Measure Up?

1. *Integrated Information Technology Systems*: All Centres on the CDE Network are obliged to use a customized internet-based clinical management programme to enter all patient contacts, findings, diagnosed complications, key clinical outcomes, medications dispensed

and laboratory results. Several of the Private Pathology Laboratories in South Africa, serving up to half the DMP patients, are able to upload the relevant results directly into the CDE system, but Centres that elect to use other certified laboratories need to enter their results manually. Patient confidentiality is assured by a multilevel, role-dependent password system. The Central Administrative Office has real-time access to all data. This facility is utilized to download, collate and check patient and Centre compliance with the "Minimum Care Guidelines" outcomes including HbA1c trends and complication rates and to present this outcomes data to funding organizations. This ensures that all accredited providers providing care are able to access and add to a patient's data, obviating the need for file transfers. We can identify "at risk" and defaulting patients using data thresholds and follow them up.

2. *Aligned finances and responsibility*: The unique structure of the CDE doctor network allows for appropriate patient referrals to specialists as required and a patient specific specialist clinical advisory service. The CDE specialists make themselves available for telephonic/e-mail advice and face-to-face referral consultations, at no charge, for patients registered on the CDE Managed Care Programme. Because of this, complicated patients, and their attending doctors, have easy access to higher levels of expertise within the same network.

   In addition, the new CDE Managed Care Programme Model makes provision for an annual clinical review of every single patient, by a CDE specialist. For this review, the CDE specialist accesses the electronic health record of patient, and provides clinical and therapeutic advice, to the CDE treating doctor. This approach ensures optimization of every patient's therapy and care strategy in a highly cost-effective manner.

3. *Care planning*: Diabetes UK (2014) [17] defines care planning as a "continuous process, in which clinicians and patients work together to agree goals, identify support needs, develop and implement action plans and monitor progress. People with diabetes should have active involvement in the care planning process of deciding, agreeing and owning how their diabetes will be managed."

   Many of the problems surrounding the provision of adequate person-centred care for those with diabetes revolve around the pressures of clinical practice and a lack of time. Good diabetes management requires attention to a number of clinical parameters

   1. (Near) Normalization of blood glucose
   2. Control of co-morbidities and risk factors
   3. Attainment of normal growth and development
   4. Prevention of Acute Complications
   5. Screening for Chronic Complications

   To fit all this *and* a holistic, patient-centred collaborative approach into a busy general practice, the servicing doctor and other team members must understand that diabetes cannot be "dealt with" coincidently during a patient consultation for an acute condition. It requires a specific individual consultation of at least half-an-hour. This can be achieved by the doctor setting aside a specific time for a "Diabetes Clinic," be it a morning a week, a day a week, or a day a month, depending on the number of patients with diabetes being serviced. Each patient should have a pre-booked half-hour appointment. Patients should regard this as the equivalent of taking themselves in for a "routine service" every 6 months. In a resource-poor environment, one can make use of group education sessions. A Registered Nurse (ideally a Diabetes Nurse Educator) performs the vital roles of team coordinator and patient advocate, mentor, counsellor, coach and self-management facilitator. In more "stretched" settings, the DNE can also assist with measuring blood pressure, weight and abdominal circumference of the patients, ordering the relevant laboratory investigations, and providing basic foot screening. The DNE can also download and check home blood glucose monitoring records. With the average number of patients at any one CDE Centre seldom exceeding 200,

CDE healthcare providers have the time to provide individualized care to patients and the patients feel recognized as individuals.

CDE patients are also encouraged to regard their Diabetes Centre as a place where they are welcome and can present for advice or discussion with their nurse educator at short notice. Patients are always asked to present their "agenda" at every consultation so that their perspective is always respected and recognized. This practical application of the "Medical Home" concept [41–43] and the central role of the patient in the diabetes team have been an integral part of the CDE philosophy since our inception.

4. *Clinical engagement and leadership*: We founded the CDE on a robust background of healthcare provider training and clinical and academic support, which has developed continuously over the past two decades. Our Central Office Team in Johannesburg is passionate about teaching diabetes care to anyone interested and we are active in exchanging diabetes knowledge with colleagues across the world. The following mechanisms are in place to attract and retain the best-skilled and most passionate people in diabetes to our Network:
   - General practitioners who are not accredited endocrinologists, and all DNEs who wish to join the CDE Network, are obliged to attend a comprehensive and person-centred "5-Day Advanced Course in Diabetes Care for Health Professionals." We present this Course, covering all aspects of practical diabetes management, several times yearly. All practitioners interested in diabetes are welcome to attend. During the 5 days of the Course, the Faculty has opportunity to identify those attendees who show exceptional passion for and insight into diabetes. These practitioners are encouraged to take their skill and interest further, as part of the CDE network or not. Many of these practitioners choose to approach the CDE to accredit as a CDE Provider. This may be one of the reasons why practitioners in our Network are of a high standard. In the past two decades, we have trained over 6000 healthcare professionals from all over the world in the principles of best-practice diabetes care.
   - As an annual follow-up to the CDE 5-Day Course, the CDE also hosts an annual national "Postgraduate Forum in Diabetes Management" which all members of the CDE Network are obliged to attend. All other interested healthcare professionals are also welcome to attend. This weekend event, in its 18th iteration for 2016, has a busy academic programme consisting of lectures, discussion groups and workshops on current and new concepts and modalities in diabetes management. A "CDE Faculty" of senior endocrinologists in the CDE Network presents and facilitates the Programme. No honorariums are offered or paid for this service and companies involved in the provision of diabetes-related pharmaceuticals and diagnostics (although welcome to participate in a concurrent trade exhibition and offer Company-branded pre-Forum satellite events) have no say or part in the development, content and presentation of any aspect of the Forum academic programme. This assures participants that the programme will provide an objective and unbiased review of the latest in diabetes care.
   - For any healthcare professional nationwide who has demonstrated a keen interest in furthering his or her diabetes knowledge and skill we facilitate subsidized (Sponsorship is sought by CDE Central Office for a portion of the fees) attendance of Masters level Postgraduate University Diplomas in Diabetes Care (University of Cardiff Diabetes Diploma/University of South Wales Diabetes Diploma). Both are online distance learning Courses with annual face-to-face introductory lectures at the CDE Central Office in Johannesburg and can be extended for an extra year to earn an MSc in Diabetes. This initiative has

provided a major boost to diabetes care competence in South Africa. The local regulatory environment has effectively halted the development of local diabetes courses (even though the expertise exists in South Africa), so the CDE sought out international methods of up skilling our local healthcare providers. A number of CDE Faculty members have "Recognized Teaching Status" with these Universities and are Tutors on the Courses.

- In addition, all members of the CDE Network receive complimentary copies of our quarterly in-house extract of current diabetes literature, produced by one of the senior endocrinologists in the Network, as well as our "Official Journal for Diabetes Healthcare Professionals," the South African Journal of Diabetes.
- Recently, the CDE has established an online Forum, which allows any CDE Centre, or team member to post questions and cases for comment and advice from the CDE Faculty.

The main motivation for improving outcomes amongst the CDE Centres appears to be a combination of concern to demonstrate good care and outcomes with the need to avoid hospital admission at the doctors' own expense. Overall, however, most of the Centres enjoy the opportunity to become involved in long-term chronic disease management and in being part of a successful nationwide network regarded as Centres of Excellence by the medical funders.

A key aspect of the CDE Programme is that the treating doctor and not the funder, is the "gate-keeper" and is wholly responsible for all related costs. This includes employing or paying for the services of a DNE, podiatrist and dietician. The clinical diabetes care given by the DMP is closely aligned to the International Diabetes Federation definition of a "standard" level of care [44]. Although the DMP concentrates on diabetes (glycaemic) control, other risk factors such as dyslipidaemia and hypertension are aggressively monitored and treated. Each patient is seen by the same named team of allied healthcare professionals and the same doctor. A key aspect of the CDE Network is that, while outcomes and standard of care are monitored, each trained doctor and Centre is free to treat their patients in any way they prefer, with their choice of any medication or insulin, as long as adequate outcomes and patient safety are assured. Generally, insulin therapy is started early and aggressively to attain and sustain glycaemic targets.

With these interventions, our accredited practitioners are generally highly empowered, motivated, insightful and knowledgeable individuals who really understand the demands of integrated, patient-centred care.

While Diabetes UK views engaging people with diabetes in a direct role in planning education and training needs as vital in this key enabler of integration, people with diabetes in South Africa are extraordinarily apathetic in getting involved in diabetes care at a political, governance or advocacy level. As a result, we have not made any progress here.

5. *Robust clinical governance*: Diabetes UK (2014) [17] defines clinical governance as "a system through which… organizations are accountable for continuously improving the quality of their services and safeguarding high standards of care by creating an environment in which excellence in clinical care will flourish."

The overriding philosophy of the DMP is to provide total patient care for persons with diabetes utilizing a trained team of healthcare professionals, including doctors specifically trained in diabetes management and encompassing a significant component of financial risk sharing.

We assure compliance across the CDE Network to our Minimum Care Guidelines and the principles of "Good Clinical Practice" in two ways. In addition to the internet-based clinical management programme previously discussed, the CDE employs a full-time medical practitioner who conducts ongoing peer review and audit of the participating Centres on the CDE Network. This both by monitoring the data entered onto the online database and by visiting the Centres regularly and unannounced to inspect patients' written records, laboratory results and reports from outside healthcare providers. Our Auditor visits each Centre on at least an annual basis. Any Centre team found to be underperforming by not fulfilling the CDE Minimum Care Guidelines or not following principles of Good Clinical Practice is counselled, coached on improvements required and then placed on probation for 3 months. On re-audit, if the Centre has not rectified the deficiencies, it is closed. Regular peer review and monitoring are part of our ethos. This has been an accreditation criterion for our Network since its inception.

No incentives are offered to CDE Centres for improvements in HbA1c, as this is an expected outcome.

We have relatively few difficulties in implementing our Programme requirements with our Providers. We achieve this by having committed buy-in from all stakeholders before a CDE Centre is allowed to operate. This contention may be supported by a study by Pringle et al. [45], who attempted to assess variables of process of care to determine their relative effects. They report that patients who attended a practitioner with an interest in diabetes and those that saw a dietician had a marked positive effect on HbA1c values. This corresponds well to the principles inherent in the CDE DMP.

Since each team is responsible for not only the costs of hospital admission for acute diabetes-related emergencies, but also ensuring good clinical outcomes, there is little resistance from Centres to providing the best possible medication, even if it is more costly, to achieve these outcomes in a particular patient.

The CDE does not practise in a vacuum and is subject to oversight by the Council for Medical Schemes (CMS), a statutory body established by the Medical Schemes Act (131 of 1998) to provide regulatory supervision of private health financing through medical schemes. Council governance is vested in a board appointed by the Minister of Health, consisting of a Non-executive Chairman, Deputy Chairman and 13 members. The Executive Head of the Council is the Registrar, also appointed by the Minister in terms of the Medical Schemes Act. The Council determines overall policy, but day-to-day decisions and management of staff are the responsibility of the Registrar and the Executive Managers.

The CDE is registered as an Accredited Managed Care Organization with the CMS. Every 3 years we have to submit to an intensive assessment of the extent to which we meet the conditions set out for accreditation by the Medical Schemes Act, including if we are fit and proper, if we have the necessary infrastructure and are financially sound. This ensures that entities contracting with medical schemes have been duly accredited as required by the Act. It has been of interest to the CDE that the CMS have modelled their accreditation and audit criteria for Managed Care Organizations on the extensive clinical, administrative, healthcare provider training and mentoring and network commissioning, coordination and auditing competencies that exist in the CDE Network and our Diabetes Management Programme.

Part VIII: Conclusion

The CDE trains, administers and audits the biggest network of diabetes providers in Africa, providing care excellence to many people with diabetes. Our capitation-based, fully integrated care model has excellent clinical and cost-efficacy outcomes, achieved largely by a geographically and economically diversified network, run primarily by primary care physicians, with the backing and support of a small group of certified endocrinologists. This demonstrates that improved glycaemic control and better outcomes are achievable in a wider primary care setting. Primary care Practitioners *can* be trained in the core principles of diabetes management and attain satisfactory outcomes. However, to achieve this, adequate training, a holistic team approach, ongoing oversight and review and adequate financial reward are required to ensure service sustainability. Furthermore, it is apparent that Managed Care Programmes for diabetes which pass on the risk and "gate keeping" to the doctor and which focus on outcomes rather than cost-containment, are successful and cost-effective in both the shorter and longer terms. Fears that capitation-based programmes may result in under servicing are unfounded, provided the servicing doctors understand the principles of chronic disease management and are judged on outcomes and take risk for failure to attain these.

We have achieved international recognition for our work and our model of care. We are working hard to set up networks of providers and funders to ensure our continued existence and, if possible, to help make financial, clinical and moral sense to any future NHI model. We work on low profit margins, enough to sustain and grow us as a business, but not to "milk" the healthcare system of vital funds.

We have also provided diabetes education to thousands of healthcare providers through the medium of evidence-based, IDF aligned diabetes training courses since our inception. This has helped to fill a huge void in diabetes competence left open by local Universities and healthcare policies. The training of healthcare providers is also essential to the success of diabetes care in the public health sector – in this vein we have already provide free training via attendance at our 5-Day Courses for nearly 50 public health employed health professionals. In addition to our local Courses and national meetings, we are currently enabling healthcare providers to obtain Masters level diabetes qualifications at very little cost to themselves. We have changed diabetes care in South Africa and beyond.

Although we have record of more than two decades of successful community practice and steady expansion in a financially and politically hostile environment, based on sustainable business principles (no grants or government assistance) and person-centred, ethical care, much more remains to be done. As a self-aware organization, we know that we only care for a very small part of the South African population with diabetes; multitudes do not receive adequate care and support. This we believe is a tragedy. Many of the contracted medical schemes have made membership of the CDE DMP voluntary, resulting in a negative selection bias; those with newly diagnosed type 2 diabetes who perceive themselves to be "well" and whose primary care doctors consider them to be "controlled" often elect not to join. This has limited the potential growth of and influence of this model in providing better care to more South Africans that make use of private healthcare.

A recent report by the International Finance Corporation [46] noted that, while the role of the private sector in African healthcare continues to be "contentious," better collaboration between both the public and private sectors would be the most efficient way of extending high-quality healthcare across the continent and crucial to improving healthcare provision in Africa. A recent academic study by Volminck et al. [47] looked at a cost-effectiveness analysis and potential utility of applying the private sector CDE DMP capitation model to the management of type 2 diabetes in the South African public sector versus "usual practice." Probabilistic modelling showed all iterations of the CDE DMP to fall below the accepted "Willingness-to-Pay" (WTP) threshold (i.e., it was cost-effective) and that it could contribute to increased life expectancy in South Africa. The study recommended that a pilot study of the CDE DMP be done to explore the practical translation of this analysis. Currently, however, the CDE lacks the political recognition and acceptance to enable a public-private partnership (PPP) with the South African Department of Health. We trust that this status quo will change and open an exploration of the possibility of better diabetes care to our population at large.

Abbreviations

ACE-I	Angiotensin-converting-enzyme inhibitors
ADA	American Diabetes Association
ARB	Angiotensin receptor blockers
CDE	Centre for Diabetes and Endocrinology
CMS	Council for Medical Schemes
DCCT	Diabetes Control and Complications Trial
DNE	Diabetes Nurse Educator
DMP	Diabetes Management Programme
DKA	Diabetic ketoacidosis
HONK	Hyperosmolar non-ketotic coma
HQA	Health Quality Assessment
NHANES	National Health and Nutrition Examination Survey
IDF	International Diabetes Federation
NHI	National Health Insurance
PMB	Prescribed Minimum Benefits
PPP	Public-Private Partnerships
UKPDS	United Kingdom Prospective Diabetes Study
VISS	Vascular diabetic complications In Southeast Sweden
WESDR	Wisconsin Epidemiologic Study of Diabetic Retinopathy

References

1. Statistics South Africa. Mid-year population estimates, South Africa. Statistical release P0302; 2014. Available from: http://www.statssa.gov.za/publications/P0302/P03022014.pdf
2. Bridging the gap in South Africa. Bull World Health Org. 2010 Nov;88(11):797–876. Available from: http://www.who.int/bulletin/volumes/88/11/10-021110/en/
3. Annual Report of the Council of Medical Schemes (CMS) 2013/2014. Available from: https://www.medicalschemes.com/files/Annual%20Reports/AR2013_2014LR.pdf
4. The Economist Intelligence Unit Limited. The future of healthcare in Africa. The Economist. 2012. Available from: http://www.economistinsights.com/sites/default/files/downloads/EIU-Janssen_HealthcareAfrica_Report_Web.pdf
5. International Diabetes Federation. IDF diabetes atlas. 6th ed. Brussels: International Diabetes Federation; 2013. Available from: http://www.idf.org/diabetesatlas.
6. International Diabetes Federation. IDF diabetes atlas update poster. 6th ed. Brussels: International Diabetes Federation; 2014. Available from: http://www.idf.org/sites/default/files/Atlas-poster-2014_EN.pdf.
7. Li R, Zhang P, Barker LE, Chowdhury FM, Zhang Z. Cost-effectiveness of interventions to prevent and control diabetes mellitus: a systematic review. Diabetes Care. 2010;33:1872–94.
8. Department of Health Schemes Act 131 of 1998. Regulations in terms of the medical schemes act, 1998 (Act No. 131 of 1998). Chapter 3, Contributions and benefits, Regulation 8. Prescribed Minimum Benefits. Available from: http://www.selfmed.co.za/PDF/GNR1262_20_October_1999.pdf
9. Jönsson B, CODE-2 Advisory Board. Revealing the cost of type II diabetes in Europe. Diabetologia. 2002;45:S5–12.
10. Council for Medical Schemes. Chronic disease algorithms – diabetes mellitus type 2 (Undated). Available from: http://www.medicalschemes.com/files/Prescribed%20Minimum%20Benefits/DiabetesMellitus1_2.pdf
11. Council for Medical Schemes. Chronic disease algorithms – diabetes mellitus type 2 (Undated). Available from: http://www.medicalschemes.com/files/Prescribed%20Minimum%20Benefits/DiabetesMellitus2_3.pdf
12. Council for Medical Schemes. How prescribed minimum benefits help you manage diabetes. cmscript Issue 8 of 2010–2011. Available from: http://www.medicalschemes.com/files/CMScript/CMScript8Of2010_2011.pdf
13. Amod A, Ascott-Evans BH, Berg GI, et al. The 2012 SEMDSA guideline for the management of type 2 diabetes (revised). Diabetes self-management education. JEMDSA. 2012;17(2 Suppl 1):S13–4.
14. Williams R, Van Gaal L, Lucioni C, CODE-2 Advisory Board. Assessing the impact of complications on the costs of type II diabetes. Diabetologia. 2002;45:S13–7.
15. American Diabetes Association. Economic costs of diabetes in the US in 2012. Diabetes Care. 2013;36:1033–46.
16. HQA. 2012 Health quality assessment industry report. Towers Watson Actuaries and Consultants (Pty) Ltd; 2013 Jan.
17. Improving the delivery of adult diabetes care through integration. Diabetes UK. 2014. Available from: https://www.diabetes.org.uk/Documents/About%20Us/What%20we%20say/Integrated%20diabetes%20care%20(PDF,%20648KB).pdf
18. The Diabetes Control and Complications Trial Research Group. The effect of intensive treatment of diabetes on the development and progression of long-term complications in insulin-dependent diabetes mellitus. The Diabetes Control and Complications Trial Research Group. N Engl J Med. 1993. Sep 30;329(14):977–86.

19. Distiller LA, Brown MA, Joffe BI, Kramer BD, Organisation and Delivery of Care. Striving for the impossible dream: a community-based multi-practice collaborative model of diabetes management. Diabet Med. 2010;27:197–202.
20. Nordwall M, Abrahamsson M, Dhir M, Fredrikson M, Ludfigsson J, Arnqvist HJ. Impact of HbA1c, followed from onset of type 1 diabetes, on the development of severe retinopathy and nephropathy: the VISS study (vascular diabetic complications in Southeast Sweden. Diabetes Care. 2015;38:308–15.
21. The Diabetes Control and Complications Trial/ Epidemiology of Diabetes Interventions and Complications Research Group. Retinopathy and nephropathy in patients with type 1 diabetes four years after a trial of intensive therapy. N Engl J Med. 2000;42:381–9.
22. Saunders SA, Wallymahmed M, MacFarlane IA. Glycaemic control in a type 1 diabetes clinic for younger adults. Q J Med. 2004;97:575–80.
23. Holman RR, Paul SK, Angelyn Bethel M, Matthews DR, Neil HAW. 10-year follow-up of intensive glucose control in type 2 diabetes. N Engl J Med. 2008;359:1577–89.
24. Ettaro L, Songer TJ, Zhang P, Engelgau MM. The economic burden of diabetes. Pharmacoeconomics. 2004;22:149–64.
25. American Diabetes Association. Economic Costs of Diabetes in the U.S. in 2012. Diabetes Care. 2013;36:1033–46.
26. Kitabchi AE, Umpierrez GE, Fisher JN, Murphy MB, Stentz FB. Thirty years of personal experience in hyperglycemic crises: diabetic ketoacidosis and hyperglycemic hyperosmolar state. J Clin Endocrinol Metab. 2008;93:1541–52.
27. Siderov J, Shull R, Tomcavage J, Girolami S, Lawton N, Harris R. Does diabetes disease management save money and improve outcomes? Diabetes Care. 2002;25:684–9.
28. Steffans B. Cost effective management of type 2 diabetes: providing quality care in a cost constrained environment. Am J Manag Care. 2000;6:S697–703.
29. Wagner EH, Sandhu S, Newton KM, McCulloch DK, Ramsey SD, Grothaus LC. Effect of improved glycemic control on health care costs and utilization. JAMA. 2001;285:182–90.
30. Menzin J, Langley-Hawthorne C, Friedman M, Boulanger L, Cavanaugh R. Potential short-term economic benefits of improved glycemic control. Diabetes Care. 2001;24:51–5.
31. Simmons D, Yu D, Wenzel H. Changes in hospital admissions and inpatient tariff associated with a diabetes integrated care initiative: preliminary findings. J Diabetes. 2014;6:81–9.
32. Mitka M. Report quantifies diabetes complications. JAMA. 2007;297:2337–8.
33. Remuzzi G, Schieppati A, Ruggenenti P. Nephropathy in patients with type 2 diabetes. N Engl J Med. 2002;346:1145–51.
34. Klein R, Klein BEK, Moss SE, Davis MD, DeMets DL. The Wisconsin epidemiologic study of diabetic retinopathy. II. Prevalence and risk of diabetic retinopathy when age at diagnosis is less than 30 years. Arch Ophthalmol. 1984;102:520–6.
35. Klein R, Klein BEK, Moss SE, Davis MD, DeMets DL. The Wisconsin epidemiologic study of diabetic retinopathy. III. Prevalence and risk of diabetic retinopathy when age at diagnosis is 30 or more years. Arch Ophthalmol. 1984;102:527–32.
36. American Diabetes Association. Retinopathy in diabetes (position statement). Diabetes Care. 2004;27 Suppl 1:S84–7.
37. Thomas RL, Distiller LA, Luzio SD, Chowdhury SR, Melville VJ, Kramer B, Owens DR. Ethnic differences in the prevalence of diabetic retinopathy in persons with diabetes when first presenting at a diabetes clinic in South Africa. Diabetes Care. 2013;36:336–41.
38. Brown MAJ. Core concepts in diabetes mellitus. S Afr J Diabetes. 2010;3(1):10–3.
39. Brown MAJ. Changing diabetes care. S Afr J Diabetes. 2010;3(2):23–5.
40. Diabetes Control and Complications Trial Research Group. The effect of intensive treatment of diabetes on the development and progression of long-term complications in insulin-dependent diabetes mellitus. N Engl J Med. 1993;329:977–86.
41. American Academy of Family Physicians, American College of Physicians, American Osteopathic Association, American Academy of Pediatrics. Joint principles of the patient-centered medical home (PC-MH) [Internet], 2007 Mar 5. Available from: http://www.acponline.org/pressroom/pcmh.htm
42. Iglehart JK. No place like home-testing a new model of care delivery. N Engl J Med. 2008;359:1200–2.
43. Fisher ES. Building a medical neighbourhood for the medical home. N Engl J Med. 2008;359:1202–5.
44. International Diabetes Federation Clinical Guidelines Task Force. Global guideline for type 2 diabetes. Brussels: International Diabetes Federation; 2005.
45. Pringle M, Stewart-Evans C, Coupland C, Williams I, Allison S, Sterland J. Influences on control in diabetes mellitus: patient, doctor, practice, or delivery of care? BMJ. 1993;306:630–4.
46. International Finance Corporation. Healthy partnerships: how governments can engage the private sector to improve health in Africa. Washington, DC: World Bank; 2011. Available from: https://openknowledge.worldbank.org/handle/10986/2304.
47. Volmink HC, Bertram MY, Jina R, Wade AN, Hofman KJ. Applying a private sector capitation model to the management of type 2 diabetes in the South African public sector: a cost-effectiveness analysis. BMC Health Serv Res. 2014;14:444.

7 English Approaches to Integrated Diabetes Care: The East Cambridgeshire and Fenland Diabetes Integrated Care Initiative: A Multiple Provider Approach

David Simmons, Dahai Yu, and Helmut Wenzel

Background

In England, there have been several approaches to replace the hospital based, medical consultant-led diabetes clinic. The rationale behind these new models has varied. In some cases, there was a genuine desire to improve access to more specialist levels of care by reducing demand, through diversion of patients with less complex needs to other clinicians with diabetes management skills, beyond those of the average general practice. In other cases, initiatives have upskilled and supported existing practices across an area to deliver care "closer to home," and within the holistic care than can be provided by the "medical home" delivered by quality general practice. Examples have been the General Practitioner with a Special Interest (GPSI) [1], the community based diabetes specialist nurse (DSN) led service [2, 3] and intermediate services [3, 4].

D. Simmons (✉)
School of Medicine, Western Sydney University, Sydney, NSW, Australia
e-mail: Da.simmons@westernsydney.edu.au

D. Yu
Research Institute for Primary Care and Health Sciences, Keele University, Newcastle Under Lyme, UK
e-mail: d.yu@keele.ac.uk

H. Wenzel
Health Economist, Konstanz, Germany
e-mail: hkwen@aol.com

However, increasingly, another driving force has been to reduce payments to hospitals for the "tariff," the sum payable per clinic appointment under the English NHS internal market system. Essentially, the tariff is a mandatory payment for the clinical service including the facility cost (i.e., the costs of, e.g., management overheads, any underpaid activity such as diabetes inpatients [5], health professional training and safety activities). A GPSI or nursing service could therefore run a clinic in an inexpensive community facility, sometimes with the staffing costs covered by a prior "block" payment making the service itself "free" from a commissioner's point of view. Similarly, use of a private service may mean that the pure facility costs are cheaper, allowing a lower price to be paid. However, reductions in activity and income for hospitals, increases the average unit overhead costs and makes hospitals increasingly unaffordable under the constrained budgets of the English NHS. It is not too surprising that 76% of English hospitals were in deficit in 2015 [6].

The evidence that in England, GPSI and intermediate services provide equal or better services than a hospital based multidisciplinary service, is limited. Furthermore, there are no externally validated training programmes for GPSIs or diabetes specialist nurses in England (unlike diabetes educator programmes in the USA, Canada, Australia and New Zealand). In England, some DSN led community services have been associated with HbA1c reduction among patients under GP care

D. Simmons et al. (eds.), *Integrated Diabetes Care*, DOI 10.1007/978-3-319-13389-8_7

[3]. However, we now know that reducing the HbA1c too far and fast in some patients can be harmful [7]. This is a particularly important issue, where primary care is paid through the Quality Outcomes Framework (QoF), a general practice "pay for performance" programme [8]. A major item within QoF, is the proportion of patients below HbA1c criteria: such reporting is not linked to rates of hypoglycaemia, ambulance call outs or hospitalisation, i.e., a practice could receive a high payment through achieving the QoF target, but with a high hospitalisation/ambulance callout rate.

Potential consequences of the introduction of multiple service providers are fragmentation of care, reductions in continuity of care and propagation of a reluctance to refer on to a more specialist service [9]. Within this paradigm, the creation of a local health system that can integrate primary, secondary and community diabetes care, sharing the work while getting the best from each, would seem to be a sensible way forward. The East Cambridgeshire and Fenland Diabetes Integrated Care Initiative (DICI) was an attempt to create such a systematic approach [10–12]. We now describe the Initiative, its progress and the issues that were identified.

East Cambs and Fenland

East Cambridgeshire and Fenland (ECF) were selected for the intervention, as an area with a selection of historically poor diabetes outcomes [11] and a number of socioeconomically deprived communities. The area is largely rural, a 2009 population of 160,000, with a diabetes population of 7790. There are 17 general practices and no major hospital, falling within 5 (four substantial) hospital catchment areas from adjacent areas. These hospitals require at least 30 min travel time, associated with limited public transport and parking challenges. Cambridgeshire includes two other areas: Huntingdonshire and Cambridge City/South Cambridgeshire as shown in Fig. 7.1, which also

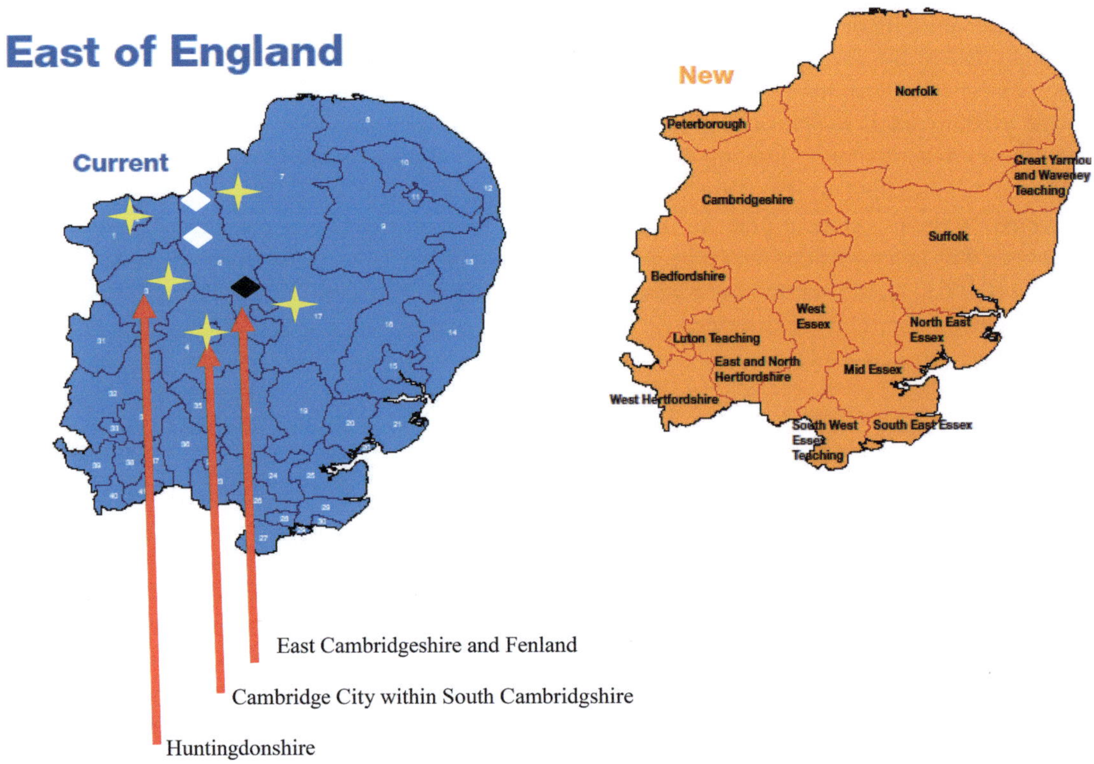

Fig. 7.1 Locations of the three areas in Cambridgeshire (*Left*). "Primary Care Trusts" in the East of England are shown on the *right*. The *stars* show the location of the five hospital diabetes clinics and the *diamonds* the location of three community hospitals: the *black diamond* is Ely hospital

shows the location of the former Cambridgeshire Primary Care Trust (CPCT), the commissioners of NHS care at the time of the DICI. CPCT paid hospitals for each patient seen as inpatients or outpatients under the national tariff, but paid the community services by a "block contract," i.e., a previously agreed single amount for services with an expectation to achieve key performance indicators (KPIs). General practitioners (GPs) were largely paid under a GP contract, with a sizable proportion of practice income derived from QoF.

A separate DSN led community service had been introduced into ECF in 2003 [2] providing type 2 diabetes education and seeing patients within general practices and their homes. The service included a health-care assistant (HCA): an unregistered practitioner, working under the governance of the two DSNs. Dietetics, podiatry and the diabetes specialist nursing service in one of the neighbouring hospitals were delivered by separate community services, within the same provider organisation. Most of the general practices had a diabetes lead GP and practice nurse who had attended additional health professional diabetes education. The ECF DSN led service provided "conferences" for health-care professional diabetes education. Relationships with hospitals services were limited, including with Addenbrookes Hospital, the local tertiary facility. Addenbrookes, and one other hospital, run the evidence based and nationally audited Dose Adjustment For Normal Eating (DAFNE) structured type 1 diabetes education programmes [13]. The three other hospitals run self-designed structured type 1 diabetes education programmes. Addenbrookes hospital also runs the major continuous subcutaneous insulin infusion (CSII) service, regional diabetes foot service and regional diabetes in pregnancy service.

The Pre-intervention Period: The Ely Clinic

The ECF DSN led service had positive relationships with most of the general practices in the area, providing a foundation upon which to build the DICI. In 2007, discussions commenced between the community service and Addenbrookes Hospital on how to address ECF needs. In April 2008, the two services established a monthly, joint community based clinic in Ely, in the heart of East Cambridgeshire. The clinic included consultant physician, DSN, registrar, HCA and dietitian. This clinic was unfunded work for the hospital, which transferred Ely patients, currently being seen in the hospital clinic, to a multidisciplinary clinic in the community hospital, i.e., the hospital had a reduction in income from tariff. The close working between Addenbrookes hospital and the community service led to the re-establishment of an ECF Diabetes Network across GPs and local specialist services in September 2008 [14]. From November 2008, Addenbrookes hospital and the community service then began unfunded work with one pilot general practice to develop approaches for a more integrated practice to diabetes care from a primary care point of view.

The East Cambridgeshire and Fenland Diabetes Integrated Care Initiative

A proposal for the ECF Diabetes Integrated Care Initiative (DICI), with an increased specialist team, was subsequently submitted to CPCT for funding. Funding (£250,000 pa) commenced on 1st April 2009, with additional staff members largely appointed by July/August 2009. The contract was additional to the DSN service contract, but was still held and managed by the community service, with the diabetes consultant subcontracted from Addenbrookes hospital. Registrar time was provided by Addenbrookes hospital at no charge. The aims of the service were to:

(a) *reduce* hospitalisation in patients with diabetes, particularly diabetic foot disease
(b) *improve* metabolic control (commencing with HbA1c/hypoglycaemia/weight control and then moving onto other measures such as blood pressure, lipids, smoking)
(c) *improve* safety and reduce medication side effects where possible (e.g., weight gain, hypoglycaemia)

(d) *increase* access to diabetes education
(e) *increase* access to diabetes specialist services (e.g., medical, nursing, dietetic and podiatric services including full multidisciplinary clinics) in ECF
(f) *reduce* the need for hospital clinic attendance
(g) *reduce* the risk of complications among those with diabetes (e.g., end stage renal failure, acute myocardial infarction and other macrovascular disease, diabetic eye disease, diabetic foot disease)

Interventions

There were six groups of interventions, discussed next.

Community Diabetes Specialist Workforce Expansion

This involved an increase in DSNs by 1.8 Whole Time Equivalent (WTE), diabetes specialist podiatrist (DSP) by 1.0WTE, diabetes specialist dietitian (DSD) by 1.0WTE, community diabetologist (CD) by 0.3WTE and HCA by 1.0WTE. This allowed allocation of one DSN to every four to six practices and the DSD, DSP and CD across all practices. There was also more time for home visits and telephone support to patients.

Increased Access to Patient Structured Education

Access to a locally developed structured, community delivered, type 2 diabetes education was limited due to low staffing levels: DICI brought more groups per month. Prior to DICI, ECF type 1 diabetes patients had limited access to DAFNE. Although reportedly, there was reluctance by some patients to travel out of the area, and for those in the north of the area, this was a long distance, the main issues appeared more to be due to a patchy reluctance to refer to Addenbrookes Hospital, where the largest programme was underway. The integrated approach established communication lines between the DICI staff and DAFNE coordinator. Addenbrookes was also able to establish a number of ECF community hospital based DAFNE sessions, making travel outside the area unnecessary for some patients.

Primary Care Support and Care Closer to Home

This included three major initiatives:

- Community/general practice based DSN and/or new DSD clinics saw patients within the general practice (locations shown in Fig. 7.2), potentially with the GP/practice nurse, otherwise in a room set aside for the purpose. The DSN/DSD had access to the within-practice clinical records but also wrote up within the community service electronic record (SystmOne). This double recording was required because, generally, the community service SystmOne did not link to the practice electronic record even if both used SystmOne. The DSD clinics ran in parallel with the community general dietitian clinics. The DSD sessions referral criteria were:
  - T2DM with HbA1c >9 %
  - T2DM initiating insulin
  - T2DM on insulin with hypos or erratic glucose
  - T2DM with chronic kidney disease IV+ seen outside a multidisciplinary clinic
  - T1DM seen outside a multidisciplinary clinic
- A second "closer to home" intervention were the multidisciplinary clinics (DSN, DSD, DC, registrar with HCA) which included an additional monthly Ely clinic and a new monthly clinic in Wisbech in the north of the county. An existing monthly clinic in Doddington with a DC from Peterborough Hospital, had a DSD added: the existing DSN continued. Criteria for the clinics were generally the same as for a hospital based clinic, but generally, those on continuous subcutaneous insulin infusion (CSII) or had undertaken DAFNE (as none of the community DSNs were DAFNE educators) were excluded.
- The third primary care support/care closer to home intervention were shared educational/clinical care sessions ("virtual clinics") where the management of 5–20 patients with either

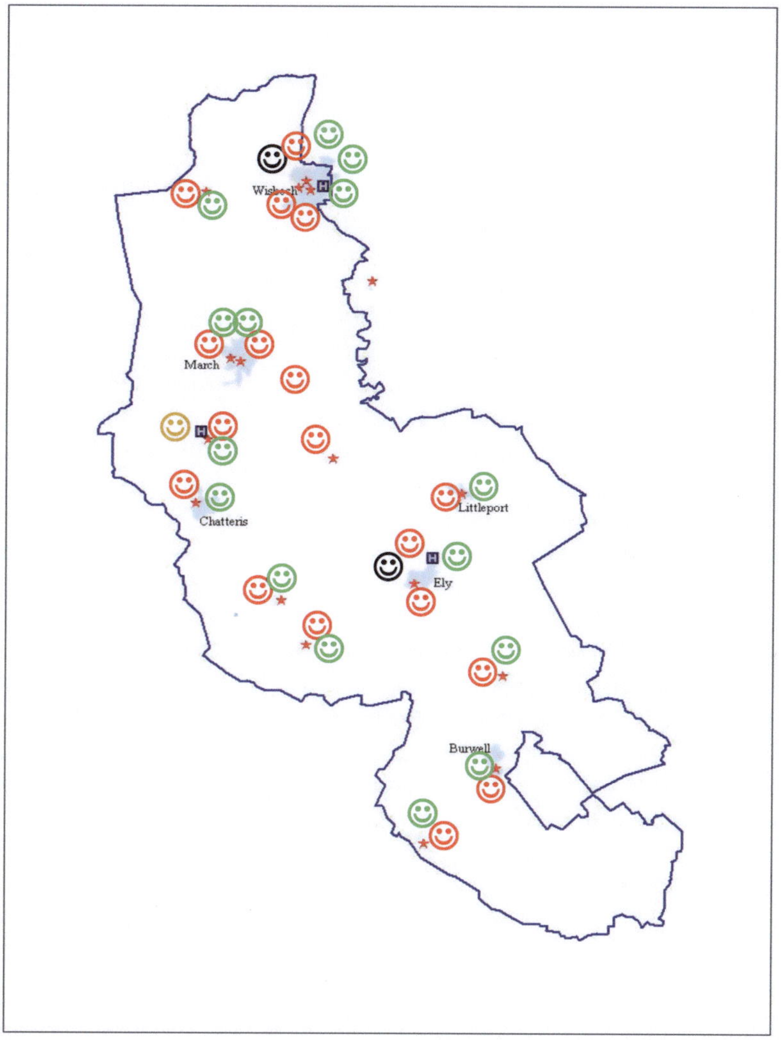

Fig. 7.2 Community/general practice based DSD/specialist podiatry clinics and consultant led community multidisciplinary (MDT) diabetes specialist clinics

Clinic key:

- New MDT clinic
- **Extended MDT clinic**
- New specialist dietitian clinic
- New specialist podiatry clinic

an HbA1c $\geq 9\,\%$, or considered at high risk of hospitalisation, were systematically discussed. The time for GP/practice nurse participation was initially covered by a countywide payment (known as a Local Enhanced Service agreement), between April 2008 and March 2010. After this time, practices received no payment for their participation and clinic frequency tailed off.

New Diabetes Specialist Podiatrist (DSP) Service

This service was created to upskill primary care, ensuring they were aware of the pathways for subacute/acute foot issues, and to be available to see patients urgently (including in their homes). Clinics were established in 14 practices and at Ely and Doddington Hospitals. Criteria for referral to the DSP were:

- foot lesion at risk of hospitalisation
- foot lesion requiring urgent attention
- foot lesion requiring higher level of knowledge/skill than community podiatrist
- recent discharge from hospital

The DSP also established "step-up step-down" clinics (i.e., clinics for patients with lesser acuity and therefore needed lesser input than the high risk foot clinics) in the three community hospitals to allow either earlier discharge from hospital clinics/inpatients or to reduce hospital clinic attendance frequency. The DSP liaised with the community podiatrists and the lead diabetes specialist podiatrists at each of the neighbouring hospitals. The podiatrist worked 1 day/month at the regional foot clinic at Addenbrookes initially to maintain and extend her skills.

Addressing Barriers to Care and Self Care in General Practice

A DSN (0.5WTE) was allocated to visiting practices and establishing a within-practice system to identify and address hurdles faced by both patients and practice staff [15]. The approach was based upon the Barriers to Diabetes Care framework (Fig. 7.3) developed and used in New Zealand and extended to use in the USA and Australia [16–18]. Table 7.1 shows the barriers and possible strategies to address them [15]. Implementation involved practice nurse training by the DSN, and use of a variety of materials/resources including referral pathways. The materials were field tested in one general practice. The practice nurse reported that the approach changed the focus of the Annual Review to being "more patient led rather than led by recording information" with care becoming more individualised with more appropriate use of local resources. However, it was "Time consuming – need at least 30 min for consultation with majority of baseline recorded prior to this, when previously would only have blood tests and blood pressure" [10].

Organisational Redesign

Organisational redesign was seen as essential to align the hospital, community and GP services provided to people with diabetes. This involved three levels of mechanisms to integrate the different services:

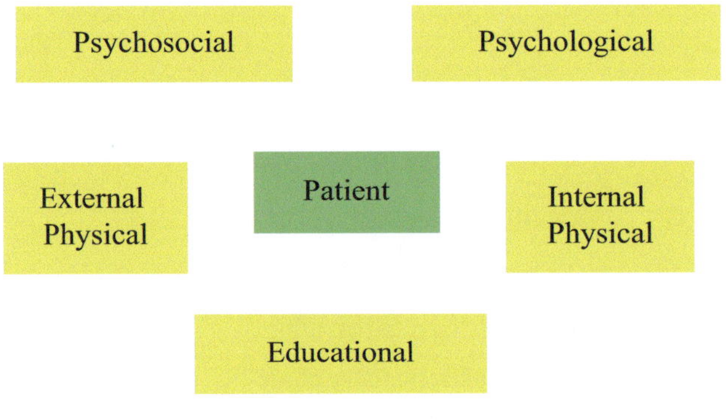

Key:

Psychosocial barriers=how patients relate to others including health care professionals, family members

Psychological=how patients behave, feel, perceive, believe

External physical=systems issues such as how the health and social welfare services operate

Internal physical=other health conditions impact on self care, e.g., blindness, obesity, disability

Educational=knowledge of diabetes, health systems and educational attainment

Fig. 7.3 Barriers to Diabetes Care major components (Data from [15, 16])

Table 7.1 Barriers to care, approaches to assessing barriers and interventions that may be beneficial in addressing the impact of barriers on diabetes care/self care

Barrier and examples	Initial assessment	External pathway
Psychological issues-normal	Detailed assessment	Health-care assistant with support from diabetes specialist nurse
Strictness of regimen (e.g. food)	Goal setting	
Motivation, "laziness," self efficacy	Motivational interviewing	
Psychological issues	Detailed assessment	Diabetes specialist nurse
Unusual e.g. needle phobia	Confirm e.g. needle phobia	Psychologist
Denial, emotional	Counselling	
Psychological issues	Detailed assessment	Finance/work related:
Priority setting	Personal time management, budgeting, social support, access to care, counselling	Citizen Advice Bureau
Time allocation	Coping skills, time management	Diabetes specialist nurse home visit if needed
Psychological issues	Personalised strategies	Discuss with psychologists
Unhelpful health beliefs	Education	
	Cognitive behavioural therapy	
Family issues	Detailed assessment-identify abuse	May need social services involvement
Inadequate support and obstruction	Make joint family involvement/ education plan	Diabetes specialist nurse home visit
	Bring partner/family member to appt	Dietician to see family
	Practice nurse home visit	District nurses can do annual reviews if trained up
Unsupportive environment	Education e.g. on how to use current local milieu/products	Discuss with diabetes specialist nurse or dietician if needed
Food, activity, insulin injections, self glucose monitoring	Meal/activity plans	Dietician to see family
	Dietician should make a plan for each area and hand to practise re: food and activity pack	
Past care unsatisfactory	Detailed assessment-	If due to patient (recurrent behaviour pattern) then psychologist
Attitudes of health workers	Identify ethnicity/gender issues	Alternative personnel (difficult in small practices) diabetes specialist nurse
	Personalised care, build trust, takes time	
	Needs staff training programme	
Communication	Assessment	Discuss with diabetes specialist nurse
Low educational status	Identify issues	Local education authority
	Personal communication plan (e.g. lower Fleisher score materials, more time, education)	
Physical co-morbidities (non-diabetes)	Assessment	Community matron, community services referral-specialist nurse,
	Identify management plan and practise nurse role	May need specialist advice and/or referral
Psychiatric co-morbidities	Assessment	Community mental health team or psycho geriatric advice/referral
Depression	Identify management plan and practise nurse role	
Diabetes management side effects	Improved diabetes tools e.g. glucose monitoring and insulin needles, different medications	Discuss with diabetes specialist nurse

(continued)

Table 7.1 (continued)

Barrier and examples	Initial assessment	External pathway
Educational issues	Practise nurse training	Discuss with diabetes specialist nurse
Diabetes	Group sessions, assessment	
	Materials, 1:1, group education	
Education issues	Assessment	Home visits, out of hours service
Accessing services	Materials	Discuss with diabetes specialist nurse
	Education	Materials
Personal finance	Practise nurse to work through	Social services
Healthy food, footwear, transport costs, time off work		Citizen Advice Bureau
Physical access	Transport	Discuss with diabetes specialist nurse/dietician/podiatry
	Care closer to home-special clinics/ visits (e.g. prison)	Annual review by district nurse
	Home visits	
Poor range of services	Evening/weekends, emergencies	Discuss with diabetes specialist nurse/dietician home visits
	Exercise/walking groups, supermarket tours	
Appointment system	Information management, Staff management	Practise to review systems
	Staffing numbers/multi-skilling	

Used with permission from Harwood et al. [15]

DSN Diabetes Specialist Nurse

- Vertical integration, i.e., bringing together the different parties to direct the DICI
- Clinical governance, i.e., the oversight of practitioners within the DICI
- Horizontal integration, i.e., bringing together the different practitioners delivering care

Mechanisms for Vertical Integration

1. ECF diabetes network: This group helped develop, and approved, the submission for the integrated care approach. It was designed to serve as a clinical reference group and provide governance over the DICI.
2. CPCT Integrated diabetes care initiative project group: Meetings provided a platform for the integrated team to report to CPCT and raise issues and link to other countywide initiatives.
3. Secondary provider reference group: This group was established to optimise communication and agreement between the hospital diabetes services in the area.
4. Patient reference group: The patient voice is crucial to allow the development within the initiative to be grounded in the patient perspective. The original plans were reviewed and commented upon by the Addenbrookes Hospital diabetes care patient advisory committee (DCPAC) which included some patients from ECF. Attempts to establish an ECF group were unsuccessful.
5. Countywide network: The countywide network was created by combining the preexisting networks from the three areas in Cambridgeshire. It provided a forum for diabetes health professionals, people with diabetes and commissioners to discuss area-specific and countywide issues, to monitor diabetes care and to formulate countywide proposals.
6. Cambridgeshire diabetes drugs advisory group: This group was established after the countywide network advised the CPCT medicines management team of the need for proposals relating to diabetes drugs and devices

to be discussed with diabetes health professionals and people with diabetes before CPCT policy was made.

7. Countywide information management working group: This working group was set up by the diabetes networks to develop and put into place a countywide approach to diabetes information management. Membership included the commissioners, national and CPCT/local provider IT staff, GP and diabetes service representatives.
8. Countywide guidelines and pathways working group: This working group collated and updated existing diabetes guidelines and pathways from across the three areas.
9. Countywide diabetes education working group: This group generated recommendations for diabetes education.

Clinical Governance, i.e., the Oversight of Practitioners Within the DICI

Governance is about "how local [public] bodies and partnerships ensure that they are doing the right things, in the right way, for the right people in a timely inclusive, open, honest and accountable manner" [19]. *Clinical governance* is the term used to describe a systematic approach to maintaining and improving the safety and quality of patient care within a health system. The day to day activities of the DICI team were under the clinical governance of the team leader (lead DSN), who reported to the community provider manager. A team meeting was held monthly for discussion of policy, key cases and incidents. Technically, the overall clinical governance for the ECF DICI was the responsibility of the DC, but this depended upon the monthly team meeting, meeting with the lead DSN and any ad hoc clinical observations. General practice teams, including practice nurses, received their clinical governance through the GPs, and GP clinical governance came from CPCT.

Horizontal Integration, i.e., Bringing Together the Different Practitioners Delivering Care

1. Integration between the community trust and CUH diabetes services: this included placement of the DC within the community team, closer working across the services including the multidiscipinary community clinics, telephone/email advisory and team meetings, professional support, upskilling and maintenance of standards for DSP and DSD. A joint approach to DAFNE, initial induction of community staff, opportunities for hospital staff to work in the community and back up staff members and for community staff to attend hospital clinics were also estasblished.
2. Integration between the community trust and other diabetes services: DSP worked with all other local hospital foot services and community podiatry, DSD worked with community dietetics and the DSN worked with Peterborough Hospital staff in Doddington. Close working with the 17 GP teams with nine practice-based activities helped integrate care. Cooperation with community matrons and district nurses was already part of the approach used.
3. Integration with other secondary services including mental health services were planned (including psychology) but did not eventuate.

Evaluation

There were three phases of evaluation:

- simple satisfaction questionnaires in the Ely clinic before the DICI commenced and evaluation of the initial practice intervention
- service evaluation with some modeling of hospitalization at the end of year 1 [11]
- full mixed methods evaluation at the end of year 3 [12]

Ely Clinic Review

Of the 207 ECF patients seen at Addenbrookes Hospital in the previous 12 months, 70 were allocated to the Ely Clinic in the first 10 months of operation. Fifty were given appointments; others either declined, had already been discharged/ died, were DAFNE graduates/awaiting DAFNE, were on insulin pump therapy, or were under the high risk foot clinic, Young Adult or nephropathy clinics. Of the 45 attending patients, 5 were discharged and 3 returned to Addenbrookes for type 1 diabetes or joint lipid management. A short patient satisfaction was distributed at each clinic and 24 were returned (0–6/clinic). All patients found the Ely clinic easier to attend, were happy with the advice given and would recommend the clinic to others. Only one negative clinical issue arose: the IT link between the clinic and Addenbrookes Hospital. Among the 21 patients attending the clinic at least twice in this period, there were no significant differences in metabolic results besides diastolic blood pressure which was significantly lower at the final Ely clinic visit (79 ± 9 vs 74 ± 8 mm Hg, $p = 0.022$, paired t-test). This was felt to be associated with the easier travel and parking arrangements.

The Specialist Registrar saw two major areas of benefit from attending the Ely clinic:

- Training
  - close consultant supervision with exemplary teaching
  - benefits from closer contact with DSD and DSN
  - easier patient follow-up: experience effectiveness of treatments, investigations
- Continuity of Care
  - patient rapport: appreciate seeing "same face," patients appear more engaged in diabetes care
  - able to follow-up results, previous discussions
  - less time spent looking through old notes and more time spent in consultation

A range of issues arose during the pilot, as noted next:

- *Organisation of appointments*: The appointments were made manually by Addenbrookes Hospital secretarial staff, but the Addenbrookes Hospital booking system, at times, continued to send appointments to patients creating confusion.
- *Management of medical records*: The limited time between filling appointments and the clinic posed problems for generating community service notes. These notes were carried in the car of the community DSN with its associated information governance risk.
- *Information management*: The electronic link with Addenbrookes worked well, but took the first one to two clinics to implement. Notes within the clinic were paper based.

Evaluation of the Initial Practice Based Intervention Including Virtual Clinics

This pilot occurred November 2008–August 2009 in a single handed rural general practice. The practice diabetes register included 87 patients in April 2009. The practice had always worked in partnership with the community DSN team, referring patients for assessment for commencement on insulin, and for advice and management of patients with a persistently raised HbA1c. The practice team members had diabetes certification through a UK University course. A practice recall system was in place. In November 2008 the practice audited its care and commenced closer work with the community team, including the DC. The practice nurse also embarked on a further diabetes qualification. Criteria for patient discussion were: HbA1c of ≥9 %, uncontrolled hypoglycaemia, blood pressure or lipids in spite medication, triglycerides >8 mmol/l, hospitalisation/CVD events in past 12 months, patients under secondary care.

At the end of the 8 month pilot, the proportion with HbA1c <7.5 % increased from 47 % to 75 % and those with a HbA1c ≥9 % dropped from 39 % to 12 %. There were various other process benefits. The barriers tool was piloted.

A second, larger practice ($n = 655$) adopted the approach once DICI was funded with six virtual clinics and increased DSN input. This practice also had a dramatic reduction in the number of patients with an HbA1c of ≥9 % from 248/655 (37.9 %) to 83 (12.7 %) over 12 months.

Outcomes Evaluation After 1 and 3 Years of Intervention [11, 12]

Methodology

De-identified electronic Cambridgeshire Secondary Uses Service (SUS) data were obtained for all patients for any past admission and hospital clinic attendance between April 2007 (i.e., 2 years before the DICI contract commenced) and November 2010 for the 1 year evaluation and March 2012 for the 3 year evaluation. Practice, patient age, elective/non-elective status, ICD10 and Health Related Group (HRG) coding were included in the datasets. Diabetes (E10–E14) was considered the primary cause of admission if coded in the first ICD field. Diabetes foot was considered the cause of admission with HRG codes of KB03A, KB03B, QZ02A, QZ04Z, QZ11A, QZ11B, QZ12Z, diabetic ketoacidosis with ICD 10 codes of E10.1, E11.1, E12.1, E13.1, and E14.1, and CVD with ICD10 codes of I20, I21, I22, I23, I24, and I25.

Because of the varying underlying patterns in admissions in the different areas, regression analysis across the whole time period was not seen as a valid approach. A novel approach to assessing the impact of the intervention was required to compare changes in hospitalisation before and after the commencement of ECF DICI. The hospital admissions were therefore summed for each month for areas/groups of practices. Each month was taken as a separate time point and the mean difference before and after each time point calculated to provide a real indication of the mean change in admissions before and after that month. A Poisson regression model was constructed to analyse the percentage change in average monthly hospital admission rate before and after each monthly cut-off point, e.g., after 1 year, 12 models were built corresponding to the 12 monthly cut-off points from July 2009 to June 2010. To allow for residual seasonality, we incorporated terms to describe an annual sinusoidal pattern in the numbers of hospital admission. The modelling of potential confounders was completed by the inclusion of indicator variables for the month. A variety of sensitivity analyses were conducted [11, 12] which showed no change to the results.

For the 1 year analysis, practices were defined as either "engaged" or "less engaged" based upon the degree of uptake of relevant ECF DICI components (referrals, virtual clinics, DSN/DSD/DSP clinics and/or barriers assessments). The lead DSN allocated the practices blind to the hospitalisation data. Analyses compared the engaged and less engaged practice hospitalisation rates.

In the 3 year analysis, the Mantel Haenszel test was used to compare the proportion of hospital episodes by patients with diabetes in ECF with those in the other two areas in Cambridgeshire (Huntingdonshire, Greater Cambridge) in 2007 and 2012. Hospital episodes and outpatient attendances were compared before and after the commencement of the DICI, between those with and without diabetes and between the three Cambridgeshire areas. Each monthly point shows the 95 % confidence intervals for the estimate of mean change.

QoF population (2008/9) data (http://www.gpcontract.co.uk/download) provided diabetes and overall population by area and the Quality Outcomes Framework metrics (diabetes overall, DM12 (BP 145/85 or less), DM17 (Cholesterol 5.0 or less), DM23 (HbA1c 7 % or less), DM24 (HbA1c 8 % or less), DM25 (HbA1c 9 % or less)) on an annual basis. Unfortunately, the HbA1c thresholds changed during this time, so that only the last 2 years are available with the same thresholds. Annual referrals for Dose Adjustment for Normal Eating (DAFNE) were obtained from Cambridge University Hospitals Foundation Trust (A Housden, personal communication). Emergency Department attendance data for hypoglycaemia were not considered adequate due to coding issues. Pharmaceutical data were not available. All analyses were conducted in STATA [STATA/SE 11.0. StataCorp, Texas] and tests are two tailed with $p<0.05$ taken as significant. Ethics approval was received from the National Research Ethics Service Committee-East of England.

Year 1 Evaluation

Those adopting the intervention fully had reduced hospitalisation and hospitalisation costs compared with those defined as less "engaged" [11]. Comparable changes in the rate of hospitalisation increase were not seen among those without diabetes or among those in other parts of Cambridgeshire.

Year 3: Summative Evaluation

Degree of Implementation

The additional staffing, clinics, barriers framework [11, 12, 15], and general practice education were implemented. Referrals to DAFNE increased from 10 to 14 per annum (2003–2009), to 25 in 2010 and 16 in 2011. Consultant virtual clinics occurred in 16 general practices: 23 in year 1 (when the LES was in place), 14 in year 2 and 9 in year 3. Conversely, the degree of implementation of the vertical integration/governance arrangements was limited (Table 7.2). A major joint effort occurred through 2010 to July 2011, including diabetes services, primary care and patients across the county, built upon the work of the ECF DICI, to create a proposal for an integrated service across Cambridgeshire. A variety of options for further investment were proposed to CPCT under their "Sustainable Health Partnership" programme, but these were all rejected. One group of GPs in south Cambridgeshire/Cambridge City (CamHealth) opted to adopt the ECF approach and invested in the additional staff. The rejection of the countywide integrated care proposal, led to uncertainty over service commissioning and an increase in competition between the different services. Identification of clinical governance issues at this time of increased uncertainty, led to the withdrawal of Addenbrookes Hospital from the DICI.

Table 7.2 Degree of implementation of the mechanisms for vertical integration/clinical governance in East Cambs and Fenland (ECF)

Governance component	Degree of implementation
ECF[a] Diabetes Network	ECF meetings were held approximately quarterly in year 1. These reduced after the introduction of the countywide network. Governance stopped after 12–18 months
CPCT[b] integrated diabetes care initiative project group	Focused on defining key performance indicators, rather than project managing and facilitating integration
Secondary provider reference group	Met infrequently
ECF patient reference group	Never eventuated
Countywide network	Did not focus on ECF
Cambridgeshire diabetes drugs advisory group	Collaborated well on countywide drug issues
Countywide information management working group	Recommendations allowing data sharing between general practice and other health services (hospitals and community services) were never implemented
Countywide guidelines and pathways working group	The recommendations were never monitored
Countywide diabetes education working group	The recommendations were never implemented
ECF team clinical governance	Clinical incidents were rarely tabled-few were placed in front of the DC

[a]East Cambridgeshire and Fenland
[b]Cambridgeshire Primary Care Trust

Impact of the DICI on Hospitalisation, Metabolic Control and Outpatient Attendance by Area

Figure 7.4 shows the weekly hospital episode rate, and Table 7.3 the monthly hospital episode rates over the 5 years for those with and without diabetes by area. The proportion of admissions by those with diabetes increased in all areas over the 5 years, but the increase was 9.2 (5.5–13.1)% and 54.1 (49.0–59.4)% greater in ECF than Hunts and Greater Cambridge respectively including a 7.4 (5.2–9.2)% and 45.5 (42.5–48.5)% greater increase in ECF over the 3 years of the intervention.

Table 7.3 also shows the mean monthly change rates in hospitalisation across the 5 years, overall, for elective and non-elective hospital admissions and for those with diabetes as a primary ICD diagnosis code: no reduction in hospitalisation was seen in ECF. Figure 7.5 shows the monthly hospitalisation change overall and for non-elective admissions by area for those with and without diabetes: in Huntingdonshire and Greater Cambridge, but not in ECF, the monthly non-elective hospitalisation change became similar between patients with and without diabetes. In ECF, the difference in monthly change in hospi-

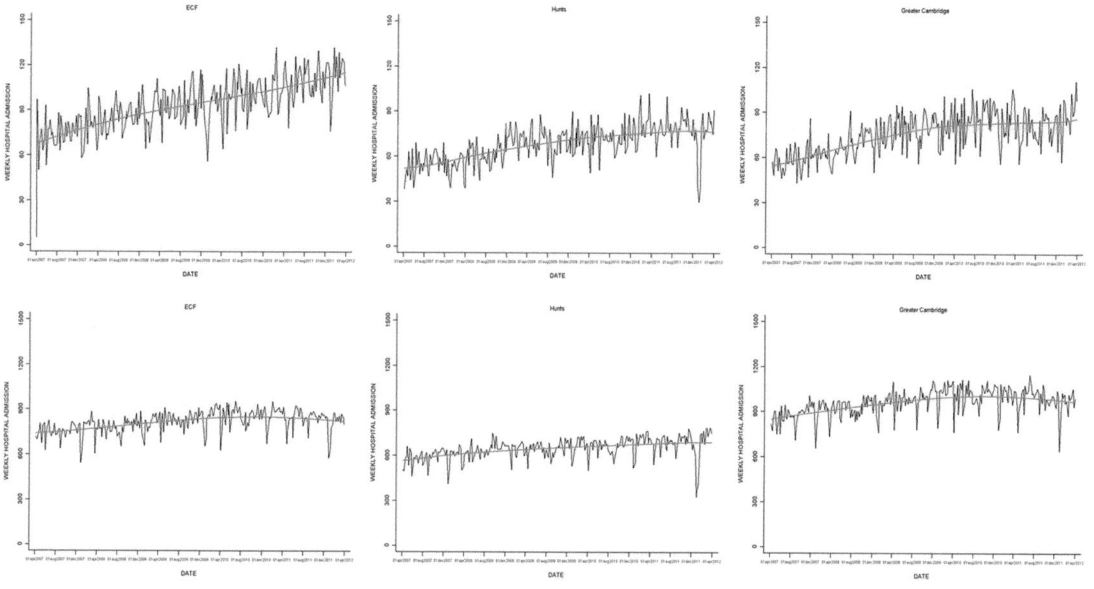

Fig. 7.4 Hospitalisation (number/week) among those with and without diabetes over the 5 years by area. Each figure is weekly hospital admission series plot with LOWESS fit line

talisation between those with and without diabetes appears to widen after the introduction of the DICI. The difference between the areas was most marked in those aged 75+ years (Fig. 7.6). The DICI was not associated with a reduction in hospitalisation rates for diabetes, diabetic foot, diabetic ketoacidosis, hypoglycaemia or cardiovascular disease in people with diabetes (Table 7.3). There was no greater achievement of diabetes QoF targets in ECF over the 5 years either overall or by individual QoF score. There was an increase in new outpatient appointments in Huntingdonshire in 2011.

There was no difference between hospitals in hospitalisation rates within ECF over the 36 months of the DICI (Fig. 7.7), besides an improvement in the Huntingdonshire hospital catchment area. Practices associated with DSN A, but not DSNs B and C, were associated with an increase in hospital admission rates over time concurrent with consistent reductions in outpatient referrals (Fig. 7.8). These changes commenced before the introduction of the DICI under the DSN led team approach. The DSNs covered practices across ECF.

Year 3: Process Evaluation

The process evaluation was conducted using the Medical Research Council guidelines for evaluating complex interventions [20].

Practice Nurse Telephone Survey

A telephone survey was undertaken with ECF practice nurses (14/16 practices – one PN was excluded as she became a member of the DICI team) including use of a barriers framework [15], confidence with insulin management, referral to diabetes specialist services, access to specialist podiatry, and how closely they felt they were now working with the community diabetes team/local hospital diabetes services. A reduction in integration between primary care and hospitals was reported by 6/14 PNs across the different hospital catchments with a parallel increase in integration with community services reported by 8/14 PNs. All PNs reported referring to the community DSN. Most PNs reported an increase in their confidence in the use of insulin (9/14, although one indicated a reduction in confidence) and 7/14 reported that they referred foot ulcers earlier to the community DSP.

Table 7.3 Hospitalisation referral by region

		2007			2008			2009			2010			2011		
		ECF	Greater Cambridge	Hunts	ECF	Greater Cambridge	Hunts	ECF	Greater Cambridge	Hunts	ECF	Greater Cambridge	Hunts	ECF	Greater Cambridge	Hunts
Population size	Registered diabetes patients	7672	6532	5077	8514	6859	5490	9052	7276	6041	9497	7658	6484	10,051	7977	6855
	Practice size	174,411	244,341	154,947	187,740	245,614	155,845	190,059	249,681	157,537	192,047	253,143	158,342	194,639	254,833	158,933
Annual diabetes hospitalisation percentage[a]		2909 (9.07 %)	2270 (6.25 %)	2134 (8.54 %)	4391 (9.74 %)	3497 (6.79 %)	3124 (8.71 %)	4801 (10.09 %)	4118 (7.52 %)	3662 (9.90 %)	5086 (10.23)	4378 (7.65 %)	3762 (9.82 %)	5589 (11.26 %)[a]	4186 (7.50 %)[b]	4091 (10.28 %)[b]
Monthly hospitalisation rate	Diabetes	327 (303, 339)	249 (238, 267)	242 (220, 251)	361 (348, 391)	284 (266, 316)	262 (238, 276)	405 (375, 427)	346 (330, 363)	311 (282, 321)	422 (410, 447)	367 (336, 395)	319 (300, 326)	466 (433, 491)	342 (331, 360)	343 (315, 359)
	Non-diabetes	3286 (3050, 3392)	3756 (3611, 3965)	2554 (2395, 2704)	3393 (3278, 3495)	3999 (3890, 4071)	2702 (2685, 2764)	3597 (3446, 3778)	4287 (4046, 4360)	2782 (2702, 2864)	3670 (3573, 3860)	4413 (4254, 4477)	2877 (2788, 3007)	3650 (3559, 3755)	4265 (4071, 4524)	2996 (2859, 3057)
Monthly change percentage -overall	Diabetes	Ref	Ref	Ref	14.3 (9.6, 19.1) %	15.7 (10.3, 21.0) %	10.1 (4.5, 15.7) %	23.2 (18.6, 27.9) %	32.0 (26.8, 37.2) %	26.0 (20.6, 31.4) %	29.0 (24.4, 33.6) %	38.1 (33.0, 43.3) %	28.7 (23.3, 34.1) %	38.4 (33.9, 43.0) %	33.6 (28.5, 38.8) %	37.1 (31.8, 42.4) %
	Non-diabetes	Ref	Ref	Ref	4.5 (3.0, 6.1) %	5.8 (4.4, 7.3) %	7.6 (5.9, 9.3) %	9.6 (8.1, 11.1)%	11.2 (9.8, 12.6) %	9.4 (7.7, 11.1) %	13.9 (12.4, 15.4) %	15.4 (14.1, 16.8) %	13.0 (11.3, 14.7) %	12.5 (11.0, 14.0) %	13.2 (11.8, 14.5) %	16.3 (14.6, 18.0) %
Monthly change percentage -Non-elective	Diabetes	Ref	Ref	Ref	13.3 (6.3, 20.3) %	11.1 (3.6, 18.5) %	12.4 (−7.3, 25.3) %	19.2 (12.3, 26.1)%	24.0 (16.7, 31.2) %	12.7 (4.3, 21.0) %	25.4 (18.6, 32.2) %	26.9 (19.6, 34.1) %	19.0 (10.7, 27.2) %	28.8 (22.0, 35.6) %	23.4 (16.1, 30.6) %	17.1 (8.9, 25.4) %
	Non-diabetes	Ref	Ref	Ref	11.6 (0.04, 22.7) %	1.0 (−1.2, 3.2) %	9.9 (7.2, 12.6) %	12.3 (1.2, 23.5) %	5.0 (2.8, 7.2) %	13.3 (10.7, 16.0) %	21.5 (10.6, 32.5) %	9.9 (7.7, 12.0) %	15.8 (13.2, 18.5) %	32.6 (21.8, 43.3) %	8.4 (6.3, 10.6) %	14.1 (11.4, 16.8) %

Monthly change percentage -elective	Diabetes	Ref	Ref	Ref	6.6 (–5.3, 18.5) %	9.1 (–3.8, 22.0) %	2.3 (–12.3, 17.0) %	9.4 (–2.4, 21.3) %	2.2 (–10.8, 15.3) %	24.4 (10.4, 38.5) %	8.5 (–3.3, 20.4) %	4.9 (–8.1, 17.9) %	19.9 (5.7, 34.0) %	17.6 (5.9, 29.2) %	–2.1 (–15.2, 11.1) %	30.9 (17.0, 44.7) %
	Non-diabetes	Ref	Ref	Ref	1.2 (–2.8, 5.2) %	–0.2 (–4.0, 3.6) %	–2.8 (–7.2, 1.6) %	0.5 (–3.5, 4.5) %	–0.9 (–4.7, 2.9) %	–6.8 (–11.1,–2.3) %	3.6 (–0.4, 4.5) %	–3.1 (–6.9, 0.7) %	–3.1 (–7.5, 1.3) %	–1.6 (–5.6, 2.4) %	–13.5 (–17.4,–9.6) %	–7.3 (–11.8,–2.9) %
Monthly change percentage -diabetes as primary code	Diabetes	Ref	Ref	Ref	–2.9 (–20.5, 14.7) %	16.9 (–3.0, 36.8) %	19.3 (–2.2, 40.8) %	20.9 (4.1, 37.8) %	34.6 (15.3, 54.0) %	19.3 (–2.2, 40.8) %	14.1 (–3.0, 31.1) %	31.7 (12.3, 51.2) %	26.7 (5.5, 47.9) %	29.3 (12.8, 45.9) %	5.2 (–15.2, 25.6) %	51.4 (31.0, 71.7) %

Rates are shown as P_{50} (P_{25}, P_{75})

Change percentage is estimated by Poisson regression model by using 2007 monthly count as reference, and is present as estimated percentage (95 %CI)

Data coverage: 9 months in 2007 (April–December); 12 months in each year of 2008–2011 (January–December)

[a]Annual diabetic hospitalisation percentage = annual diabetic hospitalisation count/annual total hospitalisation count, %

[b]Means the results of trend analysis across 5 years were statistically significant (p<0.0001)

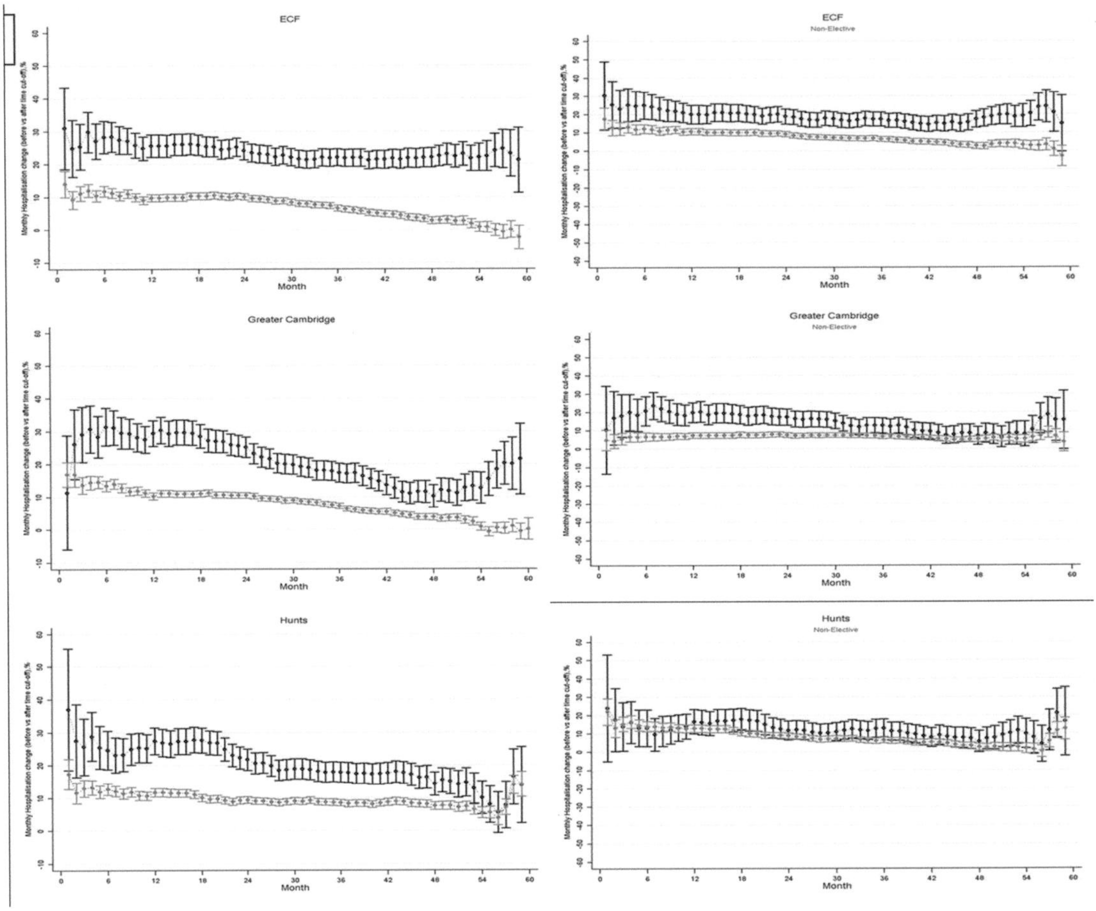

Fig. 7.5 Monthly percentage change in hospital admission rate (monthly hospital admission rate before and after the month) across areas among all patients and non-elective admissions. *Left* plots are for all-caused hospitalisation; *right* plots are for non-elective hospitalisation. *Black* (*upper*) plot represents for hospital admission change percentage for those with diabetes. *Grey* (*lower*) plot represents for hospital admission change percentage for those without diabetes. Figures above 0 % indicate that the mean monthly hospitalisation rate after the index month is greater than the mean hospitalisation rate before the index month

Degree of Integration: Multidimensional Analysis (MDS)

Multidimensional Scaling (MDS) used the practice nurse data to create a proximities matrix (similarities or dissimilarities) between health-care providers (GPs, community services and hospitals) [21]. The MDS algorithm minimises the standardised residual sum of squares ("the stress factor"): the closer to zero, the better the representation: a value <0.1 is excellent [22]. Figure 7.9 shows the mapping of health-care providers according to their dissimilarities: the stress factor is 0.18, which is acceptable.

The distances between the indicators show that they are quite dissimilar. The proximity of "working with community" and "CCS Nurse Referral" indicate increased integration between the community services and general practice, associated with increased self-reported confidence in managing diabetes. Conversely, hospital referral and working with hospitals are rated quite low, reflecting decreased integrated working between general practice and hospitals. This is in line with our observations during the project.

Figure 7.10 shows the mapping of the providers according to their dissimilarities; they form six clusters of perceived changes and the corresponding rating. The first cluster is best represented by provider (EC5) and shows

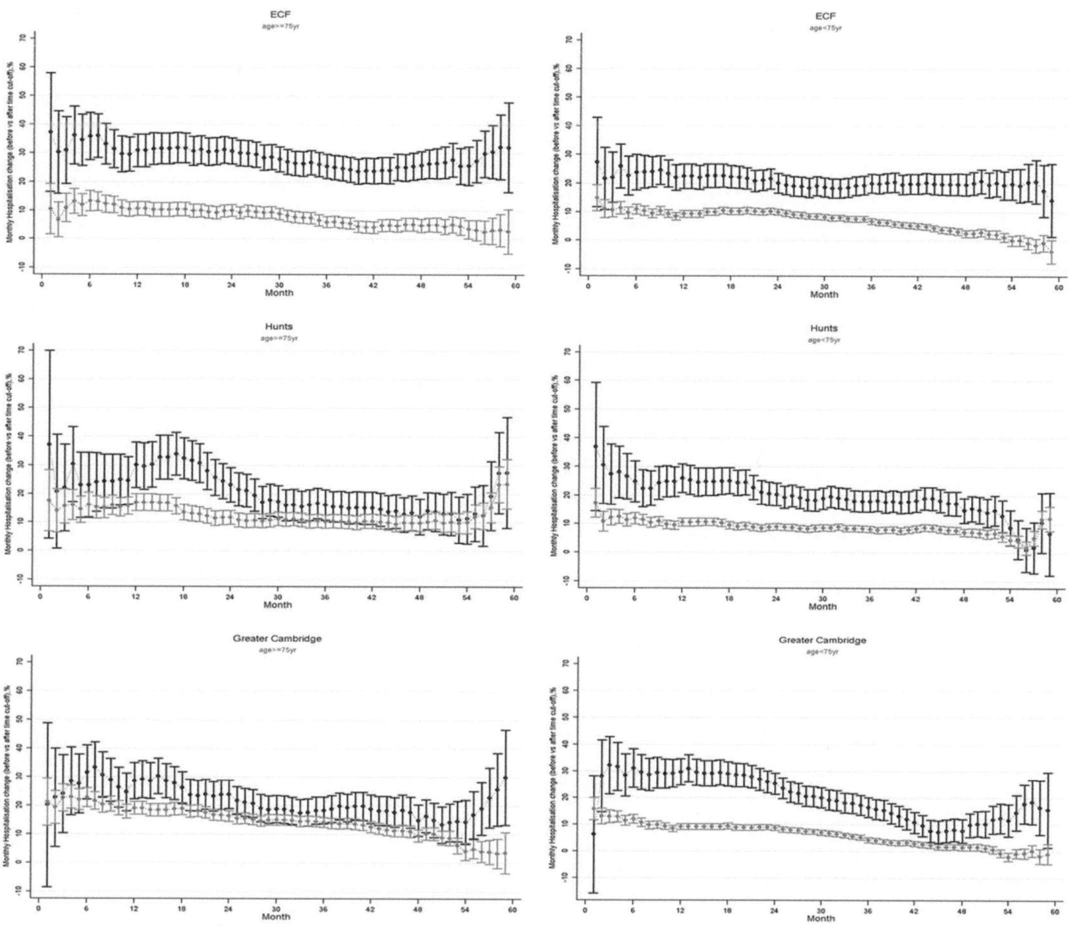

Fig. 7.6 Monthly percentage change in hospital admission rate (monthly hospital admission rate before and after the month) across areas among all patients aged <75 years and 75+ years. *Left* plots are for those aged 75+ years; *right* plots are for those aged <75 years. *Black* (*upper*) plot represents for hospital admission change percentage for those with diabetes. *Grey* (*lower*) plot represents for hospital admission change percentage for those without diabetes. Figures above 0 % indicate that the mean monthly hospitalisation rate after the index month is greater than the mean hospitalisation rate before the index month

improvements in all categories, indicating increased integration. In the second cluster provider (F5) is typical for the cluster and shows only slight improvements, i.e., in the category "CCS Nurse Referral." This means that integration was quite low. In the third cluster, best represented by provider (F2), "CCS Nurse Referral," "working with hospital" and "own confidence" were improved, but "hospital referral" was evaluated negatively. This also indicates low integration, but higher when compared to the fourth cluster. Provider (EC5) is typical for the fourth cluster; "working with hospital" and "hospital referral" worsened, but all other categories showed improvements. In the fifth cluster "CCS Nurse Referral" and "working with community" are rated positively with no changes in "own confidence." This cluster is best represented by provider (H3), integration was also very low. For the sixth cluster nothing changed, except a worsening in the category "CCS Nurse Referral." This indicates no improvement in integration.

Observations and Interviews

Ethnographic field notes were collated from observations by social scientists. Semi-structured

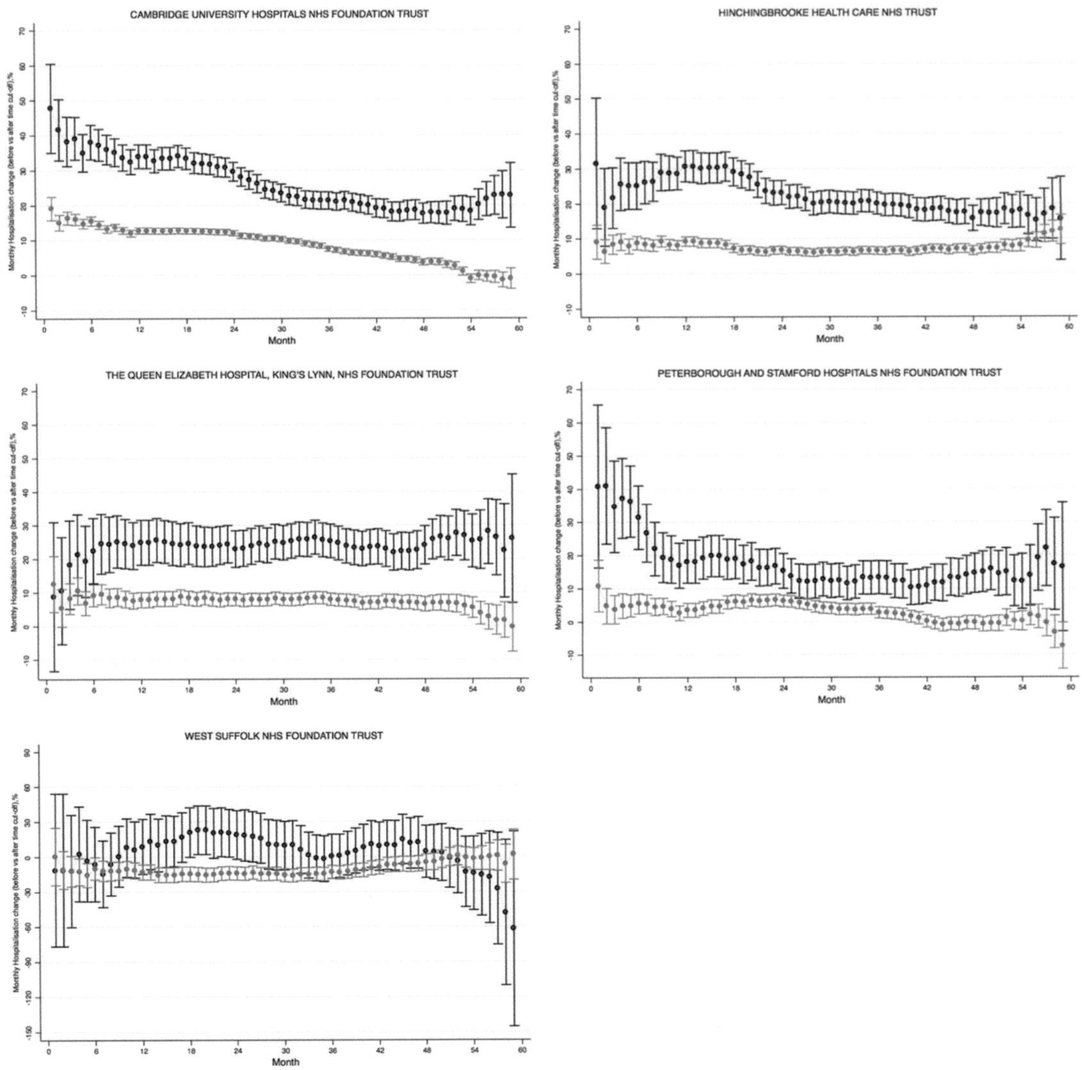

Fig. 7.7 Monthly percentage change in hospital admission rate (monthly hospital admission rate before and after the month) by hospital and diabetes status. *Black* (*upper*) plot represents for hospital admission change percentage for those with diabetes. *Grey* (*lower*) plot represents for hospital admission change percentage for those without diabetes. Figures above 0 % indicate that the mean monthly hospitalisation rate after the index month is greater than the mean hospitalisation rate before the index month

interviews, supplemented by more casual interactions, were carried out with 21 patients (primary care alone in two practices (n=7), DICI service (n=7), hospital multidisciplinary clinic (n=7)) and 20 health-care professionals (ten DICI staff, six hospital staff (three podiatrists, one consultant, one DSN, one DSD) across two hospitals and four primary care staff (two practice nurse and two GPs) across four practices). Patients (17/21) were interviewed on two occasions at least 6 months apart to obtain insight into how care and perspectives changed. Interview data and ethnographic notes were transcribed and entered into NVivo 9 for analytical coding using a grounded theory approach [23]. The datasets were cross-referenced for further refinement and corroboration.

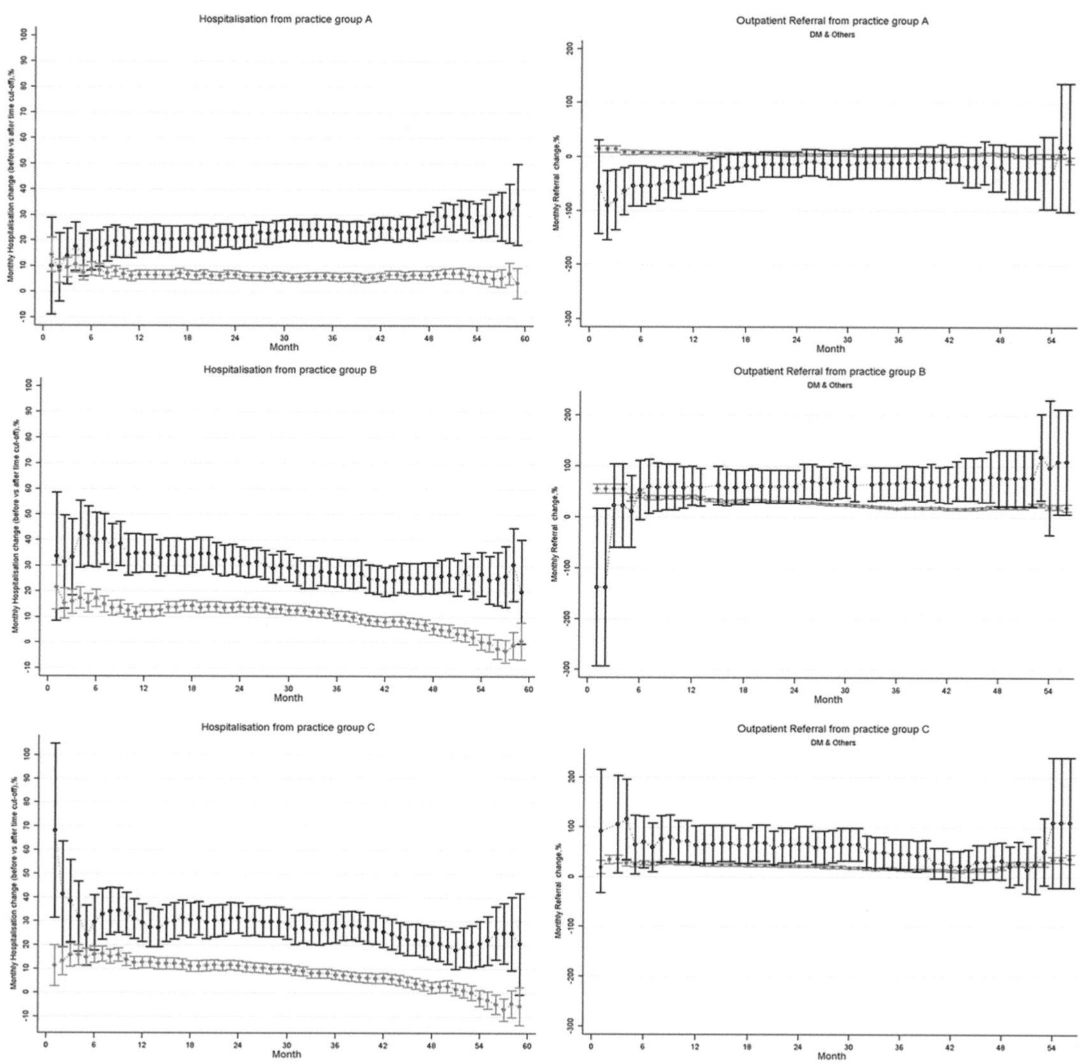

Fig. 7.8 Monthly percentage change in hospital admission rate and in outpatient referral rate (monthly hospital admission rate before and after the month) by practice group. *Left* plots are for inpatient hospitalisation; *right* plots are for outpatient referral rate. *Black* (*upper*) plot represents for hospital admission/outpatient referral change percentage for those with diabetes. *Grey* (*lower*) plot represents for hospital admission/outpatient referral change percentage for those without diabetes. Practice group A is associated with DSN A. Practice group B is associated with DSN B. Practice group C is associated with DSN C. Figures above 0 % indicate that the mean monthly hospitalisation/attendance rate after the index month is greater than the mean hospitalisation/attendance rate before the index month

Detailed comments from the interviews are shown elsewhere [12], and indicated three themes:

- Integration
- Continuity of care: the Health-care professional and patient relationship
- The need for tailored care

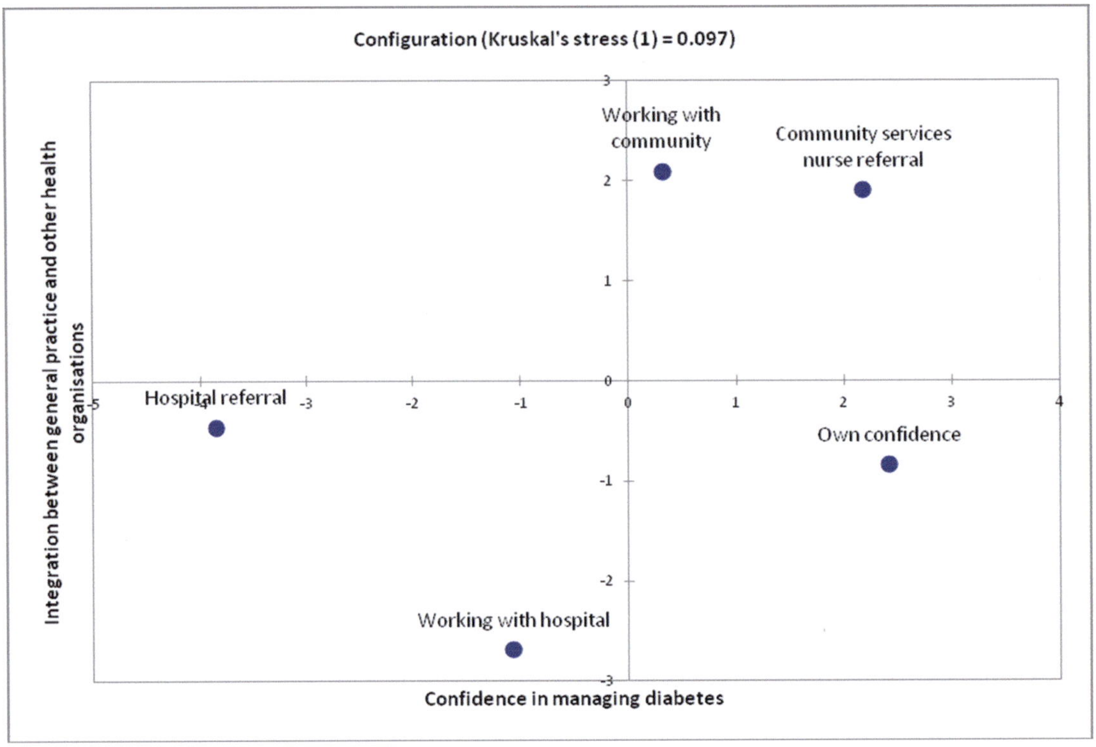

Fig. 7.9 Mapping of the questions according to their dissimilarities based upon the practice nurse survey

Discussion

The expansion of the community diabetes team was successfully implemented across ECF, patient experiences were positive, PN clinical confidence improved, and there were early reports of clinical benefit [10, 11]. The approach was seen as sufficiently beneficial for one GP group in South Cambridgeshire, CamHealth, to invest in a similar joint service. It is therefore surprising that the DICI was associated with no improvement in QoF measures and no reduction, and indeed perhaps a worsening, in hospitalisation among those with diabetes over the 3 year period. In view of the size of the investment, the acceptability of the approach to patients, primary care and the diabetes specialist services and the fulfilment of the goals of "care closer to home" and primary care support, the question has to be asked why no improvements were shown over 3 years?

Was the Time to Show Benefits Too Short?

Lower hospitalisation rates have been seen in similar interventions in other countries within 12 months within single providers [24, 25], or in contexts where multiple primary care providers work with a single specialist provider under an integrated insurance scheme [26]. Foot interventions have also been shown to have benefits on a population basis within 2–3 years [27, 28]. Although changes in some adverse outcomes (e.g., cardiovascular disease, microvascular disease) would take longer than 3 years, the absence of any positive impact on foot admissions in spite of a major increase in resource indicates that the time should have been sufficient to show an improvement in at least this key indicator of success.

Were Patients Worse at Baseline in ECF?

We wondered if the greater pre-existing morbidity and lower socioeconomic status in ECF was a major influence, particularly in those practices

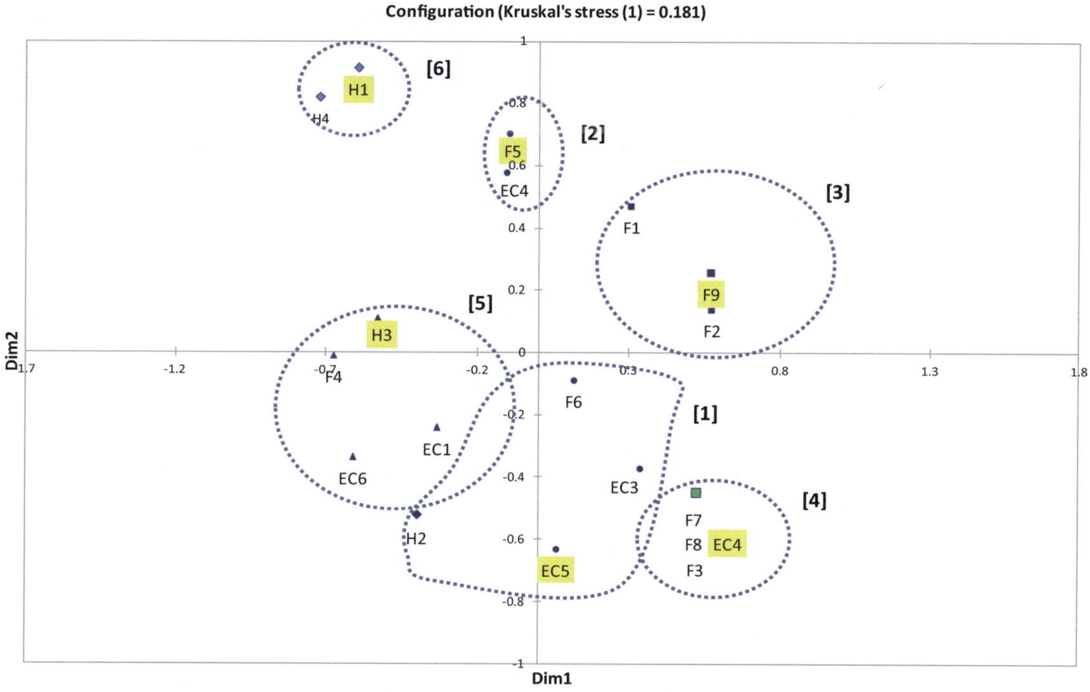

Fig. 7.10 Mapping of the health-care providers according to their dissimilarities and clusters based upon the Practice nurse survey. The typical members of the clusters are highlighted. Hospitals (H1-4), Fenland practices (F1-9), East Cambs practices (EC1-EC6), Trinity (Fenland) did not participate in the survey and Sutton had a new practice nurse at the time of the survey

associated with DSN A. However, those practices were across ECF, and the trends were not shown with DSN B or C. In fact, neither the QoF data nor the hospitalisation data support that patients with diabetes were worse off at baseline in ECF. There was evidence that the trajectory for those practices associated with DSN A was downward.

Were Benefits Obscured by Secular Changes?

One weakness of the study is that it was not a randomised controlled trial and therefore influenced by historical, secular and other changes. By comparing data between the three Cambridgeshire areas and between those with and without diabetes, we had hoped to minimise confounding: all patients were under the same commissioners (CPCT), with no differences in policies overall. We excluded possible confounders such as changes in hospital admission and diabetes coding policies, as the changes occurred independent of hospital.

The collateral data indicating no significant improvements in metabolic control in ECF also support the evidence that although the DICI was implemented, it had no major population impact.

Was the Intervention Fully Implemented and Maintained?

The clinical interventions were indeed implemented and horizontal integration occurred for most of the 3 years. It is clear, however, that the vertical integration components were not implemented successfully. The approach appeared to reduce integration between hospitals and primary care, something that is clearly at the core of successful initiatives.

The failure to implement integrated information management for putative information governance reasons, almost certainly contributed to communication and integration difficulties. Most integrated care initiatives attempt to include data sharing [29] and this was not possible within the local information governance arrangements. This was noticed by the patients and was a source of frustration.

Several interventions were not maintained. The multidisciplinary clinic in the north of the county (Wisbech) occurred only a few times, as a result of a lack of space-although a clinic was attempted within one large general practice, this had to be out of hours which was too difficult to maintain. After the rejection of the countywide approach, a more competitive atmosphere appeared to emerge. For example, the reducing numbers attending DAFNE provided by Addenbrookes Hospital in ECF and Cambridge, coincided with the community services increasing referrals to the hospital service in Huntingdonshire, run by the community services themselves. These were also associated with the recognition of defects in the clinical governance approach. Such clinical changes probably reflected reductions in the degree of vertical integration as the new GP commissioning era began to be introduced.

Was There Something Intrinsic About the Model-Lack of Vertical Integration?

We feel that the low degree of vertical integration provides a clue as to the reason for the failure of the ECF DICI to impact on hospitalisation over the 3 years. In fact, the vertical integration was never fully implemented, something the proposed countywide diabetes proposal was intended to address. The proposed plan included a pooling of the diabetes service funds and a fully integrated countywide clinical/corporate governance framework-more akin to a joint venture model.

The ECF DICI generated a closer relationship between the community services and general practice, and initially with Addenbrookes Hospital. However, the relationships between the ECF DICI and 3 of the other neighbouring hospitals remained limited and competitive. While the community Wisbech clinic was not maintained, the Wisbech clinic that was an outreach service from the neighbouring hospital was not included in the integrated care plan. Conversely, the non-medical diabetes specialist staff in the fourth hospital (Hinchinbrooke in Huntingdonshire), were already employed by the community services. During the time of the ECF DICI, Circle, a private provider took over the running of the hospital in Huntingdonshire (Hinchinbrooke) (http://www.circlehealth.co.uk/about-circle/media/circle-named-as-hinchingbrooke-preferred--bidder-nov-10, accessed 26/6/2015) through a competitive tender process. The Doddington community clinic, run with Peterborough Hospital for over 20 years, was taken over by Hinchinbrooke Hospital with the community services, again highlighting the competitive nature of the Cambridgeshire environment. Perhaps in a less competitive, more collaborative environment, ECF DICI would have successfully impacted on diabetes hospitalisation.

Was There Something Intrinsic About the Model: Piggy in the Middle?

Hints as to why this three component model (GP, hospital, community services) might not be effective come from the observation that the preceding nurse led service in ECF had reductions in referrals to hospital outpatients as one of its targets [2], and changes in outpatient appointments were included in the DICI variation in contract. Similar emphasis on reducing hospital outpatient referrals (ergo payments) was included in, e.g., Birmingham [30]. Within this context, it was perhaps to be expected that attempts at creating greater integration in information management, clinical governance, budget and overall management were agreed but not implemented: actions more achievable within a single organisation.

Interestingly, integration was perceived as happening when there was one person "fronting up" for all those involved [12]. Case management has been proposed as one approach to integration, and requires the case manager to corral and coordinate the services for a given individual [31].

Clinical inertia, a less "aggressive" approach to management under non MDT management, greater PN confidence and financial disincentives to referral to the hospital clinics, could all have delayed onward referral to the broader associated multidisciplinary team management. We wonder if the diabetes foot intervention reflects this most clearly. The DSP made major, and successful, efforts to link in with the four neighbouring hospital diabetes foot clinics. However, the interviews suggest that this was associated with delayed referral for MDT foot care, i.e., the DICI service promoted hospital avoidance rather than admission avoidance [12]. Many PNs reported that their working with the hospital services was reduced, suggesting that the placement of the DSNs between the practice and the hospital service created a barrier not a bridge to optimal care. In fact stepping back, a possible explanation for the lack of effectiveness on a population basis, may be that the community service were popular with general practices by reducing their diabetes workload (perhaps resulting in similar outcomes), while obstructing the on-referral to often more skilled, multidisciplinary, one stop shop hospital services (perhaps resulting in worse outcomes for the non-referred patients). This was further undermined by the inability of the local leadership to translate into reality, countywide agreements, across all health professionals and patient representatives, on education, information management, clinical governance and a vertically integrated approach.

Is the ECF Experience Likely to Be "Typical"?

Whether our findings are due to a unique set of circumstances or a predictable consequence of a three compartment model in a competitive local health system is unclear, but there are indications that the circumstances are not special. There are calls for more integration and less fragmentation in health-care [30], yet so far, the major integration projects in England have revealed negligible, if any, benefits [25, 32]. The latest changes in commissioning in the English NHS, with emphasis on the need to consider "Any qualified Provider" in service delivery, and associated market procurement approaches, could well impair the quality of diabetes care while increasing overall cost, if the experience here is reproduced elsewhere. Calls for more integrated care have not yet addressed the need for a competition, and in Derby, "a perceived to be successful" integrated (joint venture) care programme was not recommissioned [33].

Conclusion

In conclusion, these data show no improvement in outcomes with investment in a separate community diabetes specialist service, and increased fragmentation between primary and secondary care. While horizontal integration occurred, vertical integration was negligible.

Studies to demonstrate improvements in diabetes outcomes with alternative models of care are urgently needed.

Acknowledgements Elissa Harwood collected some ethnographic data and Chris Bunn/Simon Cohn undertook the analyses reported elsewhere [12, 15]. Tosin Daniels undertook the practice nurse interviews. We thank the patients and staff for their interviews, Michael Thoresby for extracting the PCT data, Liz Robin for her useful comments on the analysis and paper drafts. We thank The ECF Diabetes Integrated Care Team and local practices for their hard work, the Addenbrookes Hospital Diabetes Care Patient Advisory Committee for guidance.

This paper presents independent research funded by the National Institute for Health Research (NIHR) under its Research for Patient Benefit (RfPB) Programme (Grant Reference Number PB-PG-0808-17303). The views expressed are those of the authors and not necessarily those of the NHS, the NIHR or the Department of Health.

References

1. Department of Health/Royal College of General Practitioners. Guidelines for the appointment of general practitioners with special interests in the delivery of clinical services: diabetes. London: DOH; 2003.
2. Hollern H, Lunn J. Development of a primary care specialist diabetes nursing service. J Diabetes Nurs. 2004;8:344–8.
3. Hicks D, James J, Hill J, Vanterpool G. Audit of the effectiveness of nurse consultant led intermediate diabetes care services in England. Pract Diabetes. 2012;29:54–7.
4. Armstrong N, Baines D, Baker R, Crossman R, Davies M, Hardy A, Khunti K, Kumar S, O'Hare JP, Raymond N, Saravanan P, Stallard N, Szczepura A, Wilson A, ICCD Study Group. A cluster randomized controlled trial of the effectiveness and cost-

effectiveness of intermediate care clinics for diabetes (ICCD): study protocol for a randomized controlled trial. Trials. 2012;13:164.
5. Simmons D, Wenzel H. Diabetes inpatients: a case of lose, lose, lose. Is it time to use a "Diabetes Attributable Hospitalisation Cost" to assess the impact of diabetes? Diabet Med. 2011;28:1123–8.
6. Lafond S, Charlesworth A, Roberts A. Hospital finances and productivity: in a critical condition? London: Health Foundation; 2015.
7. The Action to Control Cardiovascular Risk in Diabetes Study Group. Effects of intensive glucose lowering in type 2 diabetes. N Engl J Med. 2008;358:2545–59.
8. Calvert M, Shankar A, McManus RJ, Lester H, Freemantle N. Effect of the quality and outcomes framework on diabetes care in the United Kingdom: retrospective cohort study. BMJ. 2009;338:b1870.
9. Rayman G, Kilvert A. The crisis in diabetes care in England. BMJ. 2012;345:e5446.
10. Hollern H, Simmons D. Cost saving and improved glycaemic control in an integrated diabetes service. Prim Care Diabetes. 2011;13:176–81.
11. Simmons D, Yu D, Wenzel H. Changes in hospital admissions and inpatient tariff associated with a diabetes integrated care initiative: preliminary findings. J Diabetes. 2014;6:81–9.
12. Simmons D, Yu D, Bunn C, Cohn S, Wenzel H, Prevost T. Hospitalization among patients with diabetes associated with a diabetes integrated care initiative: a mixed methods case study. Future Hosp J. 2015;2(2):92–8.
13. Elliott J, Jacques RM, Kruger J, Campbell MJ, Amiel SA, Mansell P, Speight J, Brennan A, Heller SR. Substantial reductions in the number of diabetic ketoacidosis and severe hypoglycaemia episodes requiring emergency treatment lead to reduced costs after structured education in adults with type 1 diabetes. Diabet Med. 2014;31:847–53.
14. Simmons D, English P, Robins P, Craig A, Addicott R. Should diabetes be commissioned through multidisciplinary networks, rather than practice based commissioning? Prim Care Diabetes. 2011;5:39–44.
15. Harwood E, Bunn C, Caton C, Simmons D. Addressing barriers to diabetes care and self-care in general practice: a new framework for practice nurses. J Diabetes Nurs. 2013;17:186–91.
16. Simmons D, Weblemoe T, Voyle J, Prichard A, Leakehe L, Gatland B. Personal barriers to diabetes care: lessons from a multiethnic community in New Zealand. Diabet Med. 1998;15:958–64.
17. Piatt GA, Songer TJ, Brooks MM, Anderson RM, Simmons D, Orchard TJ, Siminerio LM, Korytkowski MT, Zgibor JC. Impact of patient level factors on the improvement of the ABCs of diabetes. Patient Educ Couns. 2011;82:266–70.
18. Simmons D, Bourke L, Yau E, Hoodless M. Diabetes risk factors, diabetes and diabetes care in a rural Australian community. Aust J Rural Health. 2007;15:296–303.
19. Langlands A. The good governance – standard for public services. London: OPM/CIPFA; 2004.
20. Anderson R. New MRC, guidance on evaluating complex interventions. BMJ. 2008;337:a1937.
21. Rencher AC. Methods of multivariate analysis. New York: J. Wiley; 2002.
22. Backhaus K, Erichson B, Plinke W, Weiber R. Multivariate Analysemethoden. Eine anwendungsorientierte Einführung. Berlin: Springer; 1996.
23. Pope C, Ziebland S, Mays N. Analysing qualitative data. BMJ. 2000;320:114–6.
24. Jha A, Perlin J, Kizer K, Dudley R. Effect of the transformation of the veterans health care system on the quality of care. N Engl J Med. 2003;348:2218–27.
25. Ham C, Curry N. Integrated care: what is it? Does it work? What does it mean for the NHS? London: Kings Fund; 2011.
26. Distiller LA, Brown MA, Joffe BI, Kramer BD. Striving for the impossible dream: a community based multi-practice collaborative model of diabetes management. Diab Med. 2010;27:197–202.
27. Lavery LA, Wunderlich RP, Tredwell JL. Disease management for the diabetic foot: effectiveness of a diabetic foot prevention program to reduce amputations and hospitalizations. Diabetes Res Clin Pract. 2005;70:31–7.
28. Rith-Najarian S, Branchaud C, Beaulieu O, Gohdes D, Simonson G, Mazze R. Reducing lower-extremity amputations due to diabetes. Application of the staged diabetes management approach in a primary care setting. J Fam Pract. 1998;47(2):127–32 [serial online].
29. Ham C, Walsh N. Making integrated care happen at scale and pace. London: Kings Fund; 2013.
30. Hill J. Seamless diabetes care: the role of the nurse consultant. J Diabetes Nurs. 2008;12:149–54.
31. Norris SL, Nichols PJ, Caspersen CJ, Glasgow RE, Engelgau MM, Jack Jr L, Isham G, Snyder SR, Carande-Kulis VG, Garfield S, Briss P, McCulloch D. The effectiveness of disease and case management for people with diabetes: a systematic review. Am J Prev Med. 2002;22(4S):15–38.
32. RAND Europe, Ernst & Young LLP. National evaluation of the department of health's integrated care pilots: final report:full version. London: RAND Europe, Ernst & Young LLP; 2012.
33. Hussain S, Dornhorst A. Integrated care – taking specialist medical care beyond the hospital walls. London: Royal College of Physicians; 2015.

8 UK Approaches to Integrated Diabetes Care: Derby—A Joint Venture Model Under the NHS

Paromita King

Why Change?

Derby City has a population of 250,000 with 18,000 people with diabetes. It has areas of social deprivation with ethnic minority populations who have a high prevalence of diabetes with prevalence rates of 10 % compared with 6.2 % in the UK in 2014 [1, 2]. Before 2008, Derby had a traditional acute trust centred model for diabetes care, with pockets of specialist services in the community.

Acute trust clinicians felt that there were large numbers being seen for routine review, with frequent duplication of appointments compromising the capacity of the service. However, variation in provision and expertise in primary care limited the ability to discharge stable patients to increase capacity.

Primary care clinicians were overseeing the care of an increasing number of people with Type 2 diabetes, often with complex co-morbidities. Difficulties in communication with the secondary care team was not only frustrating, but patients struggled to access care in a timely manner resulting in preventable admissions.

People with diabetes stated that they valued the expertise of the specialist team; but we provided poor continuity of care resulting in them having to tell their story repeatedly. The frustrations are exemplified by Mrs, Smith (Case) and her experience summarised in Fig. 8.1.

P. King (✉)
Department of Diabetes and Endocrinology, Medical Specialties, Derby Teaching Hospitals NHS Foundation Trust, Royal Derby Hospital, Derby, UK
e-mail: Pking2@nhs.net

> **Case** Mrs Smith, age 46, has insulin treated type 2 diabetes and is overweight with poor glucose control. Her GP has sent her to the hospital diabetes team. Each time she attends she sees a different doctor who tells her to lose weight. The last doctor was uncertain how to help her as she has forgotten to bring her list of medication with her but refers her to a nurse for help with insulin management and a dietitian to lose weight. In the last 2 months she has had four appointments to see the consultant, nurse and dietitian as well as attended for retinal screening and a foot check. She has to take two buses to attend hospital and has found that her glucose control has not improved and that she has gained rather than lost weight. At her last appointment the nurse referred her back to the consultant who said he would write to the GP and sends her back to the nurse. Her GP feels unable to help as he has not received any communication from the hospital as the secretary is off sick. Frustrated at the lack of progress and her time consuming journeys she disengages and does not attend.

D. Simmons et al. (eds.), *Integrated Diabetes Care*, DOI 10.1007/978-3-319-13389-8_8

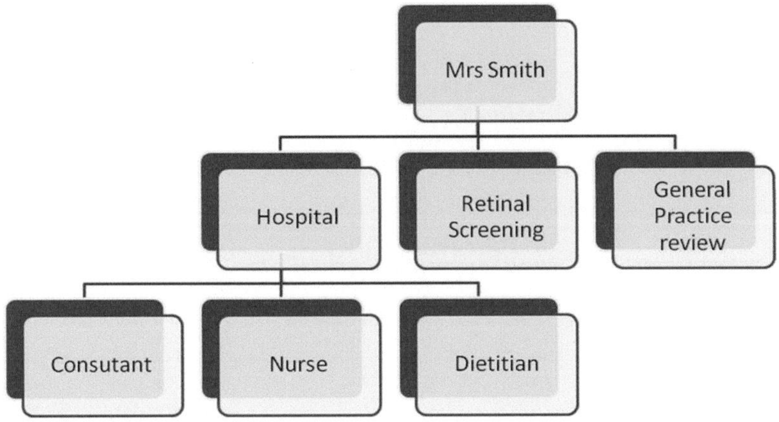

Fig. 8.1 Traditional model-duplication of specialist appointments, inaccessible service and poor communication resulting in a disengaged patient

All involved in the care of people with diabetes and the users felt that the service was fragmented, with variation of provision and expertise, and that there was a clear case to redesign the service to better meet our user needs.

Our Vision

Inspired by the 2008 Royal Colleges' publication "Teams without Walls" [3], our vision was to move away from the silos of the traditional model, where each professional works diligently in relative isolation delivering their part of the pathway, to designing seamless pathways around the user rather than location, where they were seen by the right person at the right time. In addition, we wanted to reduce variation and duplication, improve outcomes across the whole health community and improve communication as well as the user experience. Our aim was to achieve this through an integrated approach. While there are many definitions of integrated care, our vision is succinctly summarised by The King's Fund/Nuffield Trust [4] as:

> An approach that seeks to improve the quality of care for individual patients, service users and carers by ensuring that services are well co-ordinated around their needs.

How Did We Approach the Problem?

Acute trust clinicians and managers, general practitioners and the primary care trust worked collaboratively to develop a whole system approach to the patient's journey that was integrated at organisational, financial, technological (IT) as well as clinical levels. The model was underpinned by a single clinical governance structure [5]. This involved a monthly multidisciplinary team meeting of clinicians, managers and users with the remit to continuously improve the standard of clinical practice. This is the first diabetes model in the UK that has successfully integrated at all these levels, and these principles are included in the five pillars of integration or key enablers in national documents recommending best practice for commissioning [6] and clinical practice [7]:

1. A single IT system or integrated IT
2. Alignment of finances
3. Care Planning
4. Clinical Engagement
5. Single Clinical Governance Structure.

The Derby Model

Like "evidenced based medicine," integration is a term currently much in use, but not always with a full understanding of what it means in practical terms, and so an appreciation of the different aspects of integration is important to gain an understanding of the Derby model.

Organisational Integration

It was felt that an organisation equally owned by primary *and* secondary care was fundamental to fostering the shared responsibility and clinical ownership that is essential when working across organisational boundaries. In addition, it would allow services that were needed to deliver seamless pathways centred around the user to be brought together under one umbrella. There are a number of legal frameworks available in the UK that could have potentially achieved these objectives [8]. The options considered included Social Enterprises and companies limited by guarantee. A Social Enterprise is an organisation whose members share the same core values and where the business has "primarily social objectives whose surpluses are principally reinvested for that purpose in the business and community" [8]. In a company limited by guarantee, members who run the company are bound by a guarantee rather than shares which require them to pay for debts up to an agreed maximum amount. Ultimately, a joint venture company limited by shares was chosen as the best vehicle to obtain a Specialist Provider Medical Services (SPMS) contract while retaining the flexibility to diversify within and beyond diabetes services [9].

Two joint venture organisations, First Diabetes and InterCare Health, were commissioned by Derby City Primary Care Trust in 2009 to deliver NHS services for the patients with diabetes in the two practice based commissioning groups that covered Derby City. These were both not for profit National Health Service Companies limited by shares.

First Diabetes was established to support the First Provider group of practices which comprised five practices with 2500 people with diabetes. The company had only two shares; one owned by the First Provider group and the other by the acute trust, and was overseen by a Board comprising two Directors one from First Provider group and one from the acute trust.

The second practice based commissioning group comprised 29 GP practices with 15,000 people with diabetes and was supported by InterCare Health Limited. InterCare was briefly piloted in seven practices before rolling out to the 29. InterCare was also jointly owned by primary and secondary care, but there were six shares held by three GPs and three by the acute trust, two senior managers and a consultant. These shareholders comprised the Board of the company which had contractual, governance and financial responsibility of the InterCare diabetes service. The services provided by the two companies were similar, but further description of the model relates specifically to the InterCare diabetes service.

Financial Integration

All diabetes care was delivered using a single pooled budget with the exception of complex services requiring cross speciality working. These exceptions included: inpatients, multidisciplinary foot care, antenatal (not preconception), joint renal clinics and transition.

A single budget allowed us to deliver seamless pathways across organisational boundaries without the competition imposed by Payment by Results, the payment system in England by which commissioners pay providers a nationally agreed tariff for each patient seen depending on the type and complexity of the case [10]. It also allowed the clinical team to own problems as well as solutions and invest profits from efficiencies into new areas of care. For example, InterCare funded the innovative community based integrated preconception care model PROCEED [11] after the end of its funded pilot until its business case was accepted by Southern Derbyshire Clinical Commissioning Group.

Information Technology Integration

In Derby City 85 % of practices use The Phoenix Project (TPP), SystmOne, which was used by InterCare and First Diabetes to provide a single shared record. As part of the referral process to specialist services, the patient consented to their record being shared. Access to the record at the point of referral ensured that they saw the most appropriate clinician to meet their needs avoiding duplication as well as being able to provide holistic and safe care. The electronic communication system using Tasks (similar to messaging) enabled instant communication between clinicians and organisations. For example, a GP and nurse specialist were able to view each other's consultations and clinicians were able to ask for advice or agree a plan of care. In addition, the specialist team could make recommendations to changes in the treatment which could be implemented without waiting for letters or the need for the user to make an additional appointment with their GP.

Clinical Integration

Core Care

For the majority who have Type 2 diabetes, core care was undertaken in the primary care setting, with care seamlessly escalated to and de-escalated from the specialist team across organisational boundaries as needed. The terms "escalation" and "de-escalation" reflect the fact that the whole team of clinicians were responsible for the care of people with diabetes either directly or indirectly through raising standards of care through the support and training outlined below. In addition, the terms reflects the lack of financial (payment by results) or technological (multiple patient records) thresholds that have to be crossed, as might be understood by the traditional terms "refer" and "discharge."

Supporting Primary Care

Practice support was designed to improve standards of care and reduced variation. A nurse specialist and consultant provided satellite support to the practices tailored in accordance to their needs. This ranged from supporting clinics in surgeries to case based discussion. In addition, educational courses were provided for all practices, which included sessions on improving the psychological literacy of consultations through the promotion of motivational interviewing techniques, the promotion of shared decision-making and care planning as well as sessions on complications of diabetes and glucose management. Visits to practices were mutually beneficial as it also allowed members of the specialist team to gain an understanding of some of the pressures of working in primary care and the visits were also invaluable for building relationships and partnership working.

Education for People with Diabetes

Fragmentation of commissioning of educational initiatives meant delivering equitable education for type 2 diabetes was challenging. Through subcontracting arrangements, the different educational resources were brought together to provide equitable access to structured education for Type 1 and 2 diabetes at diagnosis and other points of the users' journey. These included DAFNE (Dose Adjustment for Normal Eating) for Type 1 diabetes, and a range of locally developed initiatives to address the needs of those with prediabetes, newly diagnosed Type 2 diabetes, people on maximum oral hypoglycaemic agents and those on a basal bolus insulin regimen.

Specialist Care

When targets were not being met or where there was a need for specialist team support, care was escalated to the multidisciplinary team where the user could be seen in one of the four community based clinics of their choice. As stated above, a single record meant the user saw the right clinicians to meet their needs or access the most appropriate educational initiative. They were also able to have other aspects of their care such as retinal screening at the same time as seeing the diabetes clinicians. To promote shared decision-making, mutually agreed targets such as HbA1c or weight were set in consultations and recorded on templates that were visible to the primary care team. When targets were achieved, care could be de-escalated back to the primary care team. The user was given a contact number for the service or clinician so that if support or advice was needed in the future, they were able to directly access the specialist team and retain continuity of care. The de-escalation allowed the service to maintain sufficient capacity to see users urgently if needed but did not leave patients and colleagues feeling isolated and unsupported.

Services requiring horizontal or cross speciality integration in the acute trust were outside the integrated diabetes contract, and financially supported by Payment by Results rather than the single integrated care budget, and included transition, multidisciplinary foot care, antenatal and renal services. Clinical pathways in integrated care were extended beyond these contractual limits so that the user journey could be continued seamlessly in and out of secondary care services. For example when a woman attending the integrated care preconception service became pregnant, her care would be transferred to the antenatal clinic. While this service was outside integrated care, the same clinicians worked in integrated care and the antenatal clinic, maintaining continuity of care for the user. Postnatally, she would be transferred back to integrated care and if appropriate her care could be de-escalated to Primary care.

In addition to these core principles, there were a number of initiatives to meet the needs of specific groups.

Type 1 Diabetes

Users with Type 1 diabetes described the importance of seeing clinicians who understood the principles of intensive glucose management such as carbohydrate counting and basal rate testing for those on pumps. Most felt that the primary care team did not have these skills and that it was important to maintain contact with the specialist team, not so much for routine review, but to support them at times of crisis. As the skills of the primary care team improved, many were comfortable to attend primary care for their annual review but to have a telephone consultation from the specialist team to support any care planning issues that arose from their review. With the technological advances in the management of Type 1 diabetes, these users were offered a Consultant appointment every 2–3 years as an opportunity to review their medication, and discuss new technologies such as advances in glucose meters and pumps. When a preference was expressed for traditional care, the annual reviews were undertaken by the specialist team.

Hard to Reach Groups

Practising in community based settings gave clinicians the opportunity to develop other partnerships to improve care for those who are traditionally hard to reach. For example, by working with the community matrons (advanced nurse practitioners with clinical and a case management role coordinating care in the community for those with complex needs [12]), who also use SystmOne, housebound users could be supported at a distance.

Derby has a large South Asian Community and we have worked across organisational boundaries to bring services together to meet their needs through a Community Engagement Project. For example, bilingual educators and interpreters supported the delivery of structured education, and public health colleagues attended these sessions to promote their lifestyle initiatives, in particular local walking groups. The dietitian leading the project established links in religious and community venues to deliver healthy eating and cooking sessions in Hindu temples, gurdwaras and Pakistani community centres. In addition, she supported the local community pharmacists who were undertaking diabetes awareness events where a risk calculator was used to discuss individual risk. The dietitian and pharmacist could then discuss lifestyle changes at an individual level.

Clinical Governance

All these measures were supported by a single clinical governance structure. A multidisciplinary clinical board of managers, administrators, primary and secondary care clinicians and users met monthly to address issues of clinical governance such as:

- Staff competencies and mandatory training (supported by annual appraisal).
- Plan Do Study Act cycles, case reviews and audits to drive efficiencies to continuously improve quality and look for new opportunities for service development.
- Discuss safety issues.
- Review pathways.
- Review agreed outcomes including user experience.

The chair of the clinical board reported monthly to the InterCare Health Limited board of directors, who carried ultimate responsibility for the governance of the service.

Summary

In summary, the five pillars of integration have allowed people with diabetes in Derby City to access a model of care that has pathways centred around them rather than location and is delivered by a team working together across organisational boundaries committed to delivering the best care.

Mrs. Smith in Integrated Care

Returning to Mrs Smith, the case account below and Fig. 8.2 describes a different experience in a system where diabetes care is integrated.

Case The Practice is struggling with Mrs Smith's diabetes and has referred her to the specialist team for help with glucose control and weight. The practice has been trained and the nurse is aware that GLP-1 analogues may be the best way forward for her, but she has not yet had much experience in the use of GLP-1 analogues with insulin. At the time of referral, Mrs Smith consents to sharing her record. The GP lead who is reviewing referrals is able to see the reason for referral and the whole GP record. It is clear that she has been on insulin for a number of years, but is struggling with weight and her glucose control remains poor. It is also clear that there are no other medical issues and that Mrs Smith is not at risk of pancreatitis, has normal liver and renal function. He can see that the practice regularly undertake her review but she is due her retinal screening. He recommends that Mrs Smith has a single appointment with the nurse specialist and dietitian and then follow up with the nurse.

(continued)

The administrator contacts Mrs Smith who chooses to attend at a community based venue within walking distance of her home. Her retinal screening is arranged on the same day. When she attends, she sees the dietitian and the nurse specialist together to ascertain her priorities and set mutually agreed targets in terms of glucose control and weight loss and the practice is sent a Task to prescribe the GLP-1 analogue. Further appointments with the nurse specialist are face to face and by telephone where her progress and targets can be reviewed. As she begins to lose weight, and glucose control improves, she is empowered to adjust her own insulin and is able to reduce the dose herself, thus reducing the number of appointments needed. When she achieves her targets, her care is de-escalated to the practice, but she has the nurse's mobile number and telephone as well as e-mail and telephone contacts for the service so she can call or request an appointment if she has problems in the future.

Service Evaluation

Outcome data for First Diabetes are published elsewhere [9]. InterCare Health was commissioned for 3 years, so a comprehensive service evaluation was presented to commissioners as we approached the end of the contract in 2012/2013, although aspects of service evaluation were regularly evaluated as part of Plan Do Study Act cycles to continuously improve quality.

The Donabedian principles [13] of improvements in structure, process and outcome were core to the service design. The changes in structure are described above and the service evaluation concentrated on process and outcome measures. In addition, indicators were chosen to reflect all six domains of quality improvement as described in the 2001 National Institute of Medicine/National Academy of Science publication "Crossing the Quality Chasm" [14]:

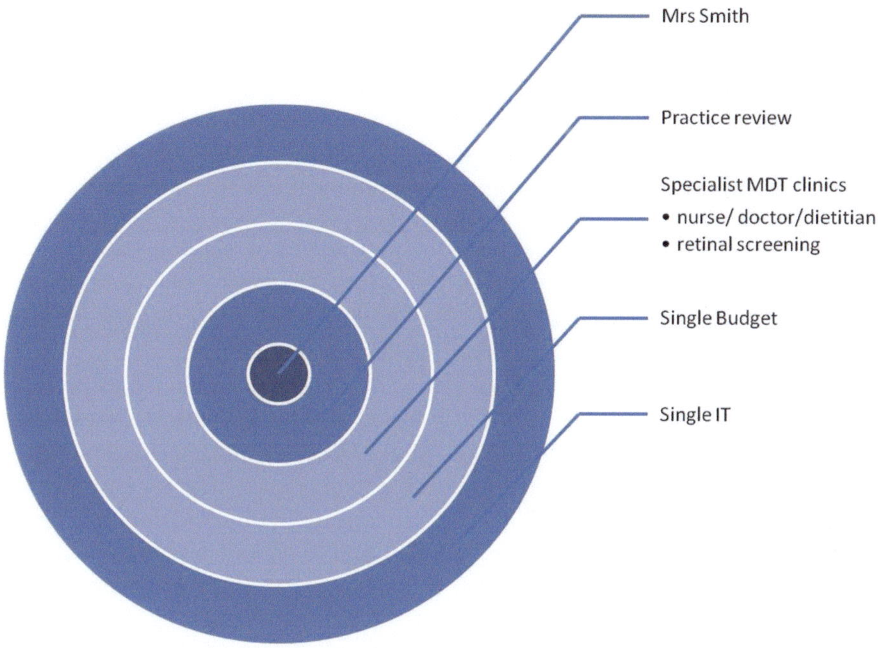

Fig. 8.2 Integrated care with care centred around the user, with routine review at the practice but additional care at one venue using a shared record and free of financial restraints allowing flow of care across organisational boundaries

- *Effectiveness* was assessed though evaluating changes in individual and service level glucose and blood pressure control, and also looking at the impact on admissions with a primary diagnosis of diabetes.
- *Efficiency and Timeliness* was evaluated by auditing the referral and assessment system.
- *Equity* was improved by implementing the measures to improve access and provision for hard to reach groups, and evaluated through user feedback.
- *Safety* was evaluated in plan do study act cycles, changes in glucose, blood pressure control and ascertaining whether there was a reduction in admissions due to diabetes.
- The provision of a *Person Centred Service* was assessed through the implementation of target setting reflecting shared decision-making as well as staff and user experience.

Methodology

A Care Bundled approach was used to systematically appraise the quality of the service in 2012–2013. This means that the entire care pathway was evaluated using a whole group of endpoints rather than individual items. The approach is described in "*10 High Impact Changes for Service Improvement and Delivery*" Change 6, NHS Institute for Innovation and Improvement, 2004 [15]. This approach, particularly when used in conjunction with Plan Do Study Act cycles, has been shown to reduce variation and is appropriate for supporting a care pathway crossing organisational boundaries.

Data from the National Diabetes information Service [9] were used to evaluate quality outcome framework targets in Derby City.

Process

Data were collected prospectively using SystmOne and reviewed monthly.

Activity

Activity in 2012–2013 was in line with our plan and there was a progressive reduction in patients attending acute trust clinics and an increase in those attending integrated care. Initially 50 % of all activity was undertaken in the acute trust, but an increasing number of users were transferred to the new service and by the end of 2012, 70 % of people with diabetes were being seen in integrated care.

In 2012, fewer patients failed to attend their appointments (DNA) in integrated care specialist clinics compared with the acute trust with rates reducing from 20 % to 11 % for nurse specialists and 16–11 % for consultant sessions. In 2013 our overall DNA rate was reduced to 7 %.

Referral and Assessment

The referral and assessment process is unique and was audited in two time periods during 2012. The components of the process were broken down and time frames allocated to each (Fig. 8.3). The aim was to process 90 % of referrals in the time period. The outcome of the audit is shown in Fig. 8.4.

Referrals were sent to the service electronically through SystmOne. The user consented to their record being released to the specialist team as part of the referral process. The GP lead triaged these referrals, and as he had access to the whole patient record was able to allocate the most appropriate clinician or clinicians for the user to see or to give advice. The target of 48 h turnaround was achieved in all but one of the referrals. The next step was contacting the user to arrange a convenient appointment and our administrative team consistently achieved this within 72 h. The last step was the time to the first appointment. In the first audit, it appears that only 84 % achieved this target, but when the reasons behind this were explored, the majority of cases the delay was due to user choice. When this was considered, the 90 % target was met as 94 % achieved the target.

These targets continued to be met. Although InterCare was not commissioned to deliver an urgent service, unlike the traditional model it was able to generate sufficient capacity to be able to see urgent referrals and promptly respond to queries, and so provide a safer as well as a more efficient service than the traditional model.

These outcomes demonstrated the efficiency, safety and timeliness of the service.

Clinical Outcomes

Target Setting

Target setting was introduced in 2012 to encourage shared decision-making and to work towards care planning. Uptake was initially slow with only two clinicians routinely using target setting in first quarter of 2012. Shared decision-making was discussed at the monthly team meetings and

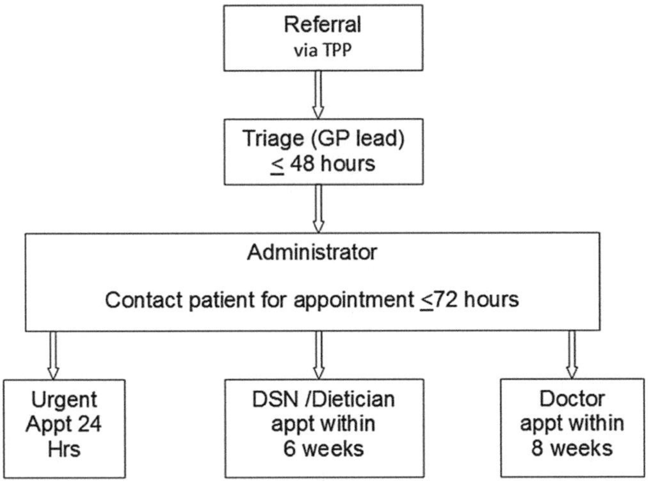

Fig. 8.3 Referral and assessment process (triage)

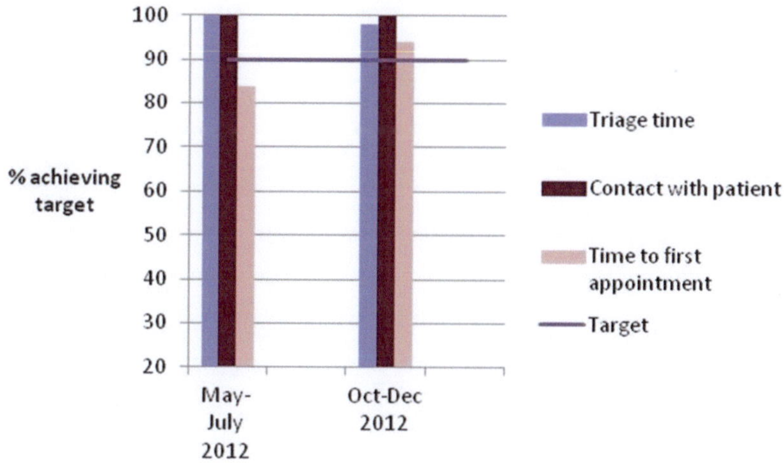

Fig. 8.4 Triage process audit

as clinicians started to understand its benefits in particular how it could be used to support care planning and review progress uptake increased, and in the last quarter of 2012, target setting and review was evident in 95 % of consultations. The majority of targets were to improve glucose control. Other targets were:

- Hypoglycaemia reduction
- Improvement of hypoglycaemia awareness
- Weight reduction
- Better blood pressure control
- Improved understanding of carbohydrate counting
- To undertake DAFNE (Dose Adjustment for Normal Eating, Type 1 diabetes structured education)
- Establishing the cause of proteinuria

The improvement in target setting reflects a more person centred approach to consultations.

Glucose and Blood Pressure Control

Improvements in glucose and blood pressure control were demonstrated at service, i.e., those referred to the specialist multidisciplinary team, and city level, i.e., outcomes for the total practice diabetes population, the real numerator of the service:

1. Glucose control as a Target:
   In March 2012 an audit of 50 patients seen in InterCare for suboptimal control demonstrated a reduction in mean HbA1c from 11.1 % (98 mmol/mol) to 8.9 % (74 mmol/l) in 6 months. In 2013 changes in HbA1c were evaluated in 50 people who had a target set for glucose and their progress reviewed after 6 months. Mean HbA1c at the time of referral was 9.7 % (82 mmol/mol) compared with a 10 % (86 mmol/mol) 12 months previously. This level of poor control was seen in patients attending acute trust as well as primary care clinics. Six months after their referral to InterCare mean HbA1c reduced to 7.95 % (63 mmol/mol); $P<0.01$ (Fig. 8.5).
2. Quality Outcome framework (QOF) targets in patients attending InterCare Health specialist team clinics:
   Changes in QOF were assessed by auditing SystmOne looking at all patients who had attended InterCare specialist team clinics. Compared to 2009/2010, in 2011/2012 there was a:
   - 62 % increase in the number achieving an Hba1c ≤7.5 % (58 mmol/mol)
   - 42 % increase in those with and HbA1c ≤8 (64 mmol/mol) or 9 % (75 mmol/mol)

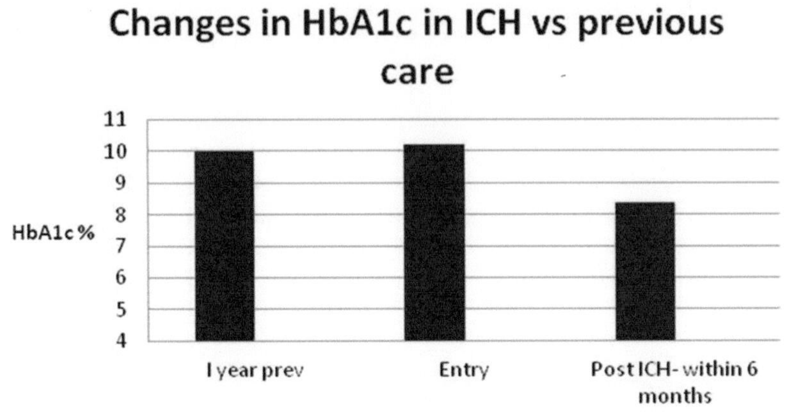

Fig. 8.5 Glucose control in patients attending InterCare (ICH) specialist clinics

- 15 % increase in the number with a blood pressure ≤150/90
- 30 % increase in those with a blood pressure <140/80

3. Changes in glucose and blood pressure targets in Derby City, i.e., the practice wide population of people with diabetes:
   The National Diabetes Information Service/Yorkshire Public Health Observatory (NDIS), now part of the National Cardiovascular Intelligence Network [16], collects diabetes outcome data at primary care trust and more recently clinical commissioning group level. As all Derby City practices were part of integrated care, comparing data serially gave an indication as to whether there was an impact on outcomes within primary care as opposed to improving outcomes in the patients seen by the specialist team as discussed above. Data from 2009/2010, 2010/2011 and 2011/2012 were examined as it was not possible to use this tool beyond 2012 as the data collection changed to clinical commissioning group level, which for Southern Derbyshire included areas that did not have access to integrated care.

   Both blood pressure and glucose outcomes improved progressively between 2009 and 2012. The data for the percentage achieving a HbA1c <7.5 % (58 mmol/mol) are shown in Fig. 8.6. Clearly factors other than clinical improvement such as improvements in data capture could have influenced these results. The 2011/2012 data were therefore compared with data from Derbyshire County (Fig. 8.6, yellow bar). Derbyshire County has a traditional model, but the majority of areas are supported by the same specialist team. NDIS took demography in to consideration, and Derbyshire County has a different demographic mix to the City, and would be expected to score better HbA1c targets than Derby City. They fact the two areas were equivalent in 2011/2012 was indirect evidence for the benefits of integrated care.

   All these measures reflected the effectiveness of the service.

4. Cost savings:
   NDIS compares outcomes with expenditure (DOVE tool). Expenditure across different areas is shown as a ranking based on 152 primary care trusts. Figure 8.7 demonstrates that in 2009–2010 Derby City ranked 16th least expensive for total spend on diabetes, but once integrated care became established, the ranking fell to the 2nd lowest, while the equivalent ranking for Derbyshire County in 2010–2011 was 14th. Data for Derby City and Derbyshire County are shown in Table 8.1.

   There was a reduction in costs for total programme spend and prescribing in Derby City as a result of implementing integrated care. Costs were consistently less than those for Derbyshire County in 2010/2011. In 2010/2011, Derby City spent £54 per patient per year less on diabetes care than Derbyshire County, as well as improving outcomes as described above. Given the diabetes prevalence for Derby City was

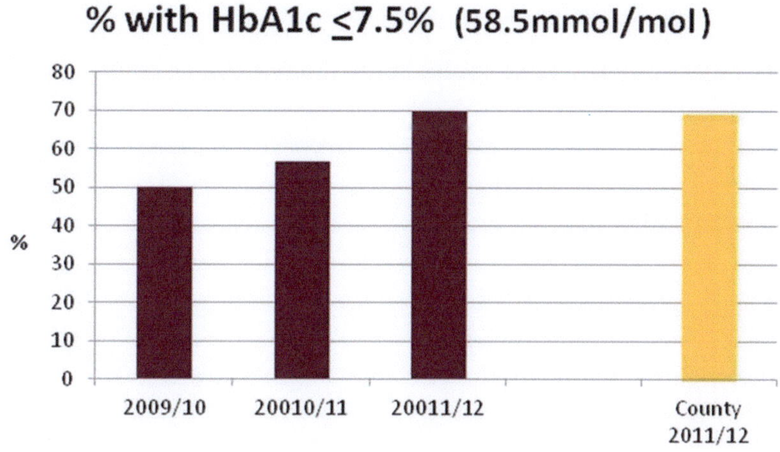

Fig. 8.6 Glucose control in Derby City

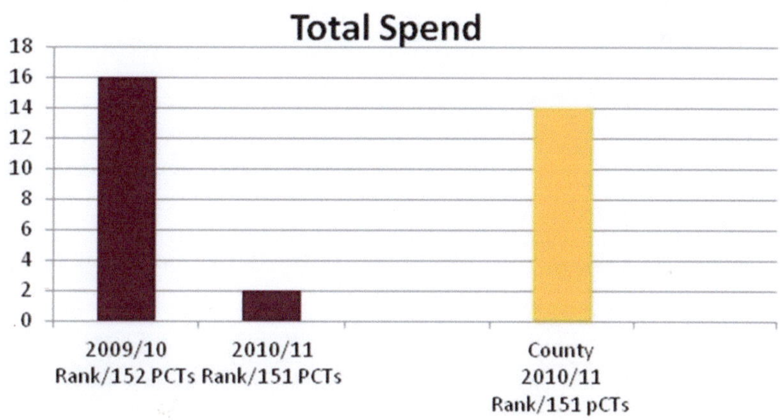

Fig. 8.7 Total programme spend/person with diabetes; Derby City and Derbyshire County Primary Care Trust (PCT) ranking (the lower the spend, the lower the rank)

£14,791, this equates to cost savings of £800,000 annually with improved outcomes.

If the model had been extended to Southern Derbyshire, the area covered by Southern Derbyshire Clinical Commissioning Group, in 2012 with 28,000 people with diabetes, the potential savings would be £1.5 million. As these figures do not include complication management, it would be expected that further savings would be seen through the reduction of complications such as sight threatening retinopathy, the number of patients on dialysis and amputation rate.

Inpatient Activity

As the InterCare service was initially provided for 7 practices before rolling out to 29, the first 6 months of the service gave the opportunity to compare admissions with a primary diagnosis of diabetes from practices in Derby City that did and did not have access to integrated care. In the first 6 months, there was a reduction of 292 bed days and a reduction of mean length of stay from 11 to 6.5 days in patients admitted from the seven InterCare practices compared with the same time period 12 months previously (Fig. 8.8).

Compared with non- InterCare practices, InterCare practice patients spent 1.8 days less in hospital (Fig. 8.9). Using a bed day cost for Diabetes and Endocrinology of £260, this equates to savings of £76,000 over 6 months.

Figure 8.10 shows unplanned admissions with a primary diagnosis of diabetes from all 29 InterCare practices. A progressive reduction in admissions and bed days is shown between 2010–2011 and 2012–2013. Using the bed day

Table 8.1 Expenditure for Derby City and Derbyshire County (£/person with diabetes)

	2009–2010		2010–2011	
	Spend	Rank/152 PCTs	Spend	Rank/151PCTs
Total spend				
City	418	16	422	2
County	411	11	476	14
Prescribing (all)				
City	234	10	240	4
County	244	17	258	14
Non-insulin prescribing				
City	50	1	61	16
County	55	3	69	
Insulin prescribing				
City	124	65	120	58
County	130	95	129	98
Glucose testing				
City	58	50	56	44
County	56	39	56	43

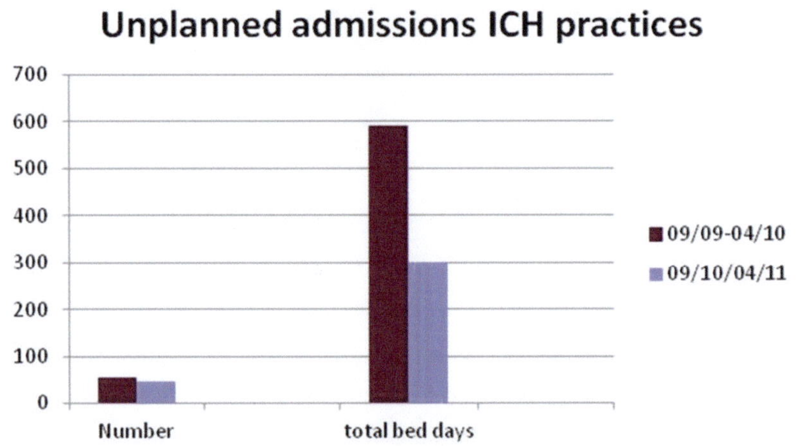

Fig. 8.8 Unplanned admissions with a primary diagnosis of diabetes; first 6 months of InterCare compared with 12 months previously

cost of £260 as above, the savings from the reduction in inpatient activity between 2010–2011 and 2012–2013 was £270,000.

These outcomes reflected effectiveness and improvements in safety.

User and Referring Staff Experience

Staff Experience

In 2012, the 29 referring practices were surveyed and asked about their experience of being part of the InterCare Diabetes Service. They received a questionnaire with seven questions. Where appropriate they were asked to rate the service from 1- very poor to 5- excellent. Twenty-one questionnaires were returned. A high level of clinician satisfaction was reported with:

- 91 % rating their experience referring patients to InterCare as excellent or very good;
- 73 % describing the experience as excellent or very good compared with referrals into hospital;
- 100 % rating their experience of tasking clinicians as very good or excellent.

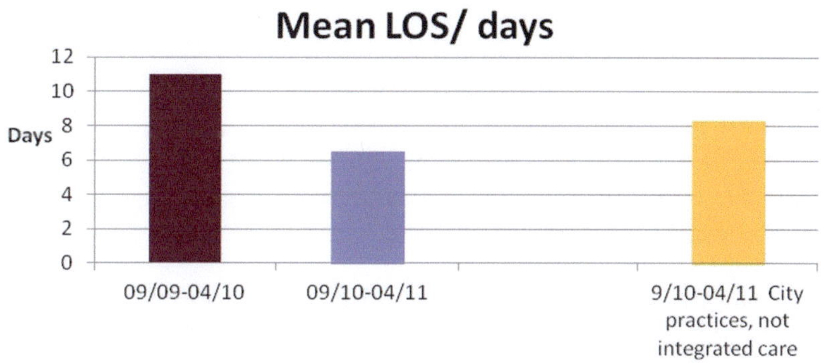

Fig. 8.9 Unplanned admissions with a primary diagnosis of diabetes; mean length of stay (LOS) in the first 6 months of InterCare Health, compared with practices that did not have access to integrated care, also compared with 12 months previously

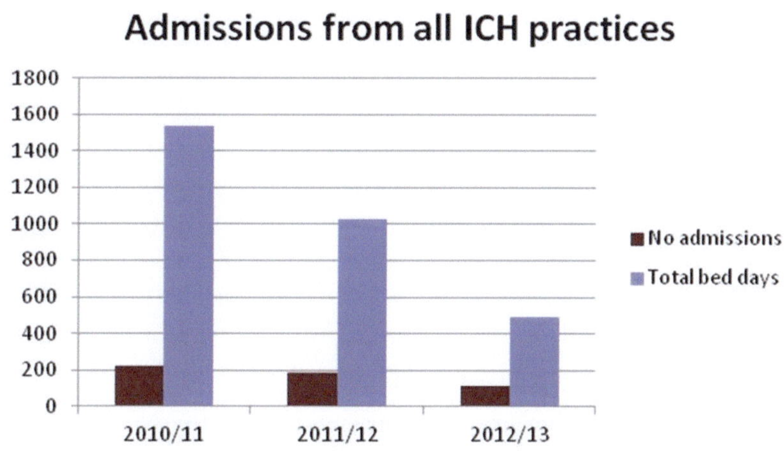

Fig. 8.10 Unplanned admissions with a primary diagnosis of diabetes – all InterCare practices

All clinicians were aware of the referral process. Twenty-eight percent received training through an accredited course, 76 % have attended courses but many requested ongoing education and training. Practice nurse comments included:

> "Joy's visits are fantastic."
> "Karen is very helpful and always sorts out any problems." "Quick response to queries."
> "InterCare is fantastic!"

GP comments included:

> "InterCare was able to help with patients who are difficult and we need another opinion."
> "Whilst there is merit in e-mail dialogues. It helps to meet face to face." (Consultant practice visit)

User Experience

A variety of methods were used to capture user experience. Users were encouraged to feedback and make suggestions for service improvement. A patient participation group helped develop aspects of the service and a focus group of users with Type 1 diabetes helped to refine the service to meet their needs as described above.

We used video to capture some user views. The video can be accessed using the following link: https://dl.dropboxusercontent.com/u/75004548/intercareviewsvideo.wmv

Formal feedback was obtained annually using a questionnaire which explored their experiences in the service using a 5 point score with 5 being excellent and 1 poor. The questionnaire was administered to 50 users in 2012. The process was repeated in 2013, but this time the survey was administered by users instead of InterCare administrators. The results were similar. Overall:

- 85 % rating the service as excellent or very good;
- 70 % felt that InterCare was excellent or very good compared with their previous care;

- 80 % felt the waiting time between referral and first appointment was excellent or very good;
- 90 % felt that InterCare was able to help them with the problem they were referred with;
- 95 % stated they would recommend the service to another person with diabetes.

Free text comments included:

"…like the services altogether, i.e., nurse, dietician and eye screening."
"…prefer the continuity in ICH…makes me feel confident."
ICH is better because I "have better control and seen quickly."

User and staff feedback provided evidence of delivering a person centred service.

Summary

InterCare was an integrated model for diabetes care, which was the first diabetes model in the UK that integrated not just clinically, but also achieved integration at a financial, organisational and information technological levels too. The whole service was supported by a single clinical governance structure.

The service was evaluated using the care bundled approach described, and showed improvements in all six domains of quality improvement: effectiveness, safety, efficiency, timeliness, equity and provision of a person centred service.

InterCare resulted in £800,000 savings in 2010–2011 with £270,000 saving as a result of reducing admissions between 2010 and 2012–2013.

This model is currently being further developed and extended to provide a single integrated service for all people in Derby City and Southern Derbyshire, the area covered by the current commissioners, Southern Derbyshire Clinical Commissioning Group.

Acknowledgement I am grateful to Dr Kyran Farrell, a GP with a special interest in diabetes, for his helpful comments. I would also like to acknowledge Dianne Prescott, Gino DiStefano, Garry Tan, Mark Browne, Stuart Holloway, and Musaddaq Iqbal who had a part in the development and running of the InterCare Diabetes Service.

References

1. Diabetes UK Diabetes Facts and Figures. https://www.diabetes.org.uk/Documents/Position%20statements/Facts%20and%20stats%20June%202015.pdf (2015). Accessed 24 Mar 2016.
2. Health and Social Care Information Centre, Quality Outcomes Framework. http://qof.hscic.gov.uk/search/index.asp (2015). Accessed 24 Mar 2016.
3. Royal College of Physicians, the Royal College of General Practitioners and the Royal College of Paediatrics and Child Health. Teams without walls. The value of medical innovation and leadership. https://www.rcplondon.ac.uk/sites/default/files/teams-without-walls-1_0.pdf (2008). Accessed 7 May 2015.
4. Goodwin N, Smith J, Davies A et al. Integrated care for patients and populations: improving outcomes by working together: a report to the Department of Health and Future Health Forum. http://www.kingsfund.org.uk/sites/files/kf/integrated-care-patients-populations-paper-nuffield-trust-kings-fund-january-2012.pdf (2012). Accessed 9 May 2015.
5. Starey N. What is clinical governance? http://www.medicine.ox.ac.uk/bandolier/painres/download/whatis/WhatisClinGov.pdf (2001). Accessed 24 Mar 2016.
6. Joint Societies. Best practice for commissioning diabetes services. An integrated care framework. http://www.diabetes.org.uk/Documents/Position%20statements/best-practice-commissioning-diabetes-services-integrated-framework-0313.pdf (2013). Accessed 7 May 2015.
7. Diabetes UK. Improving the delivery of adult diabetes care through integration. Shared experience and learning. http://www.diabetes.org.uk/Documents/About%20Us/What%20we%20say/Integrated%20diabetes%20care%20(PDF,%20648KB).pdf (2014). Accessed 7 May 2015.
8. British Medical Association. Collaborative GP networks – basic legal structures. http://www.bma.org.uk/support-at-work/gp-practices/gp-networks/basic-legal-structures (2015). Accessed 26 Mar 2016.
9. Rea RD, Gregory S, Browne M et al. Integrated diabetes care in Derby – new NHS organisations for new NHS challenges. http://www.practicaldiabetes.com/SpringboardWebApp/userfiles/espdi/file/September%202011/Rea%20online%20+%20charts.pdf (2012). Accessed 16 May 2015.
10. Department of Health. A simple guide to payment by results. https://www.gov.uk/government/uploads/system/uploads/attachment_data/

file/213150/PbR-Simple-Guide-FINAL.pdf (2012). Accessed 24 Mar 2016.
11. King P. Proceed. www.derbyproceed.co.uk (2014). Accessed 9 May 2015.
12. Lillyman S, Saxon A, Treml H. An evaluation of the role of the community matron – a literature review. https://www.wlv.ac.uk/media/wlv/pdf/nov2009_SLillyman.pdf (2009). Accessed 10 Oct 2015.
13. Donabedian A. The quality of medical care. Science. 1978;200:856–64.
14. Institute of Medicine. Cross the quality chasm: a new health system for the 21st century. https://www.iom.edu/~/media/Files/Report%20Files/2001/Crossing-the-Quality-Chasm/Quality%20Chasm%202001%20%20report%20brief.pdf (2001). Accessed 14 May 2015.
15. NHS Modernisation Agency. Change no 6. Increasing the reliability of performing therapeutic interventions through a care bundled approach in 10 high impact changes for service improvement and delivery. http://www.nursingleadership.org.uk/publications/HIC.pdf (2004). Accessed 14 May 2015. (Please note that this is a NHS Institute for Innovations and improvement publication – their website no longer exists but the publication can still be accessed through the link provided.)
16. The National Diabetes Information Service. http://www.yhpho.org.uk/resource/view.aspx?RID=102082 (2015). Accessed 14 May 2014. (Data after 2013 are part of National Cardiovascular Intelligence Network, accessible through the same link.)

Integrated Diabetes Care: Coventry and Warwickshire Approach

9

Ponnusamy Saravanan, Vinod Patel, Joseph Paul O'Hare, and Sudhesh Kumar

Introduction

The clinical and economic burden of Type 2 Diabetes (T2D) is very high across the world as the number of people suffering from diabetes is increasing rapidly, even in low-income countries. A total of 380 million people live with diabetes and health expenditures of 548 billion US dollars (USD) which is 581 (ID), were spent on the condition in 2013 across the world [1]. The vast majority of this is spent in high-income countries. The healthcare cost for managing chronic diseases such as Diabetes is increasing even in these high-income countries [2]. There has been much emphasis on reducing this cost and improving (or at least without compromising) the quality of care, over the past two decades [3]. "Case-finding" approaches [4], "care closer to home" and "pay for performance" [5] are such examples. In the UK, prior to the introduction of pay for performance as a part of the Quality and Outcomes Framework (QoF) in 2004, there was wide primary care variation in the care and prompt referral of patients with T2D [6]. Although the QoF initiative improved overall process and intermediate outcome measures, significant disparities in diabetes outcomes still exist between general practices and regions, especially among patients from ethnic minorities [7]. These intermediate improvements appear to be levelling off, which may partly be due to less challenging targets to secure the QoF points, as well as increasing use of exception reporting (proportion of patients who can be excluded by the practice team for a variety of reasons) [8]. There is now evidence that these improvements in individual risk factors have not translated into improvements in hard outcomes [9].

The majority of the practices across the UK achieved the QoF targets within a few years of the introduction of the incentive scheme. However, nationwide audit data for England 2009–2010 showed that more stringent targets for HbA1c (≤7.5 %/58.5 mmol/mol), blood pressure (BP) (<140/80 mmHg) and total cholesterol (<4.0 mmol/l) were achieved in only 67 %, 69 % and 41 % of people with T2D. Poor glycaemic

P. Saravanan (✉)
George Eliot Hospital NHS Trust, Coventry, UK

Warwick Medical School, The University of Warwick, Coventry, UK

University Hospitals Coventry and Warwickshire NHS Trust, Coventry, UK
e-mail: p.saravanan@warwick.ac.uk

V. Patel
George Eliot Hospital NHS Trust, Coventry, UK

Warwick Medical School, The University of Warwick, Coventry, UK
e-mail: Vinod.patel@warwick.ac.uk

J.P. O'Hare • S. Kumar
Warwick Medical School, The University of Warwick, Coventry, UK

University Hospitals Coventry and Warwickshire NHS Trust, Coventry, UK
e-mail: j.p.o-hare@warwick.ac.uk; Sudhesh.kumar@warwick.ac.uk

D. Simmons et al. (eds.), *Integrated Diabetes Care*, DOI 10.1007/978-3-319-13389-8_9

control was associated with younger age and social deprivation [5]. Significant variations existed with practices that are less likely to achieve adequate levels of control, in areas of high deprivation and serving populations with higher proportions of Black and Minority Ethnic (BME) groups [7, 10] as well as those practices with lower levels of organisation [11]. West Midlands South (the Coventry and Warwickshire area) and East Midlands (particularly Leicester city) are such areas with high BME population density coupled with lower socioeconomic status among White Caucasians. In Coventry and North Warwickshire there were also significantly higher numbers of small general practices. Although geographically close and densely populated (~800 mi^2 and ~850,000 population), the Coventry and Warwickshire region has three different NHS providers (hospital trusts) and initially six different commissioning groups (which became three primary care trusts and then three clinical commissioning groups). This added further challenges in providing cohesive, integrated care within the region for the 39,000 patients with diabetes, catered for by 147 general practices.

Alternate Services to Traditional Hospital Based Clinics

Increasingly, patients with diabetes have been managed in primary care across the world. This trend was partly due to the increasing number of patients with T2D and the inability of existing specialists to cope with the demand. Our local audit data shows that approximately 85–90 % of patients with diabetes are managed by GPs and practice nurses in Coventry and Warwickshire. Only a small proportion of newly diagnosed patients with T2D (typically around 5–10 %) who attend the DESMOND (Diabetes Education and Self-Management for Ongoing and Newly Diagnosed) education programme come into contact with some aspect of the specialist services [12]. Apart from this group, patients with T2D come into contact with a member of the specialist services, usually when there is evidence of complications. There is no structured educational support for the primary care team that provides regular update on diabetes knowledge. In addition, Payment by results (PBR) has also actively, *albeit* indirectly, disincentivised primary care to seek opinion from specialist services [13]. GPs with a special interest in Diabetes (GPwSI) were thought to offer a solution to this problem and were rapidly adopted across the UK between 2004 and 2006. The GPwSIs either on their own, or in collaboration with hospital diabetes specialists, set up alternative services to hospital-based services across the UK. These clinics are called "Intermediate Care Clinics for Diabetes" (ICCD). The very first ICCD set-up was in Bradford in 1998, based in 19 clinics across the city, and led by GPwSIs, supported by a community diabetologist, diabetes specialist nurses, dieticians and podiatrists. An evaluation conducted between 1999 and 2001 found high levels of uptake, with over 2000 referrals [14]. During this period, hospital attendance fell by 25 %, but overall attendance (hospital and ICCD) increased by 35 %. Intermediate care clinics were popular with patients and practitioners and their cost was similar to a hospital outpatient clinic. Problems identified included inequity in referrals between practices in which the clinics were based and other practices, and lack of communication and strategic planning [14]. Similarly, several other regions (Southampton, Lambeth in London, and Wales) had their own model of ICCD clinics with varying success [15–17]. Although recent evidence has suggested that the most effective interventions in Diabetes include the trial of team changes, case-finding and management and patient education and empowerment [18], none of these models had a unifying methodology. In addition, none of the ICCD services that have been set up were evaluated in randomised clinical trials or had their cost-effectiveness assessed with appropriate health economic evaluations. This has raised serious questions about the validity of the clinical and cost-effectiveness of ICCD clinics.

Inefficiency Due to Lack of Integrated Services

Large volumes of data are collected by various services ranging between primary care, local laboratory facilities, ambulance services, hospital clinics (of varying specialties), retinal screening services and several allied healthcare professionals. However, the majority of these systems are not unified and therefore result in duplication of data collection and lack of data utilisation beyond the purpose of collection. This can result in missed opportunities, delayed communication, inability to use electronic solutions (prompts, alerts, algorithms etc.), inefficient use of resources and patient fatigue (repeated testing but no apparent benefit). Thus, in the majority of the regions in England, the delivery of diabetes care is disjointed and lacks integration. Each service collects and utilises data for their own "narrow" purpose, which could be used in a holistic way with the patient at the centre of the care (Fig. 9.1a, b).

A meta-analysis that assessed the effectiveness of 11 strategies to improve HbA1c in patients with T2D managed in primary care showed that only three strategies resulted in improvement (team changes, case-finding and management, and patient education and empowerment) [18, 19]. Intensive management can also reduce complications such as retinopathy, nephropathy and neuropathy, as well as reducing the risk of cardiovascular disease [20]. Benefits are gained from improved glycaemic control, lower blood pressure and better management of lipids [21–23]. Patients with improved glycaemic control also consistently report better functional status and wellbeing [24–26]. Studies showed that intensive control of risk factors can be achieved in the UK at comparable cost. However, detailed cost-effectiveness of this strategy was not discussed [27]. The challenge for diabetes services across the UK and the world is how to translate these interventions into individualised patient care. Whilst the QoF has raised the standard of cardiovascular risk factor data collection (HbA1c, BP and Cholesterol), these have been primarily used as cross-sectional data in patient management, which is probably one of the reasons for the lack of improvement in hard outcomes [9]. Although available data have been more complete since the introduction of QoF in 2004, they have not been utilised for aggressive "case-finding" or "individualised" cardiovascular risk management. Trends in deterioration could potentially be identified by electronic solutions at individual patient level for each risk factor and used for proactive risk management.

To improve the local services in diabetes care in Coventry and Warwickshire, two studies were set up. First was a cluster randomised controlled trial to evaluate the effectiveness and cost-effectiveness of the ICCDs based in three primary care trusts (PCT) in Coventry, North Warwickshire and Leicester [28, 29]. The second was an innovation project funded by Department

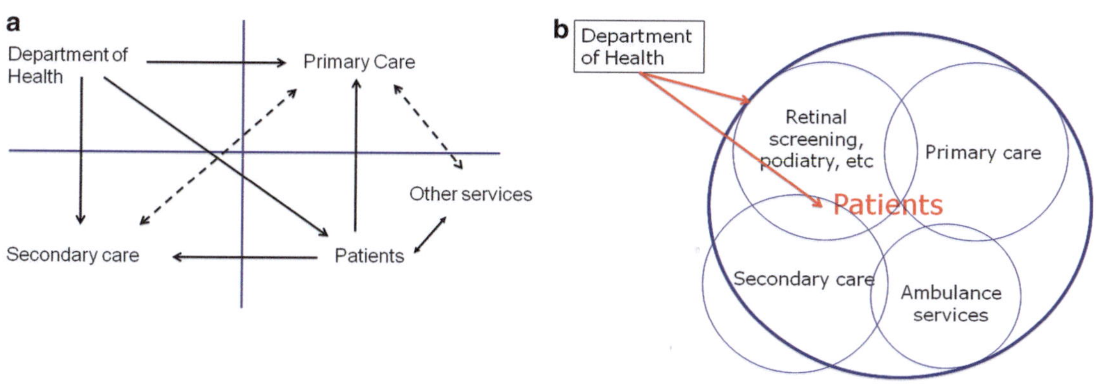

Fig. 9.1 (**a**) Current disjointed services. (**b**) An integrated service model

of Health (Health Innovation Education Cluster), with a view to digitally integrate diabetes data across 12 GP practices. These two projects are discussed in this chapter.

Intermediate Care Clinics in Diabetes Study

Detailed protocol, study design and results have been published [28, 29].

Aims and Objectives

The overall aim was to evaluate the effectiveness and cost-effectiveness of community based intermediate care clinics in the management of T2D.

Specific objectives were to:

1. Compare the following in patients with T2D registered with practices that have access to ICCD with those that have access only to usual care:
    - Glycaemic control,
    - Control of blood pressure and dyslipidaemia,
    - Quality of life,
    - Satisfaction with services and continuity of care,
    - Referral patterns,
    - Annual cost per patient with diabetes.
2. Estimate the difference in the cost of the resources used by patients in each arm of the trial, and the cost-effectiveness of the ICCD intervention.
3. Explore the views of users and service providers participating in the study.

Methods

Study Design

It was a pragmatic two-arm cluster randomised controlled trial in three different PCTs (Coventry – PCT1, North Warwickshire – PCT2 and Leicester city – PCT3). Randomisation was stratified by PCT and GP practice size. Practices recruited to the study were randomised to either (i) usual care or (ii) intervention, with the latter having access to the new ICCD clinics. Practices randomised to usual care were issued with local guidelines and were advised to manage their patients in the usual way.

Inclusion and Exclusion Criteria

Inclusion criteria were kept broad. All T2D patients aged 18 years or over were eligible to participate. Patients with following characteristics were excluded:

1. Severe cognitive impairment
2. Severe mental illness
3. Receiving terminal care

Outcome Measures

Primary Outcome

Proportion achieving ALL the targets – HbA1c (<7.0 %), blood pressure (<140/80), cholesterol (<4 mmol/l)

Secondary Outcome

1. Proportion achieving individual risk factor targets:
2. Mean HbA1c
3. Mean Systolic and Diastolic Blood Pressure
4. Mean Total Cholesterol,
5. Ten year CVD risk score by UKPDS risk engine [30]

Other Assessments

Health status assessment – EQ-5D [31]

1. Problem Areas in Diabetes (PAID) [32]
2. Continuity of Care questionnaire [33]
3. Economic outcome measure – data on NHS resource use and personal costs [34]

Sample Size Calculations

Percentage of patients achieving control in the usual care group in a UK survey prior to funding application were: median practice performance in achieving HbA1c <7.5–48 %; blood pressure <145/85–59 %; and cholesterol <5–60 % [35]. We used HbA1c for our primary sample size calculation as this is the outcome variable for which there is the most robust information on intra-class correlation (ICC) which has been estimated as 0.047 [36]. To detect a difference between percentage well controlled of 50 % in the control group and 60 % in the intervention group (alpha = 0.05 Power = 0.8), not allowing for clustering, required a sample size of 408 subjects in each arm. Using an ICC of 0.047, and with 72 patients in each cluster, the necessary sample size in each arm was 1770, a total of 3540 patients. This number is also adequate to detect a 10 % difference in total cholesterol control (from 60 % to 70 %) and blood pressure control (from 60 % to 70 %). Estimates of ICC for blood pressure and cholesterol were taken from UKADS, a study of care provision for people of South Asian ethnicity with diabetes [37]. Assuming the ICC for our combined primary outcome (adequate control of HbA1c, blood pressure and cholesterol) was 0.05 and achievement was at 20 % (from a baseline of 15–20 % as suggested by local audit data) in the control arm and 30 % in the intervention arm, we would need a total of 2848 patients.

The study was successful in recruiting 49 practices (11, 13 and 25 in PCT 1, 2 and 3 respectively). A total of 1997 patients were enrolled with an average of 42 per practice. This sample size had 80 % power to detect a 12 % difference in the combined outcome measure, if 75 % follow-up was achieved.

Results

Of the 49 practices, 24 were randomised to intervention and 25 to the control arm. Of the 1997 patients recruited 64 % were followed up. Two practices declined to allow the research team to undertake follow-up assessments. The consort diagram (Fig. 9.2) shows the recruitment, follow-up rates and numbers analysed.

Table 9.1 shows the baseline characteristics by trial arm. It shows although the intervention and control groups were similar at baseline with respect to gender, smoking status, co-morbidities and achievement of blood pressure, HbA1c and cholesterol targets, there was a substantial difference between groups with respect to the "combined control" (primary outcome), with 11.2 % in the intervention and 8.7 % in the control arm.

Table 9.2 shows there were large differences between PCTs in levels of control at baseline, in particular, in the rates of achievement in the "combined control" and cholesterol control between PCTs 1 and 3.

In PCT 1 and 2, the ICCDs that existed at the time of funding application were closed due to lack of adequate referrals. Therefore for the purpose of the study, at study initiation two clinics were set-up. These were agreed between the local consultants, GPs and PCT. The consultants provided their time for the ICCDs at no charge, community Diabetes Specialist nurses provided their time as a part of their community role and one GP (PCT 1) provided her time at no charge for the purpose of the study in order to work alongside an experienced consultant. All these clinics (all three PCTs) ran for 18 months. In PCTs 1 and 2, only trial participants were referred to ICCD. These were 145 and 35 patients, respectively. In PCT 3, all patients of practices randomised to the intervention group were eligible for referral – this was due to the local PCT guidelines at that time. The overall recruitment rate of patients to the trial from the intervention arm was 19 %, and so we estimate that of the 101 patients who attended clinics in PCT 3, 19 (19 %) were trial participants. Thus a total of 199 (145 + 35 + 19) trial participants attended ICCD, representing 18.8 % of trial participants. The proportion of participants referred to ICCD varied across the three PCTs: 145/431 (34 %) in PCT 1, 35/240 (15 %) in PCT 2 and 19/386 (5 %) in PCT 3.

Follow-up data was available for 1280 patients. Last observation carried forward method (LOCF) was applied for missing values: primary outcome variable (combined control), individual secondary outcome variables, and each of the covariates used in the primary analysis. Thirty-three patients were excluded from the final analysis due to missing data, with no possible LOCF. The baseline characteristics of the final 1247 patients are shown in Table 9.3.

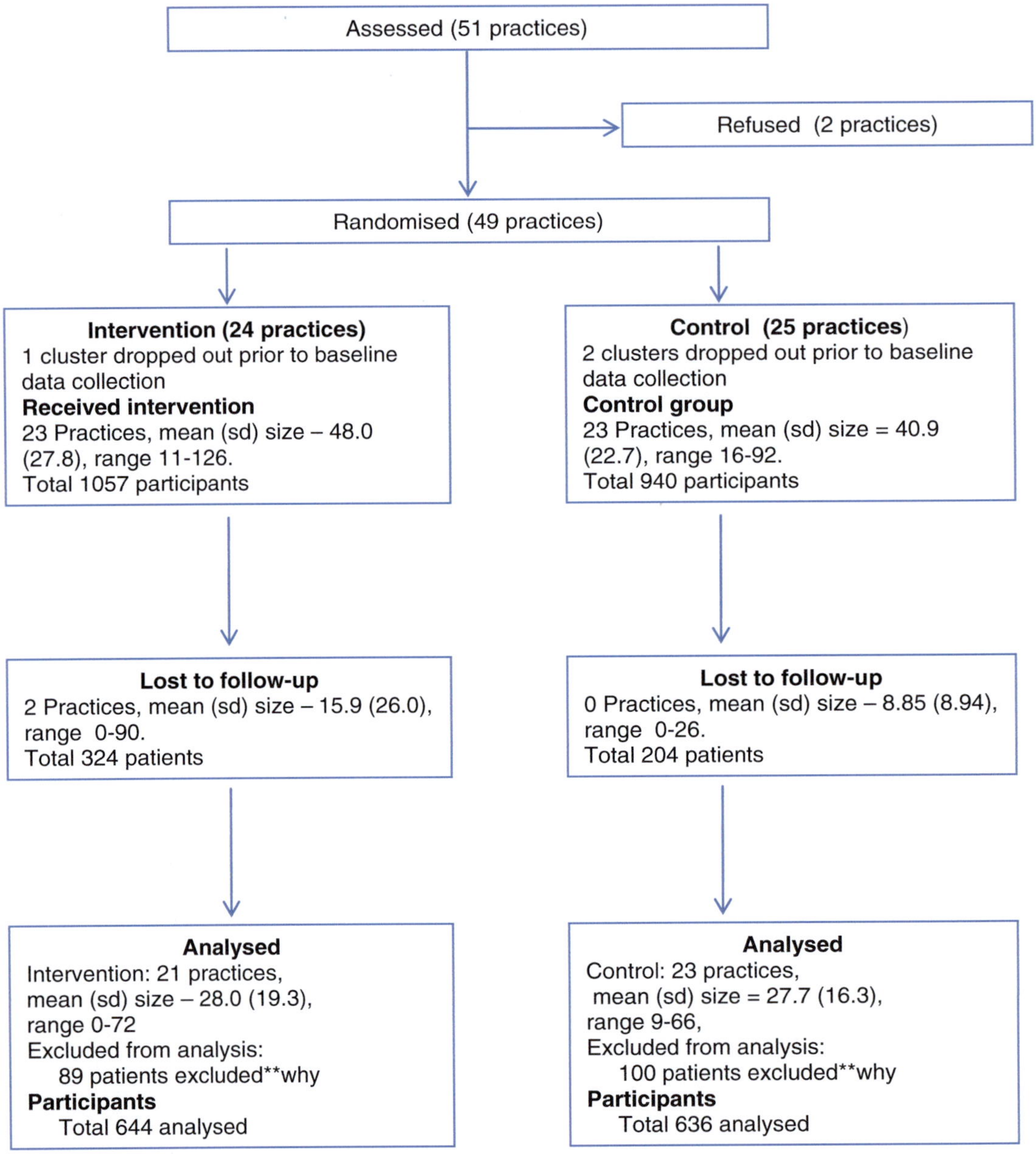

Fig. 9.2 GP Practice and patient recruitment and progress through the study

Primary Outcome

A series of analyses were performed for the primary outcome using logistic mixed effect models. Such models compensate for variations at the GP practice level by modelling the contribution of the practices as a random variable with a normal distribution. In effect, this allows the model to have multiple intercepts, one for each practice, where the intercept's variation from a fixed point is normally distributed. Equivalently, a separate linear regression model is calculated for each practice, but the coefficient for each covariate is the same in each of those models. This approach allows consideration of the effect of group-level variance separately to the effect of individual-level variance between groups.

In the first, main analysis, general practice was included as a random effect, with the following covariates included as fixed effects:

Table 9.1 Baseline characteristics by trial arm

Variable	Control (n=940) n (%)	Intervention (n=1057) n (%)
Achieved combined control	81 (*8.7*)	116 (*11.2*) *
Controlled HbA1c (<=7.0%)	497 (*53.9*)	536 (*51.7*)
Controlled blood pressure (<140/80)	304 (*32.8*)	398 (*38.3*)
Controlled cholesterol (<4 mmol/l)	442 (*48.2*)	519 (*50.2*)
PCT 1	242 (*25.7*)	431 (*40.8*)
PCT 2	225 (*23.9*)	240 (*22.7*)
PCT 3	473 (*50.3*)	386 (*36.5*)
Male	543 (*58.1*)	613 (*58.4*)
Smoker	118 (*12.7*)	116 (*11.1*)
Hypertension	505 (*55.6*)	612 (*59.1*)
IHD	161 (*17.7*)	149 (*14.4*)
CVD	35 (*3.85*)	28 (*2.72*)
Heart failure	25 (*2.75*)	35 (*3.38*)
PVD	10 (*1.10*)	15 (*1.45*)
Renal failure	24 (*2.63*)	24 (*2.31*)
Ethnicity: White	614 (*65.3*)	554 (*52.4*)
Asian	257 (*27.3*)	405 (*38.3*)
Black	32 (*3.40*)	55 (*5.20*)
Other	37 (*3.94*)	43 (*4.07*)

Table 9.2 Baseline characteristics by PCT

Variable	Coventry (n=673) (PCT 1) n (%)	Nuneaton (n=465) (PCT 2) n (%)	Leicester (n=859) (PCT 3) n (%)
Achieved combined control	48 (*7.2*)	42 (*9.4*)	107 (*12.6*)
HbA1c (<=7.0%)	323 (*48.5*)	256 (*58.3*)	454 (*53.2*)
Blood pressure (<140/80)	228 (*34.2*)	170 (*38.0*)	304 (*35.6*)
Cholesterol (<4 mmol/l)	270 (*40.5*)	190 (*44.1*)	501 (*58.7*)
Male	383 (*57.2*)	290 (*63.2*)	483 (*56.6*)
Smoker	74 (*11.1*)	53 (*11.8*)	107 (*12.5*)
Hypertension	393 (*59.2*)	351 (*78.0*)	373 (*44.9*)
IHD	92 (*13.8*)	88 (*19.6*)	130 (*15.7*)
CVD	20 (*3.00*)	35 (*7.78*)	8 (*0.97*)
Heart failure	19 (*2.86*)	12 (*2.67*)	29 (*3.50*)
PVD	6 (*0.90*)	14 (*3.12*)	5 (*0.60*)
Renal failure	15 (*2.25*)	24 (*5.33*)	9 (*1.08*)

Table 9.3 Baseline characteristics of patients used in the final analysis

	Control (n = 636)	Intervention (n = 591)	
Variable	N (%)	N (%)	p-value
PCT 1	164 (25.8 %)	166 (28.1 %)	0.399
PCT 2	339 (53.3 %)	237 (40.1 %)	<0.001
PCT 3	133 (20.9 %)	152 (25.7 %)	0.054
Male	370 (58.2 %)	347 (58.7 %)	0.894
Smoking	77 (12.1 %)	66 (11.2 %)	0.672
Co-morbidity			
Hypertension	341 (53.6 %)	335 (56.7 %)	0.307
IHD	115 (14.9 %)	95 (16.1 %)	0.392
CVD	22 (3.46 %)	15 (2.54 %)	0.438
Heart failure	15 (2.36 %)	17 (2.88 %)	0.697
PVD	7 (1.10 %)	9 (1.52 %)	0.690
Renal failure	13 (2.04 %)	12 (2.03 %)	1.000
Ethnicity			
White	365 (57.4 %)	271 (45.9 %)	<0.001
Asian	98 (15.4 %)	202 (34.2 %)	<0.001
Black	20 (3.14 %)	33 (5.58 %)	0.050
Other	20 (3.14 %)	22 (3.72 %)	0.690
Baseline assessment of outcome measures			
Primary outcome (combined control)	61 (9.59 %)	76 (12.9 %)	0.084
HbA1c (<=7.0 %/53 mmol/mol)	347 (54.6 %)	326 (55.2 %)	0.878
Blood pressure (<140/80 mmHg)	354 (55.7 %)	324 (54.8 %)	0.812
Cholesterol (<154 mg/dl/4 mmol/l)	305 (48.0 %)	308 (52.1 %)	0.162
Individual factors (mean/sd)			
HbA1c (%)	7.22 (1.24)	7.18 (1.23)	0.470
Systolic BP (mmHg)	137.5 (17.3)	137.0 (18.0)	0.528
Diastolic BP (mmHg)	80.6 (10.0)	79.3 (10.7)	0.005
Total cholesterol	4.05 (1.04)	3.99 (1.18)	0.231

Intervention arm, combined control and age at baseline, gender, ethnicity, smoking status at follow-up, PCT, deprivation and presence of co-morbid conditions such as hypertension, ischaemic heart disease, cerebrovascular disease, heart failure, peripheral vascular disease and renal failure. Intervention arm was considered the main exposure variable, estimated as a fixed effect.

The achievement of combined and individual risk factor control by trial arm is shown in Table 9.4. The odds ratio (OR) of achieving the primary outcome (combined control) was significantly better in the intervention arm at 1.62 (95 % CI: 1.04, 2.43) though when adjusted for covariates, it lost significance. The adjusted OR (aOR) was 1.59 (95 % CI: 0.983, 2.49). Not surprisingly, only the baseline levels of "combined controlled" was a significant contributor to this OR but not the other covariates (as highlighted earlier), including deprivation index. Similar effects were seen when intention to treat analysis was carried out (n = 1910, aOR 1.60 (95 % CI: 0.984, 2.60).

Secondary Outcomes

The mean values of individual risk factors achieved at the baseline and follow-up by intervention and control group are shown in Table 9.5. The OR of the primary outcome and these key secondary outcomes are shown in Table 9.6.

Table 9.4 Proportion of patients achieving risk factor control at the end of the study

	Intervention (644)		Control (636)	
Baseline (B) or follow-up (F)	B	F	B	F
% Achieved combined control (n)	12.9 (82)	14.3 (92)	9.7 (61)	9.3 (59)
% Controlled HbA1c (n)	54.9 (349)	57.5 (370)	55.3 (347)	51.1 (325)
% Controlled blood pressure (n)	40.0 (254)	39.8 (256)	33.2 (209)	32.0 (203)
% Controlled cholesterol (n)	52.9 (335)	61.8 (397)	48.8 (305)	55.2 (351)

Table 9.5 Mean risk factor control at baseline and follow-up

	Intervention		Control	
Baseline (B) or follow-up (F)	B	F	B	F
HbA1c % (n = 1249)	7.18	7.17	7.22	7.28
Systolic BP mmHg (n = 1251)	137.0	136.9	137.5	138.0
Diastolic BP mmHg (n = 1251)	79.3	79.1	80.6	80.5
Cholesterol (n = 1245) mmol/l	3.99	3.79	4.05	3.90

There were no differences seen in the UKPDS risk score between the groups. Similarly, there were no differences in any of the four domains of the "Continuity questionnaire" or the "PAID questionnaire."

Economic Evaluation

Cost of Consultations in ICCD

Separate data were collected through direct contacts with the ICCD sites independent of the trial. These data were used to estimate the cost of seeing a patient in each of the IC clinics. As described earlier, in PCTs 1 and 2, clinics were available only to trial participants, and so the total cost of these services has been included. In PCT 3, only a minority of clinic attenders were trial patients (19 %). In this PCT the cost per consultation was based on 2010/2011 figures. Average costs per consultation and patient attending at the three sites are shown in Table 9.7.

Table 9.6 Odds ratios for primary and secondary outcomes

	Odds ratio	95 % confidence interval
Primary outcome (composite)	1.56	(0.983, 2.49)
Secondary outcome measures		
HbA1c control (<=7.0 %)	1.45	(1.07, 1.96)
Blood pressure control (<140/80)	1.23	(0.88, 1.73)
Total cholesterol (<4 mmol/l)	1.48	(1.08, 2.03)

Questionnaire responses at follow-up were used to derive patient costs in terms of NHS resources used. This is referred to as the "resource use" element of the study questionnaire.

Analysis of Direct Costs

For calculating the direct healthcare cost clean dataset of n = 1322 is used. Patients in the intervention group did not have a statistically significant difference in total resource use costs (p = 0.101). However, breaking the data down into the cost headings, in the intervention group, the cost of primary care and community clinic consultations were higher than for the control group (184.98 vs. 76.82; p < 0.001). This is likely to be because some of the ICCD attendances are included in this category and/or because ICCD input triggered more primary care consultations. The detailed breakdown of the direct costs is shown in Table 9.8.

Indirect Costs

Only around 50 % of the participants responded to the "sickness rates." This is probably partly the reflection of the age group studied (retired). Therefore, sickness was not included in the indirect cost in the economic analysis.

Cost Utility Analysis

The QALY gain during the baseline to follow-up period was calculated by using the following formula:

Table 9.7 Average cost per ICCD consultation/patient attending at each site

PCT	Total costs	Total consultations/patients attending ICCD	Average cost per consultation/ patient attending ICCD
1	£43,553	442/145	£98.54/300.37
2	£8881	120/35	£74.01/253.74
3	£14,701	95/19	£154.75/773.74
Total	£67,135	657/199	£102.18/337.36

Table 9.8 Direct cost spent according to resources utilised

	Intervention (n=665)		Control (n=657)		
Resource item	Mean	(SE)	Mean	(SE)	P value
ICCD					
Intermediate care clinic for diabetes	60.18			N/A	
Cost of consultations					
Primary care doctor and nurse costs	37.25	2.335	31.19	2.044	0.051
Community clinic staff	1.46	0.381	0.49	0.201	0.025
Hospital doctor and nurse costs	26.13	3.876	32.03	5.272	0.366
AE staff	1.02	0.525	0.59	0.295	0.476
Optometrist, podiatrist and dietician	11.65	1.047	12.51	0.907	0.534
Sub total	**137.70**	**5.53**	**76.82**	**6.25**	**<0.001**
Cost of care					
Diabetes tests	58.27	2.27	62.74	2.63	0.199
Hospital inpatient costs	155.71	75.60	98.96	58.67	0.554
Total costs	**351.68**	**76.51**	**238.52**	**60.70**	**0.247**

$$\text{QALY} = \begin{pmatrix} 0.5(\text{BL Quality} + \text{FU Quality}) \\ * \text{No. of months between BL and FU} \end{pmatrix} / 12(\text{BL} = \text{Baseline}; \text{FU} = \text{Follow up})$$

[38]. Individual scores for patients were summed to give a total QALY gain for each trial participant, and also summed at the level of the two cohorts. As there was no significant difference in baseline Quality of Life scores between two groups (0.69 vs. 0.70, p=575), the QALY analysis was not adjusted for baseline QALYs [39]. The incremental cost-effectiveness ratio (ICER) was calculated using the usual formula $(C_1 - C_0)/(E_1 - E_0)$, with C being costs and E the clinical or QALY outcome. Using this formula, the following calculations were performed:

$$\text{Cost} - \text{utility} = (\text{Control cost} - \text{Intervention cost}) / (\text{Control QALY} - \text{Intervention QALY})$$

The incremental cost-utility ratio focused on the costs per QALY gained. Bootstrap resampling with 1000 replications was performed. Scatter plots of 1000 bootstrapped ICERs on the cost-effectiveness plane were generated. The cost-effectiveness results were presented as Cost-Effectiveness Acceptability Curves (CECA). These show the probability that the intervention group is cost-effective relative to the control, given varying values of ceiling ratios, i.e., the willingness to pay (WTP) for one quality-adjusted life-year. In this analysis we used the threshold amount of £30,000 based upon the threshold figures usually employed by NICE [40]. For the QALY data and ICER analysis, as per NICE recommendation these values were discounted at 3.5 % [40]. Table 9.9 show the summary data used in ICER analysis.

This suggests that the intervention group had a higher average cost per patient, primarily because of the higher hospital cost utilised by a small number of patients. Therefore, sensitivity analysis was carried out by removing these outliers. The cost was estimated by matching the sample to those completed the EQ-5D. By this method the median cost for QALY gained was marginally higher in the intervention group (£7912 vs. £7778) after applying 1000 replicated bootstraps.

Cost-Effectiveness

Due to the uncertainty around ICER estimates, cost-effectiveness acceptability curves (CEACs) are often used within the economic evaluation of clinical trials [41]. The CEAC curve below indicates the probability that the intervention group is cost-effective relative to the comparator group for a range of possible societal valuations of a QALY. If, for any given valuation of a QALY, the CEAC reaches or exceeds a 95 % probability, then it is possible to conclude that this intervention is cost-effective relative to the control group. Sensitivity analysis was carried out by removing outliers who had hospital admission stay of more than 10 days. CEAC were recalculated and shown in Fig. 9.3. This demonstrated that there is a high probability (>95 %) that the intervention group was more cost-effective than the control group above the cost per QALY threshold (£20,000–30,000). However, these data should

Table 9.9 Summary data for ICER

	QALY		Cost	
	Intervention	Control	Intervention	Control
Mean	1.274	1.219	1041.14	418.58
Standard error	0.001	0.001	6.92	1.54

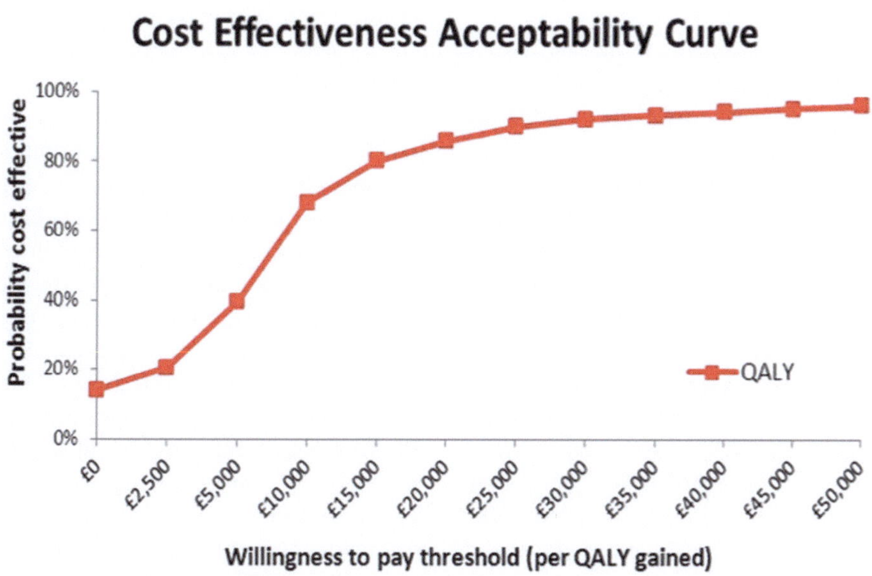

Fig. 9.3 Cost-effectiveness acceptability curve

be interpreted with caution as the data were still skewed despite the sensitivity analysis. In addition, although only a small number of patients were excluded from the cost analysis (those not completing the Resources Use questionnaire), a much larger number were excluded from the QALY analysis because they had not completed their EQ-5D questionnaires at both baseline and follow-up. As economic evaluations do not attempt to test a specific hypothesis, sample size is less important. However, a reduction in the sample may affect the reliability of the results. This should be kept in mind in interpreting these economic analyses.

Qualitative Study Summary

Previous studies that focused on community-based care in chronic diseases such as diabetes have shown that patients prefer care closer to home. This has resulted in several initiatives by the Department of Health in the UK to drive chronic disease management to be carried out in the community, although many did not show any clear clinical benefit. Therefore a qualitative study was carried out alongside this randomised trial to focus on the stakeholders' perspectives. The study results are briefly summarised below.

There was general agreement among participants across both primary and intermediate care that most T2D care should take place within primary care, but that this was currently not always possible as general practices varied in terms of their capacity and levels of expertise. Intermediate care was seen as providing useful support to primary care, especially for those practices not currently able to provide comprehensive diabetes support in-house. Two main types of support were identified: that ICCDs can help to upskill primary care professionals; and that patient care may be temporarily taken over by intermediate care professionals. Both formal and more informal opportunities for upskilling were provided across the three sites, and include formal training sessions, telephone support, and case discussions. Primary care staff appeared keen in principle to take advantage of these opportunities, but in practice the time available for them to do this was often limited (this particularly seemed to be the case for GPs). Intermediate care professionals' temporarily taking over patient care seemed to work well, and was regarded as offering important benefits for patients such as the opportunity to have a fresh look at an ongoing problem and/or for them to consult a professional with a higher level of expertise.

Whilst these two key forms of support were valued, there was, however, general agreement that they should lead to genuine capacity building within primary care and that practices' need to rely on intermediate care to take over patient care should reduce accordingly. Participants reported that, if an intermediate care service is to work well, then two main factors are important: close coordination with primary care (both when the service is being set-up and on an ongoing basis); and making the intermediate care service accessible and appropriate for patients.

Discussion

The ICCD study was an ambitious attempt to assess the effectiveness of community-based intermediate clinics in a randomised control trial setting. The results show that provision of ICCDs did not significantly increase the proportion of patients achieving good control of hyperglycaemia, blood pressure and cholesterol. When PCT was removed as a covariate, the primary outcome measure reached statistical significance ($p=0.048$); further highlighting the baseline variations between PCTs have probably contributed to the overall outcome. Any improvement, however, in clinical terms was small reflecting the global experience of difficulty in ensuring improved healthcare in this group [18].

Although the trial was not powered to detect the differences between the PCTs, there were important differences between them both at baseline and follow-up. In addition, there were also differences in the proportion of patients attending the ICCDs in PCTs. This was probably due to the differences in the case-finding approach used in the PCTs. In PCT 1 and 2, active case-finding approach was used and GPs were prompted and encouraged to use the ICCD services whilst in PCT 3 patients were referred by the GPs as they saw fit. The active case-finding approach was carried out by one of the ICCD nurses by looking through the GP records for patients who were not adequately controlled according to their risk factors. The small changes in risk factor control may reflect low referral to ICCDs, which could have been improved by more active case management. ICCDs are one way to provide such an enhanced case-finding and more aggressive target management service in the community with specialist input. Integrated case management through "case-finding" coupled with intensive intervention within existing primary care services and settings might be equally effective. Though the ICCDs are not explicitly constructed around the proven principles of case management and work force changes [18], PCT 1 and 2 used the proactive "case-finding" approach which were led by new team members. This in part may have been the reason for better uptake for the ICCDs and improvement in the control arms in these PCTs (concomitant primary care education and upskilling), whilst the uptake was poor in PCT 3, with deterioration in the risk factor control in the control arm.

The economic analysis suggested that ICCD is cost neutral and potentially beneficial gain at QALYs (£20,000–30,000) though this needs to be interpreted with caution due to the skewed distribution of hospital cost by a small number of patients. The findings also raise the notion that "stratified management of diabetes" according to their phenotype (for example morbidly obese patients may need bariatric surgery) or co-morbidity (for example patients with mental health problems would need treatment strategies that target their risk factors as well as their mental health). Such stratified management of diabetes might be more cost-effective.

From the qualitative data, all the stakeholders, including the patients, felt the usefulness of such ICCDs, in particular the aspect of care closer to home and the benefits of working closely with primary care. Primary care appreciated the case based educational opportunities on offer. It was also perceived that digital integration of data could provide further benefits for both ease of "case-finding" as well as "individualised risk factor target setting and management." One of the regional leads (Ponnusamy Saravanan) of the ICCD study team secured an innovation grant to implement such integrated service with digital integration of data in 12 practices in PCT 1 (Coventry) and PCT 2 (North Warwickshire). This innovation project was funded by Department of Health (Health Innovation Education Cluster funding stream) and led by two of the authors (Vinod Patel and Ponnusamy Saravanan). This was considered the follow-on project to the ICCD study, albeit as a pilot study in a subgroup of GP practices. The rationale, aims and objectives, methodology and results of this study called, Community Based Integrated service and Education for Diabetes (COMBINE for Diabetes) will be discussed in the next section.

COMBINE for Diabetes: A Pilot Study of a Digitally Integrated Diabetes Care Model

Introduction

Although the ICCDs were considered a success with some aspects of the local diabetes care model, one of the key stakeholders' feedback was the lack of utilisation of the risk factor data that are being collected for the purpose of QoF. In addition, the primary care teams (physicians and nurses) feel that they do not have opportunities for high quality, ongoing education in the field of diabetes and cardiovascular disorders, despite the increasing emphasis on managing these chronic diseases in primary care. Patients are also increasingly frustrated about the lack of ability in assessing their data by the diabetes specialists in the region for improving their individualised care.

As highlighted earlier in this chapter, improvement in the process measures since the introduction of QoF in 2004 enabled cardiovascular risk factors data (e.g., HbA1c, BP, Lipids, Smoking data, presence of CKD) are collected regularly and available electronically at individual patient level. Pulling together the longitudinal data at individual patient level at real-time that can be seen electronically could offer several advantages:

(a) Can be accessed and monitored remotely by specialist services (GPwSI, practice nurse with special interest and expertise in diabetes, diabetes specialist nurses, consultant diabetologists);
(b) Identify trends in deterioration of a particular risk factor for an individual patient prior to development of complications;
(c) Proactive "case-finding" (identifying patients with worse control) before the patients presenting with symptoms;
(d) Effective use of limited specialist resources (more patients can be reviewed electronically than face-face);
(e) Setting individualised risk factor targets for individual patients, if appropriate and
(f) Developing machine learning techniques to spot the deterioration as well as alerts for inappropriate prescribing (e.g., metformin in patients with deteriorating renal function, prompting discontinuation of hypoglycaemic agents when there is no improvement in HbA1c, etc.).

This innovation project was funded based on the above rationale and the potential advantages of digital integration and remote monitoring of primary care cardiovascular risk factor data in patients with diabetes. This pilot study was implemented in six general practices in Coventry and six in North Warwickshire. The study utilised a system called Diabetes Manager [42], which was developed by a GPwSI, based in Norfolk. Details of this system, and its subsequent version, Eclipse, are discussed below. The study was led by a local diabetologist and the intervention ran for a period of 3 months.

Objectives

1. Improving cardiovascular risk factors of patients with diabetes – Individualised patient targets for various risk factors by integrated collaborative approach between primary and secondary care team.
2. Education and "upskilling" of GPs and practice nurses – specifically targeting the practices that deliver less than satisfactory quality of care (will be identified using Quality outcome Framework – QoF data).

Methods

These 12 practices were chosen from the pool of GP practices that participated in the ICCD study. The Diabetes Manager system utilised the "QoF" template for remotely extracting the "read-codes" (each risk factor, e.g., HbA1c, BP). To avoid manual input, initially the system was only able to extract the data from GP practices that did not use "web-based" systems. The practices were chosen based on their systems. The lead specialist met all the 12 practices individually to demonstrate the system and firm commitment was obtained that they will implement the plans provided by the specialist for the individual patients. This agreement included a named GP and practice nurse for individual practices. Once the agreement was in place, it took an average of 2 weeks for the system to be ready and up- and running. Each user was given a unique user name and password. The risk factor data were automatically uploaded every Sunday (so that at any given time, the data were only 6-days old). The system was fully compliant with Data Protection Act 1998, as this was anonymous and handled by the same company that extracted the data for the QoF. Only patients' age and sex was visible along with a unique id that can only be linked by the named GP and Practice nurse in a given GP practice. A simple, user-friendly interface was developed using these individualised risk factor data. For ease of monitoring this interface utilised traffic light system. Figure

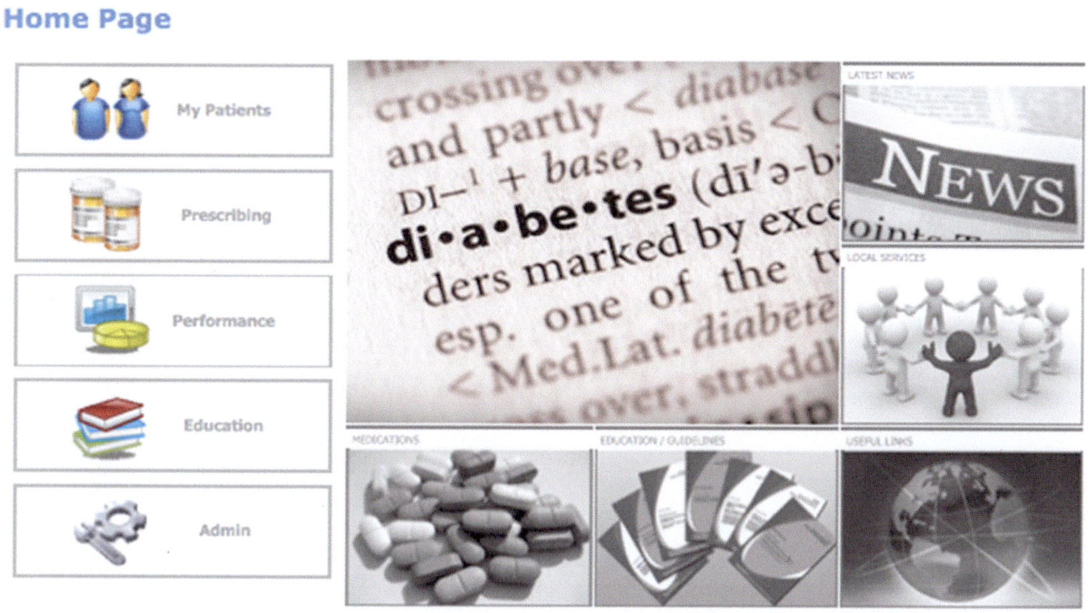

Diabetes Management Software (page 1 of 3)

Ref	Surgery	HbA1c	Chol	Chol Ratio	BP Sys	BP Dia	Weight (BMI)
2447	12806	13.8 28/09/2011			127 28/09/2011	78 28/09/2011	55.0 (20.8) 28/09/2011
1646	12806	12.3 15/12/2011	5.7 15/12/2011	2.71 15/12/2011	108 15/12/2011	66 15/12/2011	68.2 (25.7) 15/12/2011
444	12806	11.3 05/10/2010	4.4 05/10/2010	4.00 05/10/2010	133 11/10/2011	69 11/10/2011	97.9 (31.6) 11/10/2011
4403	12806	11.0 11/04/2011	3.5 11/04/2011	4.40 11/04/2011	135 03/02/2011	75 03/02/2011	64.0 (25.5) 08/07/2011
108	12806	10.7 06/12/2011	3.6 30/12/2010	2.80 30/12/2010	131 20/12/2011	87 20/12/2011	131.0 (38.3) 04/01/2012
465	12806	10.7 19/07/2011	4.1 17/01/2012	2.90 17/01/2012	120 25/10/2011	65 25/10/2011	47.0 (18.7) 25/10/2011
6478	12806	10.5 28/11/2011	5.9 17/10/2011	4.50 17/10/2011	154 14/10/2011	90 14/10/2011	95.0 (34.5) 08/03/2010
5165	12806	10.4 06/07/2011	6.4 06/07/2011	4.90 06/07/2011	158 22/06/2011	89 22/06/2011	124.0 (47.8) 20/06/2011
2436	12806	10.0 07/11/2011	4.2 07/11/2011	3.20 07/11/2011	140 14/11/2011	80 14/11/2011	87.0 (33.2) 05/10/2011
1293	12806	10.0 17/11/2011	4.5 17/11/2011	2.25 17/11/2011	123 17/11/2011	75 17/11/2011	57.0 (22.1) 17/11/2011
1277	12806	9.8 11/12/2008	4.6 07/06/2011	2.40 07/06/2011	215 11/12/2008	82 11/12/2008	74.1 (23.4) 11/12/2008

Fig. 9.4 (**a**) Diabetes Manager interphase. (**b**) Summary page, tabular form. (**c**) Single patient summary. (**d**) Single patient summary, graphical

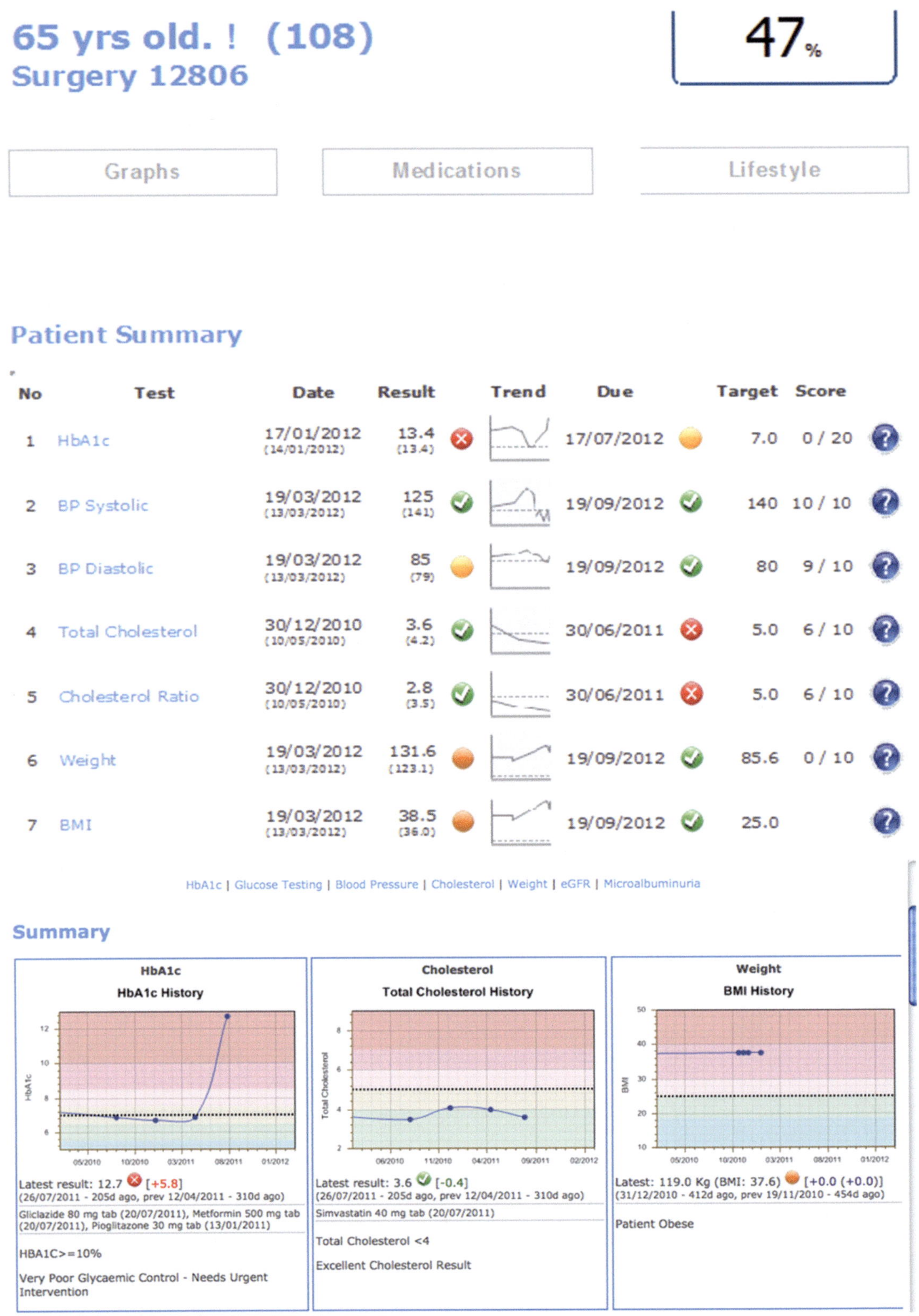

Fig. 9.4 (continued)

9.4a–d shows the screen shots of various graphs that can be generated. They can be seen either as longitudinal trend graphs (for assessing deterioration or improvement at individual level) or as tables with traffic light system (for selecting a group of patients above or below a particular target/threshold). Thus, for both the primary care team and the specialist team, it was possible to identify the patients who require attention within three to four clicks after logging to the system. Although the system allows real time referral that can be sent to the specialist (and guidance back to the primary care team), this facility was not utilised during this pilot study to standardise the process (some GP practices do not want this to be done).

Individualised Risk Factor Management Strategy

For an individual patient, the relative deterioration of a risk factor is more important than blanket threshold set by NICE. However, this is not done in routine practice. In this proposed project, patients' were set individualised targets for their risk factors by careful analysis of the longitudinal values. The specialists did this in collaboration with the patients and the GPs. Such a comprehensive approach was seen as more likely to get the "buy in" from patients and therefore result in improvement.

The specialist proactively identified the patients with poor cardiovascular risk factor management control in each of the 12 practices and devised individualised management plans for the patients. These patients were then put on the "watch list," which enabled the follow-up was done easily. Each practice had this management plan input once during the study. In addition, GPs could and did contact the specialist for asking doubts about specific patients. If the specialist felt the decision for the management plan couldn't be implemented remotely, the primary care team was recommended to send referral to the relevant specialist team (including community diabetes specialist nurses). Thus the individualised risk factor management was carried out in the following steps: (a) Risk factor screening, (b) Individualised target setting and (c) Patient consultation as and when required and appropriate.

Education Workshops

Alongside the intervention, two half-day workshops were conducted for all practice nurses and GPs. This was tailor made for the practice nurses and GPs – one on basic education and the second on advanced diabetes care. Each workshop had a maximum capacity of 20 places and was conducted by an experienced diabetes specialist nurse (DSN) and a clinician specialised in diabetes. A total of ten workshops were conducted during the 12-month period, to aid self-sustainability for developing individualised cardiovascular risk factor management plans (care plans) in patients with diabetes. Each participant therefore had to attend two half-days on two different days (a total of 7–8 h of education).

Evaluation of the Intervention

(a) Diabetes knowledge questionnaire pre and post workshops
(b) Individualised risk factor modification – change in risk factors (3 months)

Results

Cardiovascular Risk Factor Data

The total number of patients with diabetes in these 12 practices was 3400. Of these 408 patients were identified as having poor control: 353 for HbA1c; 222 for BP and 105 for Cholesterol. For the purpose of this pilot study QoF targets were chosen as this itself identified nearly 15 % of the patients (HbA1c: >7.5 %, BP: >145/85 mmHg and Cholesterol >5.0 mmol/l). Typically three-steps were given for individualised management plan for each of these patients, by the specialist to the primary care team. All patients had a follow-up period of minimum 3 months (some had up to 6 months).

The baseline characteristics of patients who were identified as having HbA1c, BP and total cholesterol above the QoF threshold in these 12 practices were shown in Table 9.10. Three-month

Table 9.10 The baseline characteristics of patients identified

	N	Mean	SD
Characteristics of patients with HbA1c >7.5 %			
Age years	353	66.17	10.1
BMI kg/m^2	347	31.7	6.5
HbA1c %	353	8.64	0.89
Systolic BP mmHg	352	138.4	19.5
Diastolic BP mmHg	352	79.8	11.1
Total cholesterol mmol/L	344	4.3	1.0
Characteristics of patients with BP >145/85 mmHg			
Age years	222	66.06	9.0
BMI kg/m^2	217	32.1	6.3
HbA1c %	220	8.32	0.94
Systolic BP mmHg	222	152.0	16.3
Diastolic BP mmHg	222	86.4	9.7
Total Cholesterol mmol/L	217	4.3	0.9
Characteristics of patients with total cholesterol >5.0 mmol/L			
Age years	105	64.45	10.7
BMI kg/m^2	104	31.2	6.2
HbA1c %	105	8.55	1.27
Systolic BP mmHg	105	136.9	18.6
Diastolic BP mmHg	105	80.6	10.8
Total cholesterol mmol/L	105	5.62	0.75

follow-up data were available for only 225/353 patients with HbA1c, whilst the data for follow-up BP (n=222/222) and total cholesterol (n=102/105) were near complete. There were marked improvements in all of these risk factors: Δ HbA1c: 0.77 % (±0.75); Δ Systolic BP: 13.43 mmHg (±20.12); Δ Diastolic BP (±13.50); and Δ Total cholesterol: 0.56 mmol/L (±0.72); all $p<0.001$.

Education Workshops

A total of 182 healthcare professionals (HCPs) attended the ten workshops. After the first set of workshop, this was opened to the whole region due to overwhelming request from the participants. At the end of the year, 91 different HCPs attended these workshops twice. Of these, 57 % were GPs, 40 % were practice nurses and 3 % were others.

The feedbacks on workshops were highly positive (4.75 out of 5 where 5 was extremely valuable; n=176). Examples of the feedback from the GPs were: "*Make sense*," "*Can we be part of the programme*," "*I will now manage patients aggressively early in the disease*," and "*We want to tap in the expertise and not be penalized at the same time*." Example feedback from the practice nurses were: "*We never get hands on practice like this*," "*Gives us confidence to manage patients – I mean the practice with real patient case histories*," "*Learnt why metformin should be prescribed*," and "*We can ask opinions quickly – especially when want to be reassured what you are thinking is right*."

Discussion

This was one of the few projects in the UK that attempted to digitally integrate the individual patient data from multiple GP practices and used case-finding approach to improve the cardiovascular risk factors in patients with diabetes. This simple, targeted case-finding approach improved the cardiovascular risk factors significantly. Although this innovation project did not have a control group and HbA1c data were not repeated at 3 months for all the patients who were identified, the marked improvement observed at 3 months supports this model of care. This project clearly showed that effective utilisation of the routinely collected longitudinal data is possible with little effort from the HCPs involved. It also showed that such data can be monitored remotely and proactively identify patients whose cardiovascular risk factors are not controlled (case-finding). Whilst the individualised management plan by the specialist may have partly helped to improve the cardiovascular risk factors, the specialist himself believes that the proactive case-finding approach played a major role and *must* become part of integrated diabetes care models. Finally, health economic analysis was not part of this pilot study. However, only a day per GP practice was spent on identifying and devising the individualist management plan (total of 12 days) by the specialist. The cost of Diabetes Manager was provided free of cost for the purpose of the pilot study and the updated version (*Eclipse*) approximately costs £600 per practice per year [43]. Therefore, this digitally integrated diabetes care model provides an opportunity for commissioning organisations across the UK to provide high quality individualised diabetes care at reduced cost. Indeed, subsequent to the completion of this innovation project, more than 30 practices in Nuneaton and Coventry (2 different clinical commissioning groups – CCGs) have incorporated the *Eclipse* system as a way to improve the diabetes services.

Conclusion and Future Directions

In this chapter, two sequential projects that were conducted in the Coventry and North Warwickshire region which has a high proportion of small and single-handed GP practices catering for multi-ethnic UK population. This region also had one of the poorest wards in the country, with severe deprivation and higher than national average prevalence of T2D [44]. Coventry also has a very high prevalence of obesity and has one of the highest incidences of stroke rates in the UK [44]. Similarly, city of Leicester (part of the cluster RCT) has the highest proportion of South Asians living in a city in the UK [45]. The first project was an ambitious attempt to assess the clinical and cost-effectiveness of ICCDs in an RCT setting in the UK. Although the study only had 64 % follow-up rates, highlighting the difficulties of conducting large-scale cluster RCTs, it enabled objective assessment of ICCDs. Prior to this RCT there were no such RCTs that comprehensively assessed the performance of the ICCDs. The study highlighted the importance of team-change (new personnel), need for local champions to drive improvement in chronic diseases such as diabetes and the need for proactive case-finding approach. The infrastructure and links developed during this RCT were utilised to conduct the digital integrated diabetes care innovation project (COMBINE for Diabetes) in a subset of these practices in North Warwickshire and Coventry.

The innovation project targeted two key issues in diabetes care models: digital integration of individual longitudinal data and proactive monitoring, case-finding and care-plan development for *all* of the patients managed by primary care. This project showed that such case-finding and proactive management might be feasible with existing resources. Such innovation, combined with locally relevant educational workshops for upskilling the primary care HCPs could also provide a sustainable long-term strategy for chronic disease such as diabetes. Success of these integrated diabetes care models will require strategic leadership, adoption by the commissioners as well as the specialist care providers in a given region. The innovation pilot has provided a strong case for working towards such an integrated diabetes care service and breaks the arbitrary boundaries not only between the primary and specialist services but also other services that cater to patients with diabetes.

Finally, to provide high quality care and reduce the cost burden of diabetes, any integrated diabetes care models must prioritise prevention *and* early aggressive intervention over downstream interventions (secondary and tertiary prevention). This can allow commissioning of services that extend from community prevention, screening, early diagnosis, strong foundations of care, and education to the treatment of complications and end of life care. We name this model as "Diabetes Matrix" which is shown in Table 9.11. This table summarises an integrated approach to prevention, care, and clinical commissioning that

Table 9.11 Diabetes matrix

Level	Target group	Recommendations
1: Community prevention	Entire local population	GP, local authority, employers, community to promote healthy lifestyle choices
2: Prediabetic screening	At risk groups within the local population	GP screening for at risk individuals: questionnaire, HbA1c%, etc.
3: Early diagnosis	Prediabetic population, known impaired glucose tolerance, newly diagnosed DM	GP: monitors and manages those with IGT, IFG and newly diagnosed diabetes
4: Forging foundations	Newly diagnosed	GP/specialist: individual's care-planning, patient education and excellent clinical care according to current best practice and NICE
5: Rolling review	5A: Well controlled with few risk factors to manage	GP: "year of care" or all main clinical needs embedded within an annual review [46]
	5B: Complicated, higher risk, poorer quality care	GP or integrated/specialist: proactive case-finding and management
6: Early escalation	Uncontrolled clinical and social factors at high risk of complications and admission	GP or integrated/specialist: aggressive management of difficult to control risk factors, consider referral or seek advice
7: Curbing complications	7A: Patients with known complications/conditions	GP and shared care: advice sought from best local advice, consider specialist referral
	7B: Patients with unpredictable complications	
8: Avoidable admissions	Hypoglycaemia, DKA, foot ulceration and infection	Specialist acute care with diabetes input: "Think Glucose" management to reduce length of stay [47]. Discharge to GP or shared care to continue
9: Unavoidable admissions	Patients with advanced disease and complications	Specialist acute care with diabetes input: "Think Glucose" management to reduce length of stay. Usually shared care with GP/specialist to continue
10. Rationalised long-term care	Patient with co-morbidities not amenable to treatment	GP or specialist or both to rationalise care: review clinical targets, outcomes and medication. Coordinate care acceptable to patients/care. Aim for symptom free, high quality end of life care

can be followed and implemented in a healthcare economy. It describes ten steps of integrated diabetes care from "community prevention" to "end of life care" with the target population at each level and recommendations for both clinicians and commissioners. It is time that proactive preventive management incorporating latest technology that can aid individualised care is implemented across the world for people with and at risk of diabetes. We should also move away from short-term goals (for example: prescribing cost of drugs) to long-term goals and strategies that can reduce the clinical and cost burden of diabetes.

Acknowledgements Authors of this invited book chapter fully acknowledge all the ICCD study group members: Natalie Armstrong, Darrin Baines, Richard Baker, Richard Crossman, Melanie Davies, Ainsley Hardy, Kamlesh Khunti, Sudhesh Kumar, Joseph Paul O'Hare, Neil Raymond, Ponnusamy Saravanan, Nigel Stallard, Ala Szczepura and Andrew Wilson.

Dr Saravanan thanks Dr Julian Brown, Founder of Diabetes Manager & Eclipse systems for providing the system free during the COMBINE for Diabetes innovation programme.

Conflict of Interest Authors declare no conflict of interest. Although Dr Ponnusamy Saravanan provided feedback regarding the Diabetes Manager system, he was not paid for this service.

References

1. Federation ID. IDF diabetes atlas. 6th ed. Brussels: International Diabetes Federation; 2013.
2. Guariguata L. Tackling the global epidemic – new estimates from the IDF diabetes atlas update for 2012. Diabetes Voice. 2012;57(3):12–5.
3. Ham C, York N, Sutch S, Shaw R. Hospital bed utilisation in the NHS, Kaiser Permanente, and the US Medicare programme: analysis of routine data. BMJ. 2003;327(7426):1257.
4. Murphy E. Case management and community matrons for long term conditions. BMJ. 2004;329(7477):1251–2.
5. The NHS Information Centre. National diabetes audit executive summary 2009–2010.
6. Khunti K, Ganguli S. Who looks after people with diabetes: primary or secondary care? J R Soc Med. 2000;93:183–6.
7. Millett C, Gray J, Saxena S, Netuveli G, Khunti K, Majeed A. Ethnic disparities in diabetes management and pay-for-performance in the UK: the Wandsworth Prospective Diabetes Study. PLoS Med. 2007;4(6):e191.
8. Calvert M, Shankar A, McManus RJ, Lester H, Freemantle N. Effect of the quality and outcomes framework on diabetes care in the United Kingdom: retrospective cohort study. BMJ. 2009;338:b1870.
9. Serumaga B, Ross-Degnan D, Avery AJ, Elliott RA, Majumdar SR, Zhang F, et al. Effect of pay for performance on the management and outcomes of hypertension in the United Kingdom: interrupted time series study. BMJ. 2011;342:d108.
10. Millett C, Saxena S, Ng A, Mainous 3rd A, Majeed A. Socio-economic status, ethnicity and diabetes management: an analysis of time trends using the health survey for England. J Publ Health (Oxf). 2007;29(4):413–9.
11. Gulliford MC, Ashworth M, Robotham D, Mohiddin A. Achievement of metabolic targets for diabetes by English primary care practices under a new system of incentives. Diabet Med. 2007;24(5):505–11.
12. Davies MJ, Heller S, Skinner TC, Campbell MJ, Carey ME, Cradock S, et al. Effectiveness of the diabetes education and self management for ongoing and newly diagnosed (DESMOND) programme for people with newly diagnosed type 2 diabetes: cluster randomised controlled trial. BMJ. 2008;336(7642):491–5.
13. Khunti K, Davies M. Glycaemic goals in patients with type 2 diabetes: current status, challenges and recent advances. Diabetes Obes Metab. 2010;12:474–84.
14. Nocon A, Rhodes PJ, Wright JP, Eastham J, Williams DR, Harrison SR, et al. Specialist general practitioners and diabetes clinics in primary care: a qualitative and descriptive evaluation. Diabet Med: J Br Diabet Assoc. 2004;21(1):32–8.
15. Halfyard C, McGowan D, Whyte M, Gayle C. Diabetes rapid access clinic: a bridge between primary and secondary care (Diabetes UK poster presentation). Diabet Med. 2010;27 Suppl 1:137.
16. Sharp PS. Glycaemic outcomes following discharge from an intermediate care diabetes clinic. Pract Diabetes Int. 2010;27(2):53–4.
17. Health in Wales. Cardiff CCM demonstrator model for diabetes intermediate care clinics-progress underway 2010 [cited 2011 29 August]. Available from: http://www.wales.nhs.uk/news/16399.
18. Tricco AC, Ivers NM, Grimshaw JM, Moher D, Turner L, Galipeau J, et al. Effectiveness of quality improvement strategies on the management of diabetes: a systematic review and meta-analysis. Lancet. 2012;379(9833):2252–61.
19. Shojania KG, Ranji SR, McDonald KM, Grimshaw JM, Sundaram V, Rushakoff RJ, et al. Effects of quality improvement strategies for type 2 diabetes on glycemic control. JAMA J Am Med Assoc. 2006;296(4):427–40.
20. Gaede P, Vedel P, Larsen N, Jensen GV, Parving HH, Pedersen O. Multifactorial intervention and cardiovascular disease in patients with type 2 diabetes. N Engl J Med. 2003;348(5):383–93.
21. Holman RR, Paul SK, Bethel MA, Matthews DR, Neil HA. 10-year follow-up of intensive glucose control in type 2 diabetes. N Engl J Med. 2008;359(15):1577–89.
22. Holman RR, Paul SK, Bethel MA, Neil HA, Matthews DR. Long-term follow-up after tight control of blood pressure in type 2 diabetes. N Engl J Med. 2008;359(15):1565–76.
23. Ray KK, Seshasai SR, Wijesuriya S, Sivakumaran R, Nethercott S, Preiss D, et al. Effect of intensive control of glucose on cardiovascular outcomes and death in patients with diabetes mellitus: a meta-analysis of randomised controlled trials. Lancet. 2009;373(9677):1765–72.
24. Ahroni JH, Boyko EJ, Davignon DR, Pecoraro RE. The health and functional status of veterans with diabetes. Diabetes Care. 1994;17(4):318–21.

25. Van der Does FE, De Neeling JN, Snoek FJ, Kostense PJ, Grootenhuis PA, Bouter LM, et al. Symptoms and well-being in relation to glycemic control in type II diabetes. Diabetes Care. 1996;19(3):204–10.
26. Papanas N, Tsapas A, Papatheodorou K, Papazoglou D, Bekiari E, Sariganni M, et al. Glycaemic control is correlated with well-being index (WHO-5) in subjects with type 2 diabetes. Exp Clin Endocrinol Diabetes. 2010;118(6):364–7.
27. Gray A, Clarke P, Farmer A, Holman R. Implementing intensive control of blood glucose concentration and blood pressure in type 2 diabetes in England: cost analysis (UKPDS 63). BMJ. 2002;325(7369):860.
28. Armstrong N, Baines D, Baker R, Crossman R, Davies M, Hardy A, et al. A cluster randomised controlled trial of the effectiveness and cost-effectiveness of Intermediate Care Clinics for Diabetes (ICCD): study protocol for a randomised controlled trial. Trials. 2012;13:164.
29. Wilson A, O'Hare JP, Hardy A, Raymond N, Szczepura A, Crossman R, et al. Evaluation of the clinical and cost effectiveness of intermediate care clinics for diabetes (ICCD): a multicentre cluster randomised controlled trial. PLoS One. 2014;9(4):e93964.
30. The Diabetes Trials Unit – Oxford. UKPDS risk engine: home page. 2010 [cited 2010 3 February]. Available from: http://www.dtu.ox.ac.uk/riskengine/index.php.
31. The Euroqol Group. EQ-5D user guide: a measure of health-related quality of life developed by the EuroQol Group. The Netherlands: EuroQol Business Management; 1995.
32. Welch GW, Jacobson AM, Polonsky WH. The problem areas in diabetes scale. An evaluation of its clinical utility. Diabetes Care. 1997;20(5):760–6.
33. Gulliford MC, Naithani S, Morgan M. Continuity of care and intermediate outcomes of type 2 diabetes mellitus. Fam Pract. 2007;24(3):245–51.
34. Drummond MF, Sculpher MJ, Torrance GW, et al. Methods for the economic evaluation of health care programmes. 3rd ed. Oxford: Oxford University Press; 2005.
35. Hippisley-Cox J, O'Hanlon S, Coupland C. Association of deprivation, ethnicity, and sex with quality indicators for diabetes: population based survey of 53,000 patients in primary care. BMJ. 2004;329(7477):1267–9.
36. Kinmonth AL, Woodcock A, Griffin S, Spiegal N, Campbell MJ. Randomised controlled trial of patient centred care of diabetes in general practice: impact on current wellbeing and future disease risk. BMJ. 1998;317:1202–8.
37. Bellary S, O'Hare JP, Raymond NT, Gumber A, Mughal S, Szczepura A, et al. Enhanced diabetes care to patients of south Asian ethnic origin (the United Kingdom Asian Diabetes Study): a cluster randomised controlled trial. Lancet. 2008;371(9626):1769–76.
38. Miyamoto JM, Eraker SA. Parameter estimates for a QALY utility model. Med Decis Making Int J Soc Med Decis Making. 1985;5(2):191–213.
39. Richardson G, Manca A. Calculation of quality adjusted life years in the published literature: a review of methodology and transparency. Health Econ. 2004;13(12):1203–10.
40. Baker R, Chilton S, Donaldson C, Jones-Lee M, Lancsar E, Mason H, et al. Searchers vs surveyors in estimating the monetary value of a QALY: resolving a nasty dilemma for NICE. Health Econ Policy Law. 2011;6(4):435–47.
41. Petrou S, Gray A. Economic evaluation alongside randomised controlled trials: design, conduct, analysis, and reporting. BMJ. 2011;342:d1548.
42. Brown J. Diabetes manager. (http://www.diabetes-manager.org.uk). 2010.
43. Brown J. Eclipse. (http://www.eclipsecolutions.org). 2013.
44. Health and Social Care Information Centre. (2015). Accessed at http://www.hscic.gov.uk on 19 Dec 2015.
45. Geographies of diversity in Leicestershire; Leicestershire City Council. (2013). Accessed at http://www.ethnicity.ac.uk/.
46. Getting to Grips with the year of care: a practical guide. (2008). Accessed at http://www.yearofcare.co.uk on 19 Dec 2015.
47. Think glucose. (2011). Accessed at http://www.institute.nhs.uk/ on 19 Dec 2015.

Integrated Diabetes Care in Germany: Triple Aim in Gesundes Kinzigtal

10

Caroline Lang, Elisa A.M. Kern, Timo Schulte, and Helmut Hildebrandt

Introduction

The German health system is based upon a compulsory, "statutory health insurance" (SHI). The contribution fee is based on income, although employees with incomes above a certain threshold, and the self-employed, can opt out of the SHI and insure themselves privately. Contrary to the terminology, the SHI is not "insurance" – where premiums are risk-based – but rather a fund, into which members have to pay. Consequently, health fund would be the more appropriate term. Three pillars make up the SHI budget:

1. Contributions based exclusively on income from gainful employment, pensions or unemployment benefits, but currently not savings, capital gains or other forms of unearned income. Since 2005, employees have been required to contribute 8.2% of their gross income; employers pay 7.3% [1];
2. Tax financed subsidies: in 2012 this was about 4.8% [1, pp 115] to 7.38% [2] of the SHI income;
3. Additional contribution fees, on average about 0.9% of gross income [1]. This effectively means that parity financing has to date been given up.

This health care funding faces an enormous increase in healthcare system expenditure as a result of a range of demographic changes. An analysis of the Robert Koch-Institute (RKI) from 2012 shows that more than 50% of German people over 65 years suffer from at least one chronic disease, approximately 50% suffer from two to four chronic diseases, and over a quarter suffer from five or more diseases [3]. This growing rate of chronic diseases and multi-morbidity in the ageing population coupled with the comparatively high life expectancy in Germany, in a setting of high-quality care standards and the universal provision (regardless of income), a broad range of medical services, medicines and medical aids have contributed significantly to an increase in Germany's public health sector expenditure [4–6]. Currently the public sector covers the majority (77%) of health expenditures in Germany [7]. An important driver of expenditure is the provision of hospital services which is about 77.0 billion € (26.04%) in 2011 rising to 82.4 billion € (26.1%) in 2013 [8]. If we take all

C. Lang (✉)
Department of Internal Medicine, Prevention and Care of Diabetes, University Hospital Carl Gustav Carus at the Technische Universität, Dresden, Dresden, Germany
e-mail: ca.lang@gmx.de

E.A.M. Kern
Gesundes Kinzigtal GmbH, Haslach, Germany
e-mail: e.kern@gesundes-kinzigtal.de

T. Schulte • H. Hildebrandt
OptiMedis AG, Hamburg, Germany
e-mail: t.schulte@optimedis.de; office@optimedis.de

D. Simmons et al. (eds.), *Integrated Diabetes Care*, DOI 10.1007/978-3-319-13389-8_10

forms of inpatient care into account it is 36.6 % of all expenditures, increasing to 37.6 % in 2013. These recent changes in healthcare in Germany are leading to new challenges requiring new approaches to healthcare. Amelung summarizes the following aspects, which should be considered in combination for the development of new forms of care [9]:

1. Competition regarding quality and financial contribution as a regulatory policy objective;
2. Opening of the healthcare market for new providers;
3. Breaking rigid structures in healthcare sectors through new forms of care;
4. Meeting new challenges in healthcare caused by chronic diseases and multi-morbidity;
5. Developing strategies against underutilization, especially in regions difficult to supply;
6. More flexible work models for female physicians;
7. Restructuring of care processes through targeted incentives to promote and reward health maintenance.

According to a survey of insured patients in Germany, which was performed by the Commonwealth Fund in 2013, 58 % of the respondents perceived that the German health system fundamentally needed to be reformed or completely rebuild [10]. The current organization of the health system is characterized by a strict sectorial segregation. This makes it difficult to implement interdisciplinary, cooperative and cross-sectoral network, efficient communication and information provision between inpatient-, outpatient-, rehabilitation care and adequate public health services. This is particularly the case in the care of the increasing number of patients with chronic diseases. To provide an efficient, effective and high-quality health system in Germany, a redesign seems to be inevitable, but depends on how to reorganize the care of patients with complex needs and diseases [5].

In recent years, various models were initiated to guarantee cross-sectoral and integrated care and to facilitate more competitive health insurance in Germany. Reorganization started with the reform of the German statutory health insurance (GKV) law in 2000, the establishment of medical care centres (§ 95 SGB V), GP-supporting care concepts and GP-centred care (§ 73b SGB V), implementation of Disease-Management Programmes (DMP; § 137f-g SGB V), the enactment for Integrated Care Solution (§ 140a-d SGB V) and the care structure law (Versorgungsstrukturgesetz; § 87b SGB V). The traditional model of collective contracts between health insurance companies and healthcare providers were superseded by allowing selective contracting between particular institutions [11, 12].

The first approaches towards integrated healthcare were introduced in Germany in 2002 through Disease-Management Programmes. These structured treatment programmes were designed to ensure integrated, cross-sectoral and evidence-based treatment and care for chronically ill people diagnosed with asthma, breast cancer, chronic obstructive pulmonary disease (COPD), coronary heart disease, Type-1-diabetes mellitus (T1DM) and Type-2-diabetes mellitus (T2DM). The DMP's aimed to avoid chronic disease complications and associated excess hospitalization, to reduce over- and underutilization of care, and thereby ensuring efficient care nationally [13]. Currently there are 7,566,191 patients registered in a DMP in Germany, of which 3,969,019 patients are enrolled in the DMP for T2DM. This programme was introduced in July 2002. Participation in a DMP is voluntary and at no personal cost [14]. Although perceived to have positive effects on DMP patient survival, evaluations has been limited and divergent [13]. Integrated care solutions have been regulated by law in Germany since 2004 and resulted from reforms of the Statutory Health Insurance (SHI) Modernization Act (GMG). Financial support was promoted from 2004 onwards by the standard care budget and by governmental regulated start-up funding for integrated care projects up to 2009 [15]. Despite the introduction of these measures and a relatively good level of healthcare provision in Germany, the treatment and care of chronically ill people is faced with historically evolved, "system resistance" that hinders optimal integrated care. This is due to strict cross-sectoral boundaries between outpatient and inpatient care, public health services and insufficient cooperation in care processes [5].

T2DM and its complications have become a growing health, social and economic burden in Europe and worldwide. An estimated number of 56.3 million people are living with diabetes in Europe [16]. According to a recent RKI study ("Studie zur Gesundheit Erwachsener in Deutschland"; DEGS), 4.6 million adults between 18 and 79 years old (7.2 %) in Germany are estimated to have been diagnosed with either T1DM, T2DM or gestational diabetes [17]. The lifetime-prevalence of diabetes has increased noticeably due to ageing. The total healthcare expenditures of diabetes are currently estimated by 30 billion € per year [18, 19]. In light of these changes and challenges, there is an urgent need for action, especially in chronic disease such as T2DM. It seems inevitable that meeting the increasing needs of this health burden will require optimized integration and coordination of chronic care [20]. Comprehensive healthcare reforms should initiate the development of integrated and coordinated care solutions, ensure good cooperation of healthcare providers and facilitate a more efficient approach to healthcare provision. One step towards a better healthcare system in Germany was the integrated care initiative "Gesundes Kinzigtal" (GK) which was launched on 1st November 2005 in Haslach, Germany.

"Gesundes Kinzigtal": A German Approach for a Fully Integrated Care System

The healthcare network and management company "Gesundes Kinzigtal Ltd" described as a "flagship-project" among integrated care approaches in Germany, is located in the affluent rural Kinzigtal region (population 69,000) that lies in the southwest of the federal state Baden-Wuerttemberg, close to Freiburg in Germany (Fig. 10.1) [21]. The integrated healthcare system GK was introduced here in 2005 [22–27].

Strategic Framework and Objectives of Gesundes Kinzigtal

The main strategic framework of GK is based on the Triple Aim Approach, developed in 2008 by Berwick et al. in cooperation with the Institute for Healthcare Improvement (IHI) [28]. Berwick et al. take a United States perspective, that a responsible, sustainable and high-quality healthcare system has to address [28]:

1. Improvement in individual experience of care;
2. Improvement in population health;
3. Reduction in the per capita costs of care for populations.

These three dimensions are displayed below (Fig. 10.2) in accordance of the Triple Aim Model of Berwick et al. [28, 29].

Derived from this approach, there are several objectives of GK [30]:

1. Financial success with an innovative shared health gain approach (see the section on Financing Model in this chapter);
2. Development of better organized healthcare for the population in Kinzigtal, in cooperation with the patient, the other local health partners and health insurance companies;
3. Increasing the attractiveness of the Kinzigtal region for the regional population through development of additional services and ensuring local long-term healthcare;
4. Securing an appropriate number of providers in the area;
5. Increasing the attractiveness of the Kinzigtal region for young health professionals in medicine and increasing job satisfaction of physicians;
6. Use of latest scientific findings for prevention and treatment created in close association with all those involved in GK;
7. Introducing innovations in the organization and delivery of healthcare.

These objectives were expected to be achieved by improved cross-sectoral management, more

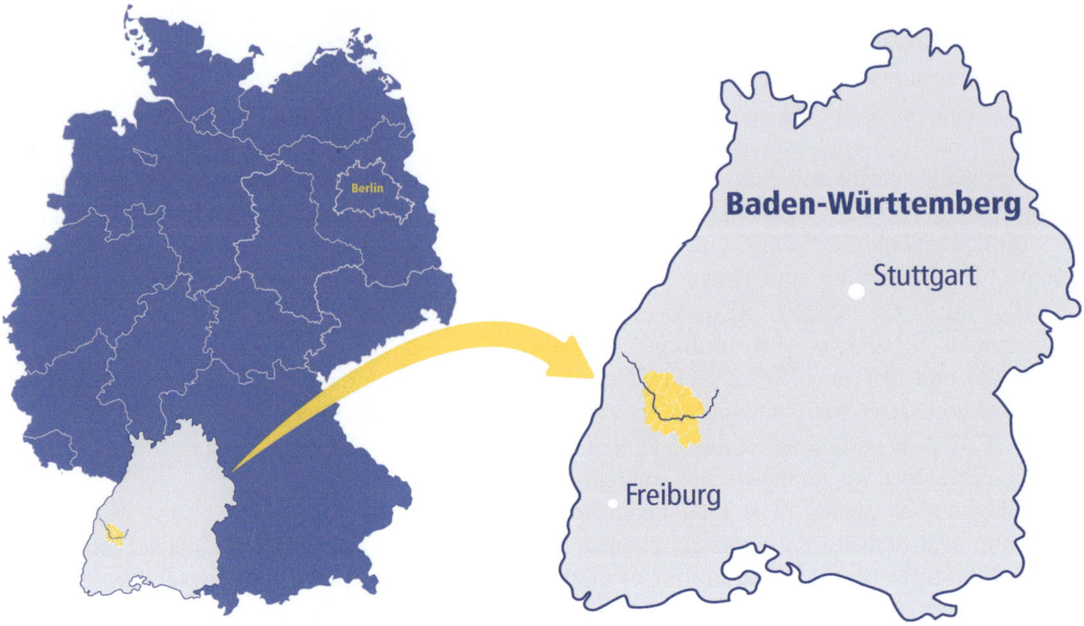

Fig. 10.1 Region of Kinzigtal in Baden-Wuerttemberg, Germany

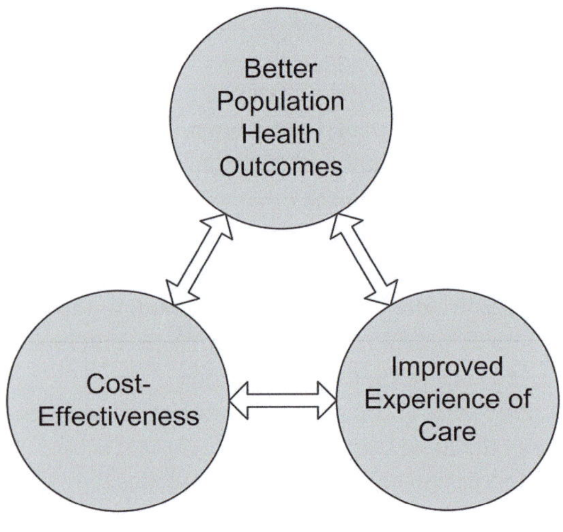

Fig. 10.2 The Triple Aim Model

efficient cooperation by healthcare providers between different care sectors, a reduction in morbidity, especially in chronically ill people, and favourable conditions for purchasing external products such as medication [22, 31]. On the one hand, the Triple Aim dimensions form the basis for the actions and decision-making processes of GK with the political authorities, the insured patients, the health insurance companies and society. On the other hand, they offer optimized leadership for healthcare in the region [32]. Combining the knowledge and experience of medical healthcare providers with those of Health Sciences and Management was expected to lead to improved cooperation and achieving the GK objectives.

Stakeholder Involvement in Gesundes Kinzigtal

GK consists of several organizations that cooperate with each other. The shareholders of this company are local physicians "Physicians' Network in Kinzigtal Region" (MQNK) and the health sciences based OptiMedis AG in Hamburg. Two health insurance companies (sickness funds) partnered with the project in 2006: AOK Baden-Wuerttemberg (AOK BW) in 2005 and the Social Security of Agriculture, Forestry and Horticulture (SVLFG; previously LKK Baden-Wuerttemberg). AOK BW and SVLFG cover the less educated part of the population who also experience higher morbidity and are more "vulnerable". A 10-year contract was in place 2005–2015, in accordance with §§140a-d SGB V. The contract is currently under renegotiation for unlimited extension. About 33,000 patients, nearly half of the Kinzigtal population, are insured either by the AOK BW (about 31,600 members) or SVLFG (about 1,400 members). Since July 2006, these patients have been invited to enrol in GK generally, or in specific healthcare programmes, to take advantage of the additional healthcare services of GK. Approximately 30 % of insured individuals (mainly the elderly and those with greater morbidity) under the two participating health insurance companies have enrolled in GK until December 2014. With the exception of dental care, all healthcare sectors are covered by the GK company [13, 22, 23, 25–27, 32, 33].

GK is also supported by several other partners covering many services including psychotherapists, physiotherapists, general physicians and specialists, paediatricians, hospitals, rehabilitation centres, nursing homes, nursing services, pharmacies and welfare centres. Sports and cultural clubs, gyms, podiatrists and wellness facilities provide further services for the wellbeing of the patient and to increase and support healthy lifestyles [34]. The insured patients enrolled in GK also have additional medical time to achieve treatment objectives and ensure intensive and patient centred outpatient care [23].

A Patients Advisory Committee (PAC) was established to strengthen cooperation in the community and to mediate between enrolled patients, the company and service providers should problems arise with GK or practices. PAC supports patients with chronic disease to develop their own vision for personal health, striving for goals with the agreement of their family doctor. The Committee consists of five patients who are participating in GK and one ombudswoman who supports the PAC if complaints arise [34].

Financing Model of Gesundes Kinzigtal

There are no incentives for risk-selection by healthcare providers under the GK contract. Instead, the cooperation agreements within GK are based on a new and innovative shared health gain approach for healthcare financing: "shared-savings" contracts similar to Accountable Care Organization (ACO)-models in the US healthcare system [25–27, 32, 33]. The intention is to create greater efficiency (balance between expenditure and health benefits) through optimizing the Kinzigtal health system. The financing of GK is achieved by the two health insurance companies making advance payments of expected savings, which are then invested into improvement activities. Savings are calculated yearly in retrospect as the financial difference between (i) the actual total costs of care of all patients in the region of Kinzigtal compared with (ii) their expected mean costs, derived from the German morbidity-oriented risk structure compensation system (morbiditaetsorientierter Risikostrukturausgleich) and income to the health insurance companies. The contribution margin (Δ, delta) of the insured patients in Kinzigtal is the defining characteristic of the financial model, and is used as the indicator of financial success (Fig. 10.3) [26, 27, 32, 33]. Remuneration for collaborating parties and for GK comes from lower healthcare costs for the regional population. Sustainable and increasing health benefits for patients is expected to be achieved by GK, through patient-centred activities, support of self-management and targeted prevention [27].

Figure 10.3 illustrates the development of the risk-adjusted expected costs in Germany (blue line – indexed in 2005), actual costs in GK (green line), the surplus contribution margin (Δ, delta) and the number of AOK BW-insured patients enrolled in GK (light grey bars) from 2005 to 2013.

Care Management of Gesundes Kinzigtal

As with other countries, there have been questions over the sustainability of the financing of the German healthcare system with the ageing population. The predominant type of financing currently is for the number of health services ren-

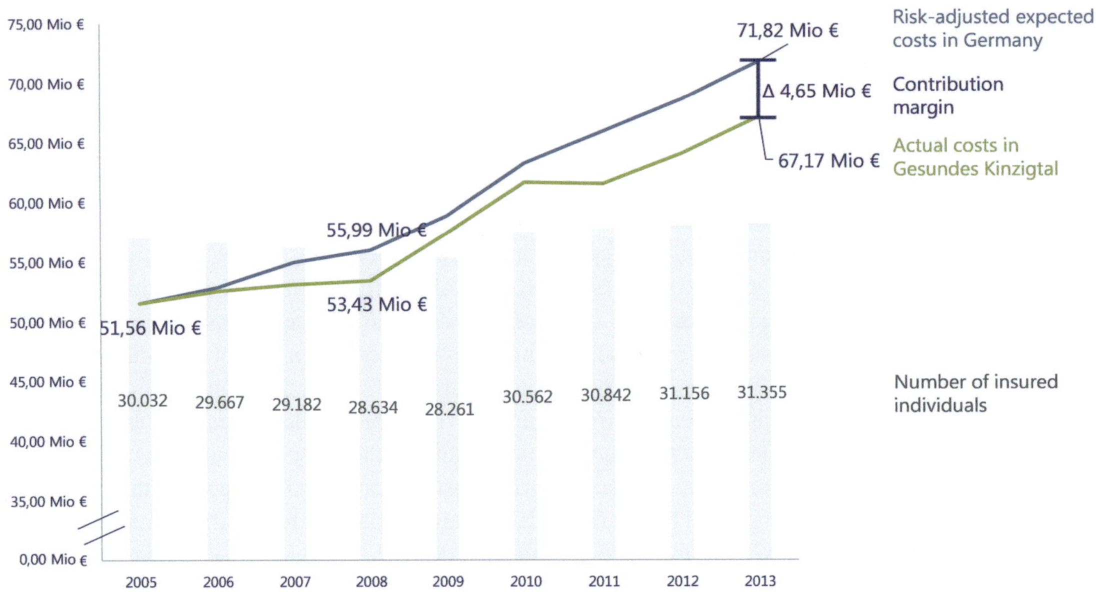

Fig. 10.3 Development of expected costs in Germany, actual costs in GK, contribution margin and number of insured individuals of the participating health insurance companies

dered (retrospective fee-for-service payments), rather than for preventive aspects of healthcare [23]. Associated partners of GK cooperate to close this gap by initiating goal-setting agreements between physicians and patients, developing individual treatment plans on the basis of a shared decision-making process and supporting self-management, through coaching and individual care (especially for those with a chronic disease). In addition, communication and patient information flow is assured through a system-wide electronic patient record. This enables all participating partners to provide effective, efficient and cross-sectoral healthcare [25].

Evaluation of Gesundes Kinzigtal

Since its inception in 2005, the GK has continuously been evaluated: externally through an independent scientific research institution, and internally by the shareholding OptiMedis AG.

The external evaluation of GK is led by the coordinating institution for evaluation of integrated care (EKIV; www.ekiv.org) which has been implemented by the Department of Medical Sociology at the University of Freiburg in Germany. EKIV is accountable for the provision of an evaluation plan, currently with four modules, which have been agreed upon from GK, AOK BW and SVLFG [25, 26]. The internal evaluation aims to show the effects of integrated care (among GK enrolled patients) on the dimensions of the Triple Aim Approach, and to assess whether the objectives of GK have been achieved through a range of parameters and quality indicators relating to, e.g., diabetes, heart failure and dementia [13, 32]. Central evaluation-relevant parameters and quality criteria for the external evaluation, which are compared with conventional care, include, e.g., improved patient empowerment, patient- and care giver satisfaction, development of patients' health status, indications for over-, under- or misutilization of health services, interdisciplinary cooperation and economic, high-quality healthcare [25, 35].

Both, the health insurance partners AOK BW and SVLFG and the shareholding OptiMedis AG in Hamburg, evaluate the financial impact of the approach. OptiMedis also provides feedback reports for providers and performs potential analyses to assess the impact of planned healthcare

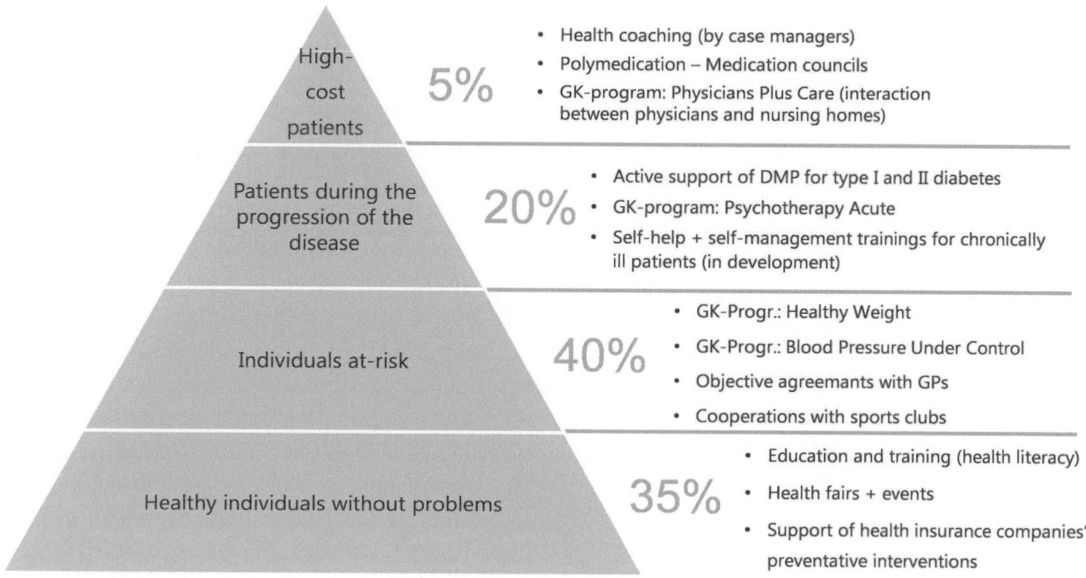

Fig. 10.4 Interventions of GK in the Context of Diabetes

programmes, health-economic evaluations of implemented interventions and several risk analyses [32].

Gesundes Kinzigtal Interventions in the Context of Diabetes

GK follows a holistic approach to optimize care for chronically ill patients with T2DM (Fig. 10.4). A whole cascade of interventions is being offered, depending on the risk level and the needs and co-morbidities of the patients. In this chapter, the development and implementation of a Kinzigtal-specific healthcare programme "Healthy Weight" for at-risk individuals is described.

Background of the Programme "Healthy Weight": The Deadly Quartet

The interaction of different factors – visceral obesity, hypertension, hyperglycaemia and dyslipidaemia-constitutes the metabolic syndrome (also known as "Deadly Quartet"). Since 2007, GK has offered a secondary prevention programme called "Healthy Weight" to reduce the development of risk factors related to the metabolic syndrome, the development of T2DM and cardiovascular diseases. The International Diabetes Federation (IDF) criteria are used by the programme to define central obesity (waist circumference: men ≥94 cm; women ≥80 cm) with at least two of the following measures [36] (Table 10.1).

Goals of the Healthcare Programme "Healthy Weight"

GK supports and motivates members to change their lifestyle through specialized comprehensive medical care, nutrition counselling and sports activities, with a special focus on obese patients. Reaching these targets is based on the biopsychosocial model, developed by Engel during the 1970s [37]. The approach involves considering the biological, psychological and social conditions involved during the development and progression of a (chronic) disease. The biopsychosocial model emphasizes the active role of the individual in the protection and promotion of their own health [37]. Supporting an

Table 10.1 The IDF consensus worldwide definition of the metabolic syndrome

Raised triglycerides	≥150 mg/dL (1.7 mmol/L)
	Or specific treatment for this lipid abnormality
Reduced high density lipoprotein (HDL-cholesterol)	<40 mg/dL (1.03 mmol/L) in males
	<50 mg/dL (1.29 mmol/L) in females
	Or specific treatment for this lipid abnormality
Raised blood pressure (BP)	Systolic BP ≥130 or
	Diastolic BP ≥85 mmHg
	Or treatment of previously diagnosed hypertension
Raised fasting plasma glucose (FPG)	(FPG) ≥100 mg/dL (5.6 mmol/L)
	Or previously diagnosed T2DM
	If above 5.6 mmol/L or 100 mg/dL,
	OGTT is strongly recommended but is not necessary to define presence of the syndrome

active patient role is a key part of the "Healthy Weight" programme.

Enrolment in the Programme "Healthy Weight"

"Healthy Weight" covers a period of 15 months and can be extended for further 15 months if the patients fulfil predefined criteria (vide infra).

Inclusion and Exclusion Criteria

The two main criteria to include patients in the healthcare programme "Healthy Weight" are registration in GK, and either a BMI of ≥30 kg/m^2 or waist circumference of ≥88 cm in women and ≥102 cm in men. A "positive risk status" is another important requirement for the participation in this programme. The following flowchart (Fig. 10.5) illustrates the enrolment procedure for "Healthy Weight." Insulin treated patients are excluded: such patients can participate in the specialized DMP for T2DM (see Chap. 1).

Risk Status and Goal-Setting Agreement

The nominated doctor fills in a risk status questionnaire for GK members during the registration process, estimates the individual health status of the patient and then invites patients to select different healthcare programmes. At the same time, the nominated doctor develops a goal-setting agreement together with the patient. This agreement is an essential tool for shared decision-making and motivation of the patient, with the intent to promote lifestyle changes and enhance self-management [32]. The agreement includes definition and steps to achieve individual goals along with a previously agreed date to ensure sustainability.

Three Standardized Programme Modules

The programme is based on close guidance of the patient and a combination of three standardized programme modules: medical care, nutrition counselling and sporting activities. "Actors" in the programme are the patient, the nominated doctor, the medical assistant, specialists, psychologists, dietitians, sports clubs, GK and the participating health insurances companies.

Medical Care in Context of "Healthy Weight"

The 15-month-intervention "Healthy Weight" includes regular contact with the nominated doctor and the medical assistant through six medical examinations: one during the enrolment, one every quarter and a final examination. At each visit, the following patient-related parameters are asked, measured and documented:

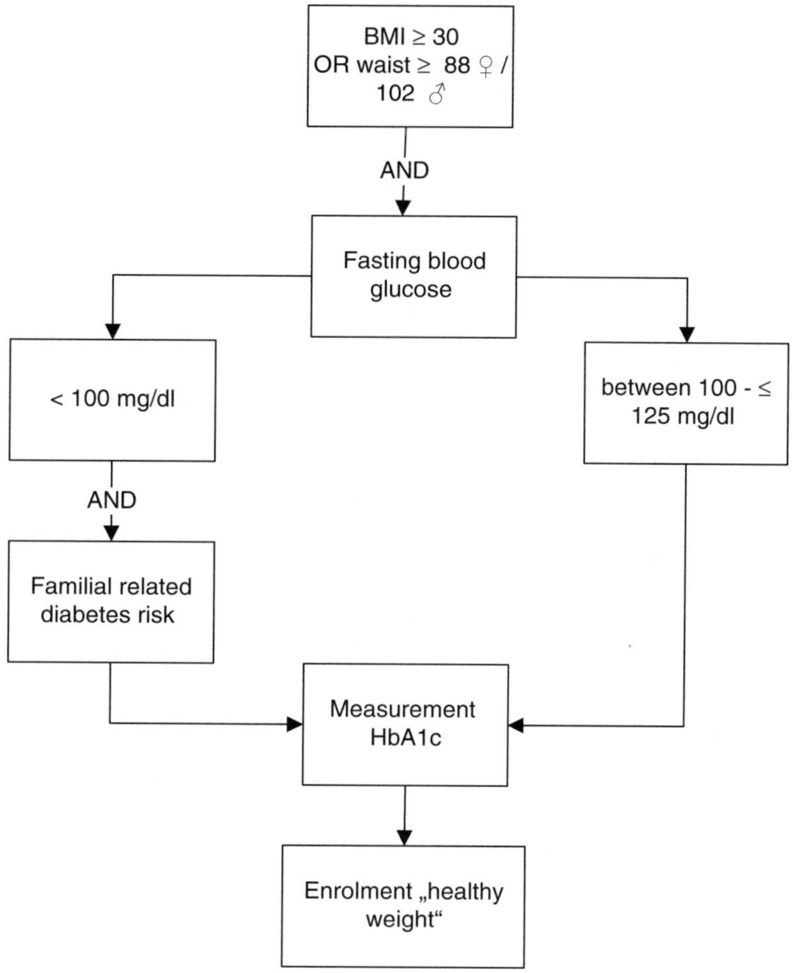

Fig. 10.5 Enrolment procedure for "Healthy Weight"

- Size and height
- BMI and waist circumference
- HbA1c, FPG, BP, Cholesterol, Triglycerides
- Diabetes mellitus (yes/no)
- Insulin treatment (yes/no)
- Oral antidiabetics (yes/no)
- Frequent hypoglycaemia (yes/no)
- Family-related diabetes risk (yes/no)

These parameters are evaluated regularly by GK (see section in this chapter on Evaluation) and used to improve and revise healthcare programmes when deemed necessary.

The medical care is also important for goal-setting and motivation of the patient. In the context of "Healthy Weight" the physician takes over the role of a coach and supports patients in achieving their individual goals (see section in this chapter on Risk Status and Goal Setting Agreement). Moreover, conversations between physicians and patients are valuable for checking the current status and the development of the programme.

Nutrition Counselling

Dietary change is an important component of "Healthy Weight." The nominated doctor strongly advises patients to participate in nutritional courses and dietary consulting. GK offers, in cooperation with AOK BW, different courses and consulting services for their members and, in particular, for "Healthy Weight" participants.

One-to-One Consultation

In cooperation with GK, AOK BW offers consultations for different subjects, e.g., dietary counselling. The GP or specialist prescribes a "prevention recommendation" for a one-to-one consultation with a dietician. The consultation is oriented towards the standards of the German Nutrition Society (Deutsche Gesellschaft fuer Ernaehrung e.V., DGE) and contains a case history, coaching and a nutrition protocol. The therapy is individually adjusted and takes four sessions on average. On top of the one-to-one consultation, AOK BW offers online programmes to support their members [38].

Nutritional Education in Groups

Group nutritional education consists of eight units, which are presented by three lecturers with different backgrounds. Nutrition training forms the basis of the course and covers four units. This part is taught by a nutritionist who is a trained diabetes advisor. Core learning includes food ingredients, different diets, causes for overweight and purchasing training. Additionally, a unit with a qualified psychologist takes place to discuss the psychological components of obesity and poor nutrition. Learning is enhanced through practice sessions during two cooking evenings. To connect nutrition and exercise, the course includes an introductory session on Nordic walking or gymnastics exercises. This session is used to introduce the participants to the topics of sports and exercise.

Sporting Activities

Another significant module of the healthcare programme involves encouraging patients to join sports activities. The aim of "Healthy Weight" is to provide ongoing courses and to integrate their members into sports clubs and societies, where they become part of a social network. GK refunds up to 150 € of the costs to enable everyone to participate in sports activities.

The built environment in rural areas like Kinzigtal, including their lack of sports activities, is a problem, especially for obese patients with severe diseases like T2DM. For this reason, GK established sports courses for the target group in cooperation with some sports clubs, a rehabilitation centre and qualified trainers. Health lectures are integrated within the sporting activities to combine theory and practice. Collaboration with self-help groups is supported by GK. The exercise programme is adjusted to the individual needs of the participants. The nominated physician observes the evolving patient health status during medical examinations.

Results of Internal Data Analysis Concerning Diabetes Care in Gesundes Kinzigtal

The results presented in this chapter are mostly part of the internal evaluation. All GK healthcare programmes are broadly supported by different datasets, including evaluations and feedback reports. The two participating SHI (AOK BW and SVLFG) provide their regional claims data to GK, which then tasks the shareholding OptiMedis AG with data analysis. These data are held within data warehouse architecture and used for different kinds of analyses. The whole GK integrated care system and most of its disease-specific interventions are also evaluated scientifically using the same data and supplementary data from another comparable region (see section on Evaluation in this chapter or www.ekiv.org).

In the following section some results from the analyses are presented, including the prevalence of T2DM in the region of Kinzigtal, the mean healthcare costs of this population and their most common co-morbidities. Some preliminary results of the evaluation of the "Healthy Weight" programme are then described, using a controlled cohort study design with matched pairs.

Potential Analysis of People with Diabetes in the Region of Kinzigtal

These analyses include inpatient and outpatient data from patients with T2DM from the region of Kinzigtal. Patients with ZIP-codes of the region and the ICD-10-GM diagnosis "E11.*: Type 2 diabetes" were selected. In 2013 (the latest year with complete claims data) the diabetes prevalence in the region of Kinzigtal was 9.2 % based upon healthcare provider consultation coding for 2860 patients who are members of the two participating SHI. This reflects a significant growth since the first year in 2006 when the prevalence was 7.0 %. The mean age of the T2DM-cohort in 2013 was 71.2 years and 53.5 % were women. In 2013 the top 5 co-morbidities of patients with T2DM were essential hypertension (78.3 %), dyslipidaemia (50.5 %), disorders of refraction and accommodation (38.2 %), back pain (33.8 %) and obesity (33.3 %). Their top 5 hospital discharge diagnoses were heart failure (3.6 %), cerebral infarction (1.9 %), T2DM (1.8 %), angina pectoris (1.6 %) and atherosclerosis (1.0 %).

T2DM in Kinzigtal was associated with mean expenditure of 5,935.70 € per person in 2013 (not necessarily only for diabetes care) including 40 % from inpatient stays, 24 % from drug prescriptions, 19 % from physician remuneration in ambulatory care and the rest from remedies and adjuvants (e.g., insulin pen systems, wheelchairs, physiotherapy, etc.), work incapacity or rehabilitation. In 2013, the net mean loss for the two SHI from all diabetes patients in the Kinzigtal region was −172.00 € per patient; however, it already improved by +299.20 € per patient per year compared to the initial year of the integrated care project in 2006. The normal improvement rate for all insured persons in the same period of time was +21.40 € per year. To put these results into perspective it has to be considered that in 2009 the German risk adjustment scheme has been changed for all patients in any SHI, allocating more money to patients having specific diseases including (among others) T2DM, so that part of the improvement of the contribution margin of the T2DM population is system-based, which is why more detailed evaluations are performed in GK concerning the intervention participants.

First Results from the Internal Evaluation of the "Healthy Weight" Programme

The GK- "Healthy Weight" programme is continuously evaluated using a controlled cohort study design with an exact matching of age, sex and programme specific inclusion diagnosis (T2DM, metabolic syndrome and obesity) in eight cost classes. People, who were not consistently insured at the time of the evaluation, including those who had died, were excluded. Each programme participant was matched in a ratio of 1:1 because of the limited data set. The non-attenders are insured persons from the two participating SHI who also live in the region of Kinzigtal, but who mainly visit providers that are not part of the integrated care system GK.

The evaluation was not performed per calendar year, but by number of years from enrolment. Controls had the same starting date as the index case in the "Healthy Weight" programme. A time period of 3 years follow-up was examined. To avoid bias, the latest date for enrolment was 31st of December 2010 because 2013 was the latest year with complete data. Analyses involved comparing the case-control difference before and after the intervention.

Of 149 individuals enrolled up to 31st of December 2010, 136 (91 %) had a matched control. The small numbers allow only preliminary insights into the achievements of the programme to date. The mean ages of cases and controls were 56.3 and 56.4 years respectively. In both groups 106 individuals (78 %) were female. One year before the start (baseline) of the programme "Healthy Weight" about 80 % of cases and controls had diabetes, about 93 % obesity and about 60 % had dyslipidaemia.

Figure 10.6 shows the hospitalization rates in the two groups. While 24 patients (17.7 %) from the "Healthy Weight" participants had been hospitalized (from any cause) in the year before enrolment, this was the case for only 12 control individuals (8.8 %). All-cause hospitalization rates were similar in the first year, but continued to decrease to 16 patients (11.8 %) in the third year of follow-up in cases, while rates remaining increased in controls. In a difference-in-difference analysis these reverse trends led to 16 less cases in the "Healthy Weight" group compared to the control group in the third year.

A comparison of the total annual difference in expenditure reveals a slower growth in the "Healthy Weight" cohort over the 3 years of follow-up resulting in −149.4 € less expenditure per

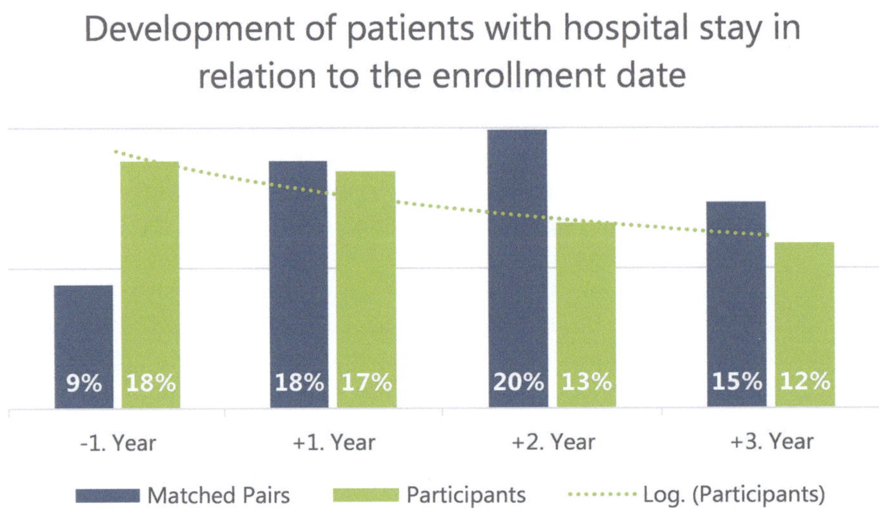

Fig. 10.6 Development of patients with hospital stay in relation to the enrolment date

capita and a difference-in-difference of −659.7 € per capita in the third year (Fig. 10.7).

Furthermore, the mean number of days off work for sickness were over 50 % lower among participants than controls, particularly in the third year of follow-up (Fig. 10.8).

Results of the external evaluation supplement the results of the internal evaluation, although they have a longer time lag and take longer to perform due to database size and methodological issues. The most recent evaluation in May 2015 supported the internal evaluation and demonstrated another improvement in diabetes care. In 2011 only 2.3 % of the GK-enrolled diabetes patients were admitted with "diabetes" compared to 4.0 % among not-GK-enrolled patients. Statistical significance is barely missed, which is shown in Table 10.2 (in accordance with [39]).

Outlook

Against the background of rapidly increasing chronic diseases and a growing burden for patients to manage their disease, innovative approaches and holistic, patient-centred interventions are needed that fit into the realities of the daily lives of patients [40]. It is important to address all dimensions of the Triple Aim (care, health and cost) and to commit all stakeholders to a process of healthcare delivery that target these dimensions as a whole. After 10 years of innovative healthcare practice, the management company GK now receives more in income than it spends. Up to 2011, all three dimensions of the Triple Aim Approach have developed positively within GK including its complex sub-interventions [41]. However, further studies are necessary before evidence of sustained success by GK can be described as proven [13, 20]. A critical success factor, already identified by the holistic, public health-related approach of GK, is the long lasting integrated care contract that is based on mutual trust between GK and the two health insurance companies. This facilitates investments in sustainable interventions with their long-term benefits, the support of a cultural change among physicians and patients, and the use of instruments like patient empowerment, shared-decision-making and coaching for the self-management of chronic conditions. Meanwhile, an ongoing sharing and analysing of data helps to identify strengths and weaknesses of interventions much quicker than in usual practice, and enables timely refinements of existing programmes.

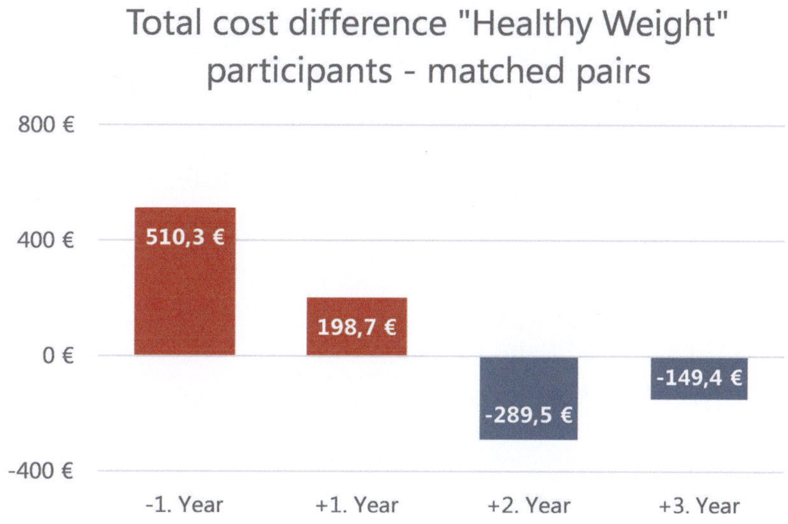

Fig. 10.7 Total cost difference of "Healthy Weight"-participants: matched pairs

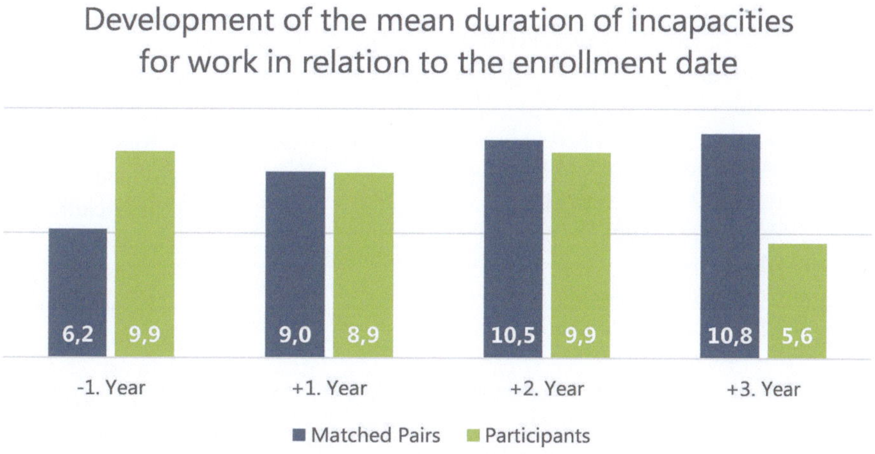

Fig. 10.8 Mean number of days off work for sickness since enrolment

Table 10.2 Comparison of enrolled (GK) and not-enrolled (Not GK) insured individuals of the AOK BW in the Kinzigtal region with diabetes and hospitalization due to diabetes (E10–E14)

Year	GK %	Not GK %	Overall %	Odds ratio	95 %-CI
2006	2.8	2.8	2.8	1.01	0.58–1.75
2007	2.3	3.5	3.1	0.61	0.35–1.08
2008	3.1	4.8	4.2	0.65	0.42–1.03
2009	2.0	3.4	2.9	0.59	0.35–1.01
2010	2.7	3.5	3.2	0.76	0.47–1.23
2011	2.3	4.0	3.3	0.62	0.38–1.02

GK has now made a "step abroad". In 2015, the Dutch subsidiary "OptiMedis Nederland B.V." based in Leiden was founded. Following the successful approach of their colleagues in Haslach in Germany, the next challenge is to improve the healthcare of the local population of 40,000 inhabitants of Nijkerk in the Netherlands [42]. Discussions with other health insurance companies are also currently taking place, in order to give other patients the opportunity to use the GK services for their healthcare and wellbeing [34]. A GK study revealed that almost all respondents (92.1 %) would be willing to recommend the GK healthcare programme [32]. We feel that an integrated care system like GK can be beneficial within the current healthcare system in Germany, especially for people with chronic conditions, through its systematic use of its population health management approaches to optimize the quality of care. The current deficiencies in the regular healthcare system to address the Triple Aim goals adequately should strengthen movement towards more intelligent solutions such as the GK programme.

Abbreviations

AG	Incorporated Company [Aktiengesellschaft]
ACO	Accountable Care Organization
AOK BW	General Local Health Insurance Company in Baden-Wuerttemberg [Allgemeine Ortskrankenkasse Baden-Wuerttemberg]
BMI	Body mass index
BP	Blood pressure
CI	Confidence interval
COPD	Chronic obstructive pulmonary disease
DEGS	German Health Interview and Examination Survey for Adults [Studie zur Gesundheit Erwachsener in Deutschland]
DGE	German Nutrition Society [Deutsche Gesellschaft fuer Ernaehrung]
DMP	Disease Management Programme
EKIV	Coordinating Institution for Evaluation of Integrated Care [Evaluations-Koordinierungsstelle Integrierte Versorgung]
FPG	Fasting plasma glucose
GK	Gesundes Kinzigtal Ltd.
GKV	German statutory health insurance [Gesetzliche Krankenversicherung]
GMG	Health modernization act [Gesundheits-Modernisierungs-Gesetz]
GP	General practitioner
HDL	High density lipoprotein
ICD-10-GM	International classification of diseases 10th revision, German modification
IDF	International diabetes federation
IHI	Institute for healthcare improvement
LKK	Agricultural Health Insurance Company [Landwirtschaftliche Krankenkasse]
LTD	Limited Company
MQNK	Physicians' Network in Kinzigtal Region [Medizinisches QualitaetsNetz Kinzigtal e.V.]
OECD	Organization for economic cooperation and development
OGTT	Oral glucose tolerance test
PAC	Patients advisory committee
RKI	Robert-Koch-Institute
SGB V	Book five of Germanys social security code
SHI	Statutory health insurance
SVLFG	Social security of agriculture forestry and horticulture [Sozialversicherung fuer Landwirtschaft, Forsten und Gartenbau]
T1DM	Type-1-Diabetes Mellitus
T2DM	Type-2-Diabetes Mellitus
US	United States
WHO	World Health Organization
ZIP-code	Zone improvement plan-code [Postleitzahl]

References

1. Busse R, Blümel M. Germany: health system review. Health Syst Transit. 2014;16(2):1–296. xxi.
2. Rosenbrock R, Gerlinger T. Gesundheitspolitik eine systematische Einführung. 3rd ed. Bern: Huber; 2014. p. 569. vollst. überarb. Aufl. ed.
3. Nowossadeck E. Demografische Alterung und Folgen für das Gesundheitswesen. Berlin: Robert-Koch-Institut; 2012.
4. Global Health Observatory. Life expectancy [Internet]. [cited 08/05/2015]. Available from: http://www.who.int/gho/mortality_burden_disease/life_tables/situation_trends/en/.

5. Amelung V, Hildebrandt H, Wolf S. Integrated care in Germany-a stony but necessary road! Int J Integr Care. 2012;12, e16.
6. Mladovsky P, Allin S, Masseria C, Hernández-Quevedo C, McDaid D, Mossialos E. Health in the European Union: trends and analysis. 2010: WHO Regional Office Europe; 2010.
7. OECD. How does Germany compare? OECD Health Statistics 2014 [Internet]. [cited 10/04/2015]. Available from http://www.oecd.org/els/health-systems/Briefing-Note-GERMANY-2014.pdf.
8. Gesundheitsausgaben nach Einrichtungen [Internet]. [cited 08/05/2015]. Available from: https://www.destatis.de/DE/ZahlenFakten/GesellschaftStaat/Gesundheit/Gesundheitsausgaben/Tabellen/Einrichtungen.html.
9. Amelung V. Neue Versorgungsformen auf dem Prüfstand. In: Amelung V, Eble S, Hildebrandt H, editors. Innovatives Versorgungsmanagement: Neue Versorgungsformen auf dem Prüfstand. Berlin: Medizinisch Wissenschaftliche Verlagsgesellschaft; 2011. p. 3–16.
10. Osborn R, Schoen C. The Commonwealth Fund 2013 international health policy survey in eleven countries. Consulté le [Internet]. [cited 21/05/2015]. Available from: http://www.commonwealthfund.org/~/media/files/publications/in-the-literature/2013/nov/pdf_schoen_2013_ihp_survey_chartpack_final.pdf.
11. Sachverständigenrat für die Konzertierte Aktion im Gesundheitswesen. Bedarfsgerechtigkeit und Wirtschaftlichkeit: Band III: Über-, Unter-und Fehlversorgung. Ausführliche Zusammenfassung. Gutachten 2000/2001 [Internet]. [cited 25/04/2015]. Available from: http://www.svr-gesundheit.de/fileadmin/user_upload/Gutachten/2000-2001/Kurzf-de-01.pdf.
12. Sachverständigenrat zur Begutachtung der Entwicklung im Gesundheitswesen. Koordination und Integration. Gesundheitsversorgung in einer Gesellschaft des längeren Lebens. Sondergutachten 2009 [Internet].[cited 25/04/2015]. Available from: http://www.svr-gesundheit.de/index/php?id=196.
13. Fuchs S, Henschke C, Blümel M, Busse R. Disease management programs for type 2 diabetes in Germany. A systematic literature review evaluating effectiveness. Dtsch Arztebl Int. 2014;111:453–63.
14. Bundesversicherungsamt Zulassungsstand. 2014 [Internet]. [cited 16/04/2015]. Available from: http://www.bundesversicherungsamt.de/weitere-themen/disease-management-programme/zulassung-disease-management-programme-dmp.html#c207.
15. Rüschmann H, Roth A, Krauss C. Vernetzte Praxen auf dem Weg zu managed care? Aufbau-Ergebnisse-Zukunftsvision. Springer; 2013.
16. Aguiree F, Brown A, Cho NH, Dahlquist G, Dodd S, Dunning T. IDF diabetes atlas: International Diabetes Federation; 2013.
17. Kurth B. Erste Ergebnisse aus der Studie zur Gesundheit Erwachsener in Deutschland (DEGS). Bundesgesundheitsbl. 2012;55(8):980–90.
18. Hall M, Felton A, Henrichs H, Barnett A. Diabetes—the policy puzzle: towards benchmaking in the EU 25. International Diabetes Federation European Region and Federation of European Nurses in Diabetes. 2005; 103.
19. Heidemann C, Du Y, Schubert I, Rathmann W, Scheidt-Nave C. Prävalenz und zeitliche Entwicklung des bekannten Diabetes mellitus. Bundesgesundheitsbl. 2013;56(5–6):668–77.
20. Hildebrandt H. Crossing the boundaries from individual medical care to regional public health outcomes: the triple aim of "Gesundes Kinzigtal"- better health+ improved care+ affordable costs. Int J Integr Care. 2014; 14(5).
21. Seiler R. Die Schwarzwaldformel-das Modell "Gesundes Kinzigtal". In: Weatherly J, Seiler R, Meyer-Lutterloh K, Schmid E, Lägel R, Amelung V, editors. Leuchtturmprojekte Integrierter Versorgung und Medizinische Versorgungszentren. Belrin: Medizinisch Wissenschaftliche Verlagsgesellschaft; 2007. p. 139–47.
22. Siegel A, Stößel U, Geßner D, Knittel R. Kooperation und Wettbewerb im integrierten Versorgungssystem "Gesundes Kinzigtal". In: Amelung V, Sydow J, Windeler A, editors. Vernetzung im Gesundheitswesen-Wettbewerb und Kooperation. Stuttgart: W. Kohlhammer; 2009. p. 145–55.
23. Hildebrandt H, Michalek H, Roth M. Integriertes Management auf Augenhöhe – Anforderungen an eine konsistente Führungsphilosophie in IV-Systemen am Beispiel von Gesundes Kinzigtal. In: Amelung V, Eble S, Hildebrandt H, editors. Innovatives Versorgungsmanagement: Neue Versorgungsformen auf dem Prüfstand. Berlin: Medizinisch Wissenschaftliche Verlagsgesellschaft; 2011. p. 215–26.
24. Siegel A, Köster I, Schubert I, Stößel U. Integrierte Versorgung Gesundes Kinzigtal: Ein Modell für regionale Prävention und Schnittstellenoptimierung. 2012. p. 148–64.
25. Hildebrandt H, Schulte T, Stunder B. Triple aim in Kinzigtal, Germany. J Integr Care. 2012;20(4):205–22.
26. Hölzel LP, Vollmer M, Kriston L, Siegel A, Härter M. Patientenbeteiligung bei medizinischen Entscheidungen in der Integrierten Versorgung Gesundes Kinzigtal: Ergebnisse einer kontrollierten Kohortenstudie. Bundesgesundheitsbl. 2012;55(11–12):1524–33.
27. Hildebrandt H, Schmitt G, Roth M, Stunder B. Integrierte regionale Versorgung in der Praxis: Ein Werkstattbericht aus dem "Gesunden Kinzigtal". Z Evidenz Fortbild Qualität Gesundheitswesen. 2011;105(8):585–9.

28. Berwick DM, Nolan TW, Whittington J. The triple aim: care, health, and cost. Health Affair. 2008;27(3):759–69.
29. Institute for Healthcare Improvement. The IHI triple aim. Available from: http://www.ihi.org/Engage/Initiatives/TripleAim/pages/default.aspx.
30. Hermann C, Hildebrandt H, Richter-Reichhelm M, Schwartz F, Witzenrath W. Managementgesellschaft organisiert Integrierte Versorgung einer definierten Population auf Basis eines Einsparcontractings. Gesundheits- und Sozialpolitik. 2006. p. 11–29.
31. Siegel A, Stößel U, Gaiser K, Hildebrandt H. Integrierte Vollversorgungssysteme und soziale Ungleichheit-das Beispiel "Gesundes Kinzigtal". Public Health Forum. 2008;16(2):e1–4.
32. Hildebrandt H, Pimperl A, Schulte T, Hermann C, Riedel H, Schubert I. Triple aim – Evaluation in der Integrierten Versorgung Gesundes Kinzigtal – Gesundheitszustand, Versorgungserleben und Wirtschaftlichkeit. Bundesgesundheitsbl. 2014. p. 1–10.
33. Hildebrandt H, Hermann C, Knittel R, Richter-Reichhelm M, Siegel A, Witzenrath W. Gesundes Kinzigtal Integrated Care: improving population health by a shared health gain approach and a shared savings contract. Int J Integr Care. 2010;10:e046.
34. Gesundes Kinzigtal im Überblick. Available from: http://www.gesundes-kinzigtal.de/die-idee-von-gesundes-kinzigtal/.
35. Siegel A, Köster I, Schubert I, Stößel U. Evaluation der Integrierten Versorgung Gesundes Kinzigtal: Konzeption, Herausforderungen, Lösungsmöglichkeiten. In: Amelung V, Eble S, Hildebrandt H, editors. Innovatives Versorgungsmanagement: Neue Versorgungsformen auf dem Prüfstand. Berlin: Medizinisch Wissenschaftliche Verlagsgesellschaft; 2011. p. 145–55.
36. International Diabetes Federation. The IDF consensus worldwide definition of the metabolic syndrome. Available from: http://www.idf.org/webdata/docs/MetS_def_update2006.pdf.
37. Pauls H. Das biopsychosoziale Modell: Herkunft und Aktualität. 2013;1(1): 17.
38. Allgemeine Ortskrankenkasse. Einzelgespräche (One-to-one consultations). In: Kern E, editor. Healthy Weight; 2015.
39. Köster I, Ihle P, Schubert I. Evaluationsbericht 2004–2011 für Gesundes Kinzigtal GmbH. AOK-Daten. Köln: 2015. p. 244.
40. Leppin AL, Montori VM, Gionfriddo MR, editors. Minimally disruptive medicine: a pragmatically comprehensive model for delivering care to patients with multiple chronic conditions. Healthcare. Multidisciplinary Digital Publishing Institute; 2015.
41. Busse R, Stahl J. Integrated care experiences and outcomes in Germany, the Netherlands, and England. Health Aff (Project Hope). 2014;33(9):1549–58.
42. Ansatz von Gesundes Kinzigtal in Holland hoch im Kurs: Gesundes Kinzigtal. Available from: http://www.gesundes-kinzigtal.de/news/een-kopie-van-gesundes-kinzigtal-en-nederland-2014.html.

11 Approaches to Integrated Diabetes Care in the Netherlands

Harold W. de Valk and Helmut Wenzel

Background to the Dutch Health Care

According to the 2014 Euro Health Consumer Index (ECHI) the Netherlands is the best country in Europe to live for health care. In a ranking of 37 countries the Netherlands was top with a score of 898 out of 1000. Switzerland was second, followed by Norway, Finland and Denmark. The UK, excluding Scotland, landed in 14th place (718 points) with Spain 19th, Italy 22nd, and Germany in 9th place [1]. By 2014, the Commonwealth Fund placed Netherlands 5th (tied with Germany) out of 11 countries: ranked second in timeliness of care, but ranked 7th–8th in safety, efficiency and equity and 10th (before the USA) in per capita cost [2].

A survey from 2010 from the "Dutch Ministry of Health" comparing 125 performance indicators across several countries, drew a more precise picture of "getting access, varying quality, and rising costs" [3]. Challenges that were revealed, dealt with timely access to ambulatory and hospital care, varying quality of care between providers, "value for the money," with rising expenditures and an ageing society. Health expenditures reportedly grew by 6–7 % per year 2007–2009, with data from the Organisation for Economic Co-operation and Development (OECD) demonstrating that the growth in health expenditure was above the OECD average. Their analysis indicated that this growth was due to increasing volumes of care. Whereas prices increased on average by 1.6 % per year, the volume of services from Dutch hospitals grew by 4.2 % per year, inpatient admissions by 3 % annually and day-patient admissions by 10 %. In order to get a more complete picture they stated that the volumes for outpatient care grew substantially (5.5 % on average per year), while the price of medicines had fallen significantly even though the number of prescriptions had increased (about 15 % in 2008) [3].

The Netherlands has the highest per capita spending in Europe [1]. In order to evaluate the affordability of health-care financing, expenditures are set in relation to the economic performance of the national economy – the Gross Domestic Product (GDP). Health expenditure, as a percentage of GDP, increased from 7.4 % in 1980 to 11.9 % in 2011 [4, 5]: a share which is higher only in the US health-care system (18 % of GDP). In the Netherlands, 1.7 % of the expenditures are privately, and 10.2 % publicly, financed in 2011. In the US the corresponding numbers are 8–9.1 % [4]. Experts expect a dramatic

H.W. de Valk (✉)
Internist-endocrinologist, Department of Internal Medicine, University Medical Center Utrecht, Utrecht, The Netherlands
e-mail: h.w.devalk@umcutrecht.nl

H. Wenzel
Health Economist, Konstanz, Germany
e-mail: hkwen@aol.com

D. Simmons et al. (eds.), *Integrated Diabetes Care*, DOI 10.1007/978-3-319-13389-8_11

increase in expenditure so that by 2040, one quarter of GDP will be needed to provide care [6]. Ageing of the population, medical and therapeutic progress and global economic distortions have made it necessary to assess whether the Dutch health system organisational principles will be able to meet future challenges.

Growing Burden of Diabetes

Diabetes prevalence in 2014 was about 7.24 % [7] and it is expected to increase to 9.5 % by the year 2035 [8]. Diabetes is an expensive disease, for example, the American Diabetes Association observed that the medical expenditures of people with diabetes, on average, are "approximately 2.3 times higher than what expenditures would be in the absence of diabetes" [9] (p1). In a disease model Zhang et al. [10] calculated the burden of disease. They reported that globally, 12 % of health expenditures and USD 1330 (Diabetes induced expenditures (ID) 1478) per person were spent on diabetes in 2010. The expenditure varies by region, age group, gender, and country's income level. Looking at Europe, the Netherlands was in the top 7 countries with expenditures of 3,793,953,000 USD (the underlying assumption in these analyses was that a patient with diabetes is twice as expensive as a comparable person without diabetes: this is conservative). Furthermore, IDF estimates expenditure of about 4113 USD per person with diabetes (Fig. 11.1), and this was expected to rise to 6943.11 USD by 2014 [7]. This would mean that the Dutch performance is within the ten most expensive countries with health expenditure rising to 4,311,488 USD by 2035 [10].

Basic Principles of the Dutch System

Prior to the health-care reforms of 2006, Dutch health care was characterised by extensive government regulation and a dual insurance system of public and private insurance, which had been perceived to be inefficient. By 2005, roughly two-thirds of the Dutch population had entered the public programme (known as the "fund for the sick") and stronger expenditure control was required [12]. The reform that was introduced was in response to a number of problems: a two-tier system of private health insurance for the people with a good income – (approximately one third of the population at that time) and state coverage for the rest; an inefficient and complex bureaucracy; lengthy waiting lists and a lack of patient-focus [13]. The Dutch health-care system was, and still is, made up of three branches, so-called compartments. The "*first compartment of care*" emphasises care and support for those people who have to cope with irreversible damage to physical or mental integrity [12]; the "*second compartment of care*" focuses on recovery and includes hospital care and visits to a primary care physician. The "*third compartment of care*" is defined *as* "*luxury care*," such as "cosmetic surgery" [13]. Care for conditions covered by the first compartment is given regardless of an individual's financial situation and is regulated by the "Algemene Wet Bijzondere Ziektekosten (AWBZ)," or "Exceptional Medical Expenses Act." Both before and after the reforms, contributions to this fund were taken from income-related salary deductions, supplemented by a general government revenue grant [13]. The AWBZ was and continues to be applicable to all Dutch citizens. Before 2006, the provision and funding of insurance for second and third compartment care were determined by an individual's total income. In 2005, the wage ceiling was set at a gross annual income of €33,000 ($40,600) for employees and €21,050 ($25,900) for the self-employed. Those people earning less were determined eligible for the public system. Those who did not qualify for the public system, could purchase private insurance to cover potential short-term medical needs in the second compartment and – in some cases – also for "luxury care" in the third compartment [12]. However, the way in which the provision and financing of the first and third compartment were organised did not change. The main changes occurred to care covered by the second compartment.

Preceding the 2006 reforms, the second compartment combined Social Health Insurance (SHI) – the so-called Fund for the sick (ZFW) –

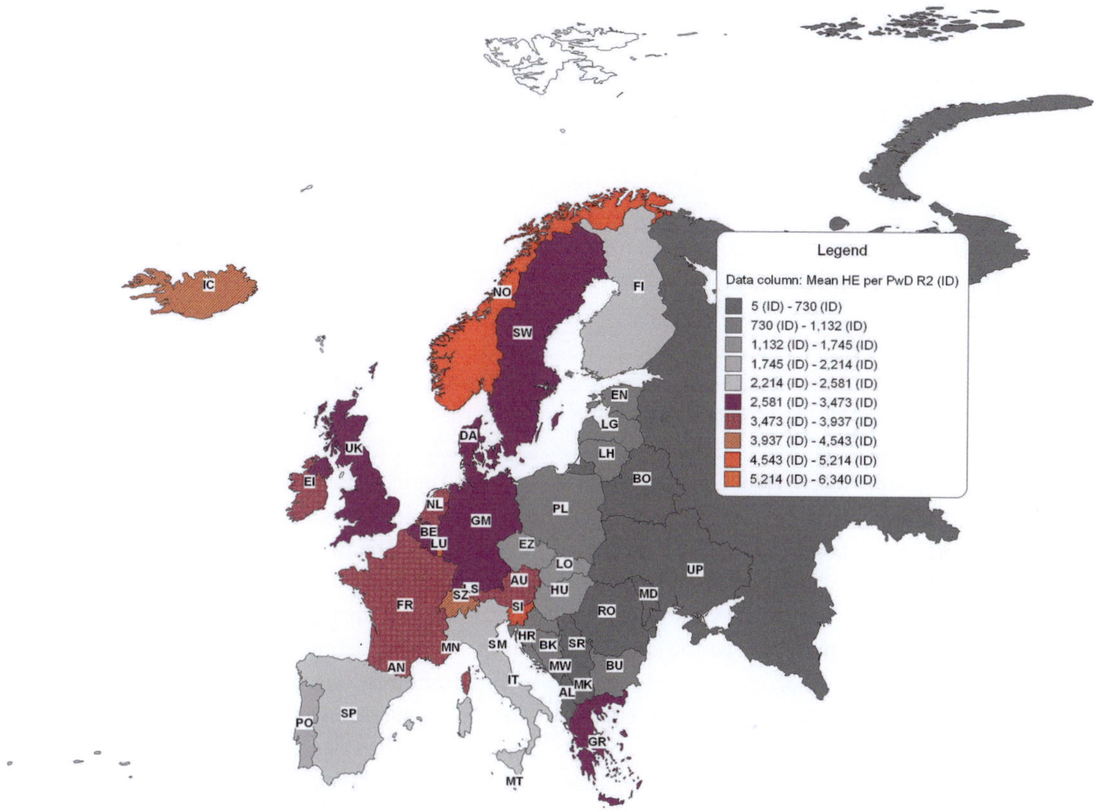

Fig. 11.1 Diabetes induced expenditures [ID] per person and year in Europe (Data are from [10], the classification limits are based on [11])

with a Private Health Insurance (PHI) scheme. SHI was compulsory for people below a certain income, funded through payroll contributions and managed by the government. The amount paid by each individual was unaffected by their medical situation. Resources were paid into a "Central Sickness Fund" which provided a mechanism for redistributing funds to compensate insurers for those considered "high risk." Along with the ABZW, the Fund allowed universal medical coverage. PHI was funded by employers or individuals with higher incomes and insurers were allowed to take the risk of an individual into account, meaning that premiums varied widely. The 2006 *Dutch Healthcare Act* (ZvW) overturned the division between SHI and PHI in the second compartment, thus creating a universally compulsory Social health Insurance scheme. Instead of being managed primarily by the government, it is now the *private health insurance market* which is responsible for providing the basic package of health insurance to all Dutch citizens. Extra government finance schemes ensure that universality of care is maintained, no matter what your income, as well as providing a safety net for illegal immigrants [13].

The original idea was to limit costs by stimulating competition between the rival insurance companies. But with ongoing mergers of companies, there seems to be limited competition. However, critics point out that large health insurance companies are said to squeeze health providers in order to lower their expenditures [14]. Adjustments to the Health Insurance Act currently being promoted will prevent patients from choosing their own medical specialist. Presently insurers have to reimburse a certain amount to patients who go to a specialist or facility that is not partnered with the insurance company, offsetting at least part of the cost of treatment for the patient [15]. Furthermore, the monthly premium for Dutch health insurance will rise by around €9.5 in 2015. This means people will spend roughly € 114 extra per year, taking the annual cost of basic health insurance to € 1215 in 2015 [16]. Moreover, the amount of money for mandatory excess deductibles (eigen risico) increased from € 360 to € 385 per year in 2016 [17]. The "eigen risico zorgverzekering" or "own risk insurance" is the amount which an individual has to pay out of pocket before health insurance coverage sets in [16]. Some insurance companies offer larger excess deductibles (up to € 900) combined with a lower annual standard price. You are better off when you do not need your deductible but when you do, you are worse off financially, This depends on your own calculation of personal risk.

The *Primary Care Provider* (PCP) plays the leading role in providing care, acting as gatekeeper and the first point of contact (except in emergencies). Every Dutch person has to register with a primary care provider (PCP) [4]. Patients must obtain a PCP referral prior to a specialist visit, except for acute conditions such as trauma or acute myocardial infarction. Nevertheless, this also depends on the insurance package; with more expensive policies, no referral is needed. Nurse practitioners are employed to perform check-ups on the chronically ill. PCPs can deal with routine health issues, perform standard gynaecological and paediatric examinations, and refer onto other services [13]. Most *specialists* work within a hospital setting.

Managed Care in the Netherlands: Integrated Chronic Care and Bundled Payments

The reform of the Dutch health-care system has been characterised as managed competition, or as "...an experiment in how far you can get with a system in which there is almost no direct government involvement" [18]. The Government executes its responsibility indirectly, only. The leading principle of this reform (theory) was that the government should stimulate competition rather than regulate the supply of health care: making the Dutch system the most extreme application of market mechanisms to stimulate efficiency in a European health-care system.

In order to achieve this, the Dutch came up with a system of "managed competition" that included a statutory general insurance provision [12]. The basic concept demands that every Dutch citizen has to buy health-care and pharmaceutical insurance from one of several private providers [19]. The extent of coverage under these policies is government-mandated and identical, including a deductible, depending on the specific insurance policy. This means that the insured patient has to pay additional expenses, ranging from the governmental fixed mandatory amount of € 385 in 2016 per year [17] to any reasonably calculated amount balancing the contribution fee against the expected expenses [20]. Insurers must also charge the same premium to all, including those with pre-existing conditions. The only exception is that group discounts (e.g., for an employer) are permitted [18] where persons are collectively insured. This could mean that the insured person of such a group can profit from a broader package at lower premium and at lower own risk. A special payroll tax also funds the government's health regulator, which provides insurers with payments to help pay expenses related to high cost policy holders. Basically, health care embraces three overlapping markets as Fig. 11.2 shows: the acquisition of insurance contracts between individuals and insurers; the provision of health-care services between individuals and providers and between insurers and providers for the pricing of those services [18].

Over the years many approaches were introduced to improve the quality and continuity of care for chronic diseases. However, fragmented funding made it difficult to establish long-term programmes [21]. Therefore, the Dutch minister of health approved, in 2007, the introduction of bundled-care (known is the Netherlands as a 'chain-of-care') approach for integrated chronic care, with special attention to diabetes. This bundled-payment approach was firstly introduced on an experimental basis, accepted in 2010 and subsequently implemented nationwide for diabe-

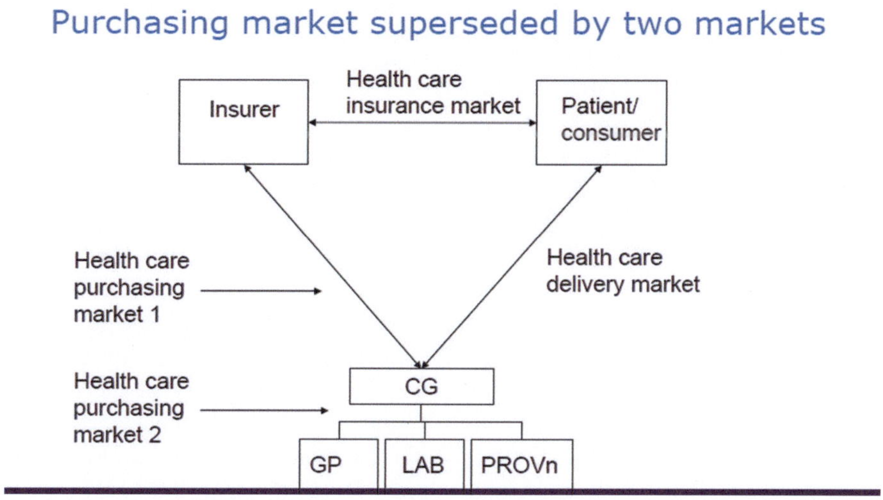

Fig. 11.2 Medical specialist are rarely part of the Care Group and only provide treatment advices or suggestions without actually treating the patients themselves. Dutch health-care market. *CG* Care Group, *GP* General Practitioner, *ProVn* Health-Care Provider, *LAB* Laboratory (From Struijs [23])

tes, chronic obstructive pulmonary disease (COPD), and cardiovascular risk management [21]. Insurers negotiate and pay a single remuneration [21] (lump sum) to a principal contractor (the "care group") to cover a full range of care services for specific chronic diseases, like diabetes, COPD, or vascular diseases for a fixed period. Care groups (CG) are new legal entities which are formed by health-care providers at local levels on a regional scale [22]. Very often they are general practitioners (GPs). As a principal contractor they negotiate with the insurers on price and products. Finally, the care group takes on both clinical and financial responsibility for all assigned patients in the particular diabetes care programme. The care group either delivers services itself or subcontracts to other care providers [21].

With the bundled-payment approach, the market is divided into two segments: one in which health insurance companies contract care from the principal contractors (i.e., care groups) and one in which care groups conclude service contracts from individual providers [23]. These providers could be general practitioners, specialists, dietitians, or laboratories. Both, the price for the bundle of services by insurers and care groups, and the fees for the subcontracted care providers by the care group and providers, are freely negotiated [21]. As Struijs et al. [21] point out, the aims of these care groups are similar to those of "Accountable Care Organizations" (ACOs), as currently designed in the United States or "Clinical Commissioning Groups" in the UK [24]. However, there are some essential differences: first, care groups (as with clinical commissioning groups) are dominated by GPs, whereas ACOs may comprise a wide range of providers, at least primary care physicians, specialists, and one or more hospitals; second, patients are to be assigned to ACOs on the basis of their patterns of service use, whereas patients here are assigned to a care group on the basis of their disease (e.g., onset of diabetes). Moreover, the care groups bear the full financial risk for the expenditures of care [21], whereas ACOs will not take over the risk of higher expenditures than expected [25].

Integrated Diabetes Care

With a bundled payment approach – or episode-based payment – multiple providers are reimbursed a single sum of money for all services related to an episode of care (e.g., hospitalisation, including a period of post-acute care). This is in contrast to a reimbursement for each individual service (fee-for-service), and it is expected that this will reduce the volume of services provided and consequently lead to a reduction in spending. Since in a fee-for-service system the reimbursement is directly related to the volume of services provided, there is little incentive to reduce unnecessary care. The bundled payment approach promotes a more efficient use of services [26].

For example, the Washington State Hospital Association [27] identified three areas where bundled payments should show progress: (1) Quality improvement and cost reduction by reducing administrative/overhead costs, sharing risk, eliminating cost-shifting, outcomes management and continuous quality improvement, reducing inappropriate and unnecessary resource use, efficient use of capital and technology; (2) consumer responsiveness, i.e., seamless continuum of care and focus on the health of enrollees; (3) community benefit by improving community health status, and addressing the prevention of social issues which affect community health. Most integrated networks include a team-based approach, as well as an emphasis on patient participation.

Furthermore, with the set-up of a bundled payment model, it is reasonable to expect that multidisciplinary cooperation between health-care providers will be facilitated insofar as existing financial barriers between care sectors and disciplines will be eliminated [28]. Under this condition so-called 'standard' diabetes care can be offered, i.e., purchased, delivered and billed as a single product [29]. From the point of view of the Dutch Diabetes Federation (NDF) this scheme mainly serves people who have recently been diagnosed with diabetes, people whose condition is well controlled and those who have no serious complications [30, 31]. Bundled payment contracts also cover consultations with secondary care specialists. However, this consultation opportunity does not include referral to and treatment by those specialists. Accruing expenditures (overhead costs) which are caused by the coordination and interaction of the integrated care processes such as management, coordination and office space may also be included; nevertheless, these are difficult to budget under the existing bundled health-care model [28].

Organisation and Coverage of Care

Care groups are a core element of the bundled payment approach. Struijs et al. [28] outline the role of the principal contractor of the bundled payment scheme in such a way that the groups are legally or contractually responsible for the coordination, consistency and quality of the diabetes care. In compliance with this role they can either contract or coordinate health-care providers for the actual provision of the specified health-care services or they even provide certain or all of the care components themselves. To ensure the required quality and efficiency of care they have the option to selectively contract health-care providers.

The coverage of care offered by groups based on a bundled payment scheme is based on standards of care (CS). These standards are defined by the Dutch Diabetes Federation (NDF), build on evidence-based guidelines and are updated regularly [32]. However, a care group may have a specialist for internal medicine under contract for consultations. If such a specialist is consulted, an outpatient hospital treatment bundle for "diabetes mellitus without secondary complications" may not be claimed. As soon as the treatment responsibility for a patient is transferred from the PCP to a specialist, a patient is no longer "under the care" of the care group; this means that the bundled payment for this patient is terminated. The specialist then bills the health insurer directly for that patient. During that time, when the specialist activates the hospital payment scheme, the care group cannot claim a bundled fee for that patient [28].

Care Based on Bundled Payment Contracts

The extent to which care is provided to a diabetic patient is defined in the NDF care standard and is approved by all national providers and patient organisations [21, 33]. However, it sets in only from the moment a diagnosis of diabetes mellitus is made [30]. Any activity which is needed to diagnose diabetes falls outside a bundled payment system. Struijs et al. [28] therefore stated that in their study of "tangible effects of bundled payment" formal diagnosis was not included in any of the contracts they reviewed. Initial risk assessments, even if part of the diagnostic phase, were included in all the contracts. Table 11.1 gives an overview of the performance of the group contracts with respect to the NDF standards.

In the contracts they reviewed, they found that periodic check-ups as well as specialist consultation were included in all bundled payment contracts. Laboratory testing was also included by nine care groups. Nevertheless, group nine, which was the exception, had a separate contract with a medical laboratory. Support in smoking reduction or cessation was not included in the payment in five groups. Exercise counselling was included in all contracts, but supervised exercise counselling was mentioned in the bundled payment contracts of group nine. Because the patient had to pay €5 per year, it is unclear whether this claim is part of the bundled payment. Medication and psychosocial care were not included in any of the bundled payment contracts. These services were not mentioned in the NDF standards either. A supplementary foot examination was covered in four contracts.

Table 11.1 Content of the bundled payment contracts by diabetes care group

	Diabetes care group									
	Required by NDF Health-Care standard	1	2	3	4	6	7	8	9	10
Diagnostic phase										
Formal diagnosis	No	–	–	–	–	–	–	–	–	–
Initial risk assessment	Yes	+	+	+	+	+	+	+	+	+
Treatment and standard check-ups										
12-monthly check-ups	Yes	+	+	+	+	+	+	+	+	+
3-monthly check-ups	Yes	+	+	+	+	+	+	+	+	+
Eye examinations	Yes	+	+	+	+	+	+	+	+	+
Foot examinations	Yes	+	+	+	+	+	+	+	+	+
Supplementary foot exams	Unclear	–	+	+	–	+	–	–	+	–
Foot treatment	No	–	–	+	–	–	–	–	–	–
Laboratory testing	Yes	+	+	+	+	+	+	–	+[b]	+
Smoking cessation support	Yes	–	+	–	–	+	–	+	+	–
Exercise counselling	Yes	+	+	+	+	+	+	+	+	+
Supervised exercise	No	–	–	–	–	–	–	–	+[c]	–
Dietary counselling	Yes	+	+	+	+	+	+	+	+	+/–[d]
Medication	No	–	–	–	–	–	–	–	–	–
Psychosocial care	No	–	–	–	–	–	–	–	–	–
Medical aids	No	–[a]	–	–	–	–	–	–	–[a]	–
Additional GP consultations (diabetes-related)	Unclear	–	+/–	+/–	+/–	–	+/–	+/–	+/–	+/–
Additional GP consultations (non-related)	No	+/–	–	–	–	–	–	–	–	–
Specialist consultations	Yes	+	+	+	+	+	+	+	+	+

From Struijs [28]

[a]Medical aids limited to blood glucose strips and billed at a maximum additional fee of €4.50 per patient per year

[b]Supplementary fee paid for laboratory testing (€27 per patient per year) via a module additional to the bundled fee

[c]Exercise programme mentioned in contract at additional fee of €5 per patient per year

[d]Dietary counselling contracted for new patients only (module 1) and for those in insulin adjustment phases (module 3) but available to other patients on specific GP referral

It was also not clear whether any extra GP consultations were covered by the bundled payment contracts. Even when distinguishing between "diabetes-related" and "non-diabetes-related" visits there was no consistent picture. As Struijs et al. [28] show, the interviews indicated that some insurance companies interpreted the coverage more broadly than the care groups.

Provision of Care

Type of diabetes, and associated treatment requirements, decide the place where care is given and by whom. Care usually comprises all aspects of diabetes care. In some cases, patients are for example referred temporarily or permanently for podiatric care to the hospital while the usual diabetes care remains provided in community care. Table 11.2 summarises the location of care.

Table 11.2 Location of care

Type 2 diabetes mellitus:
Community care (1st line in our terms)
Specialised care
General hospitals (2nd line in our terms)
University care (3rd line in our terms)
Type 1 diabetes mellitus
Specialised care
General hospitals
University care
Diabetes and pregnancy (including GDM)
Specialised care
General hospitals
University care
Secondary diabetes
Community care (selected individuals with stable diabetic disease and primary morbidity (like renal transplant, steroid related disease)
Specialised care (genetic cases, syndromes, drug-related, HIV-(drug)- related)
General hospitals
University care
Specific centres for CFRD and lung transplant, other solid organ transplant, bone marrow/stem cell transplants)

Management of Type 2 Diabetes

The great majority of patients have type 2 diabetes. All professionals agree that many patients with type 2 diabetes can be treated well enough under community care (Dutch estimation: 80 %). The Netherlands is a small country and generally distances are no issue (except for traffic jams and, for some, public transport fares). There is a national consensus (LTA: national transmural agreement [34] – between 1st and 2nd/3rd line) that describes which patients would logically be treated in the community care and which ones in specialised care. In general terms, many patients are therefore treated under community care, the GPs can consult the hospital-based specialist and others are referred temporarily for a specific problem (some of them stay under hospital specialist care however) or are referred permanently. Referral back to the GP is guided by the nature and severity of the diabetic condition, nondiabetic morbidity and the wish of the patient. In modern terms "shared decision-making." Very generally outlined indications for (permanent) referrals are:

- Intensive insulin therapy or those having trouble achieving adequate control
- Insulin treatment and (recurrent) hypoglycaemia
- Severe hypoglycaemia in any patient
- Difficult hyperlipidemia
- Difficult hypertension
- Severe obesity
- Renal impairment (eGFR <45 in patients <60 years, <30 in those >60 years) and/or macroalbuminuria/proteinuria
- Difficult neuropathy
- Complicated diabetic foot
- Pregnancy-related issues

The LTA is then translated into a RTA (regional transmural agreement) with local adaptations. Good implementation requires good communication and human relations. The personal factor(s) is/are essential to make this scheme work. The essential issue for the government is to provide the best care near the patient, but basically they appear to be seeking the cheapest care by health-care professionals with the minimally-required level of expertise (in theory).

There are some important issues diabetes professionals are confronted with:

- There is little room for innovation (costs money)
- Restricted access to new medications
- Safeguarding adequate referral to secondary care.

Evaluation of the Bundled Payments Approach

As mentioned above, changes or improvements should occur most likely in three areas: (1) Quality improvement and cost reduction by reducing administrative/overhead costs, sharing risk, eliminating cost-shifting, outcomes management and continuous quality improvement, reducing inappropriate and unnecessary resource use, efficient use of capital and technology; (2) consumer responsiveness, i.e., seamless continuum of care and focus on the health of enrollees; (3) community (e.g., whole village/town) benefit by improving community health status, and addressing the prevention of social issues which affect community health. As the RAND Corporation states, the evaluation should cover at least: changes in consumer financial risk, waste reduction (as a consequence of reduced (unnecessary) services), reliability through focus on key processes and improved coordination, patient experience, health, coverage, capacity, operational feasibility [26].

Dutch integrated diabetes care, induced by the bundled payment approach, affects both horizontal and vertical integration of providers. So far, goals like multidisciplinary care and seamless care (especially seen from the patient's viewpoint) seems to have been reached. In a recent study de Baker et al. came to the conclusion that "the bundled payment led to important changes in the financing and delivery of chronic care in the Dutch health-care system. In a relatively short period of time, care groups were created throughout the country, providing integrated, multidisciplinary care for patients with diabetes …." [35] (p430). They also identified improved organisation and coordination, better collaboration among the providers and better adherence to care protocols. On the other hand they also recognised a dominance of the Care Groups by GPs. Furthermore, prices varied to a large extent among the care groups, and, as they state, "this could not be fully explained by differences in the services offered. Moreover, outdated information and information technologies led to an increased administrative burden. Nevertheless, the introduction of bundled payments might turn out to be a useful step in the direction of risk-adjusted integrated capitation payments for multidisciplinary provider groups offering primary and specialty care to a defined group of patients" [35].

As far as efficiency of care is concerned, after 3 years of evaluation, several changes in care processes have been observed, including task substitution from GPs to practice nurses and increased coordination of care [31, 36], thus improving process costs. However, Elissen et al. [31] concluded that the evidence relating to changes in process and outcome indicators, remains open to doubt, and only modest improvements were shown in most indicators. Struijs et al. [36] present a more differentiated picture. Process indicators like measurement of HbA1c, body mass index, blood pressure, cholesterol, kidney tests and foot examination have shown improvements. On the other hand, this improvement was accompanied by a decrease in annual eye testing. Some intermediate outcome measures like blood pressure and cholesterol level have improved slightly as well. Body mass index remained unchanged, and the average HbA1c has increased. Struijs et al. found that patients in a bundled payment diabetes care programme, used less specialist care than patients receiving usual care [37]. However, there has been no improvement in outcome parameters like efficiency outcomes to date.

During the first year, the expenditure per patient was actually higher than for patients receiving usual care. In their comparison of integrated care outcomes in three countries, Busse et al. identified an increased annual cost of $388 per patient in the Dutch model. This was associated with mixed clinical outcomes but better experiences for patients and providers (Tables 11.3 and 11.4) [38]. More than 90 % of the

Table 11.3 Quality of diabetes care in terms of process indicators in second and third years after bundled payment implementation, percentages by care group and for total sample

	1		2		3		4		6		7		8		9		10		Total	
Care group	year 2	year 3	year 2	year 3	year 2	year 3	year 2	year 3	year 2	year 3	year 2	year 3	year 2	year 3	year 2	year 3	year 2	year 3	year 2	year 3
Patients with:																				
At least 4 check-ups	58.3	70.3*	45.2	57.4*	52.9	68.7*	59.7	70.7*	–	38.1	–	–	–	66.1	–	–	–	–	54.5	66.3*
Eye examination in past 12 months	–	38.4	32.6	31.3	60.1	69.1*	45.5	41.4*	–	27.1	52	42.8*	–	63.6	42.8	54.2*	77.3	73.5*	48.1	44.6*
Eye examination in past 24 months	–	–	–	44.8	–	88.0	–	54.5	–	–	–	72.7	–	–	–	71.6		92.4		63.0
Foot examination	–	63.7	68	79.2*	67.2	84.4*	92.9	91.7*	–	58.9	65.1	70.8*	–	73	76.3	77.8	88	84.8*	78.4	82.4*
HbA1c test	74.2	97.0*	89.7	93.2*	93.6	94.3	94.9	94.8	–	89.2	82.6	81.3*	–	77.6	93.9	95.2	99.3	99.0	90.8	91.4*
Blood pressure measurement	98.5	97.3	91.1	91.8	96.7	96.9	99.2	99.2	–	89.9	86.8	85.4*	–	94.5	88.8	82.2*	98.7	98.2	93.9	93.4*
BMI measurement																				
	99.4	97.3*	92.1	92.1	96.6	96.9	99.1	99.1	–	90.6	79.9	83.1*	–	94.3	86.9	81.4*	91.6	91.5	91.7	92.3*
Creatinine clearance calculation or test	71.8	80.8*	91.2	94.2*	60.8	75.0*	86.5	86.8	–	83.6	75.9	73.0*	–	60	90.8	91.2	92.5	92.1	83.8	84.6*

Urine test (spot sample) for albumin or albumin-creatinine ratio	69.1	46.8*	63.8	74.7*	55.2	69.1*	–	–	–	68.6	65.6	68.9*	–	45.8	86.8	88.4	74.2	72.6	66.6	71.8*
LDL test	71.5	78.7*	83.7	87.6*	66.2	83.0*	88	88.5	–	81.5	75.2	71.8*	–	63.1	90	93.0*	96.3	95.7	83.3	84.4*
HDL test	72.1	79.0*	86.5	90.6*	66.8	84.2*	–	–	–	83.8	77.7	73.9*	–	66.1	92.5	94.4	96.5	94.3	82.7	83.9*
Total cholesterol	72.7	80.5*	87.3	91.3*	66.8	84.1*	89.7	90.2	–	83.9	77.7	74.0*	–	65.9	92.7	94.4	96.6	96.8	85.4	86.6*
Triglyceride test	72.4	80.5*	87.2	91.2*	66.7	84.1*	88.5	88.3	–	83.7	77.5	73.7*	–	65.9	92.5	94.4	96.5	93.7*	84.9	85.5*
Smoking status know		100		100		96.1		78.8		100		93.7	100		98		68.5		88.5	
Dietician consultation	–	21.6	21	16.1*	–	–	5.9	3.4*	–	2.8	0.1	5.2*	–	–	–	–	–	–	7.7	7.4*
Composite indicators																				
Tested/know: HbA1c, blood pressure, BMI, total cholesterol, creatinine clearance, foot exams	–	58.3	57.8	72.9*	60.7	74.9*	83.8	84.3	–	51.1	52.5	60.5*	–	46.4	64.6	60.4	77.4	74.2	68.1	73.7*
Lipid profiling (total cholesterol, triglycerides, HDL, LDL)	71.2	78.7*	83.7	87.5*	66	82.8*	–	–	–	81.5	74.8	71.6*	–	62.7	89.9	93.0*	96	90.3*	80.3	81.3*

From Struijs et al. [36]
*Significant ($P < .05$)

Table 11.4 Quality of care in terms of outcome indicators, at T1 (first value in second year after bundled payment implementation) and T3 (final value in third year after implementation), by care group and for total sample

Care group	1		2		3		4		6		7		8		9		10		Total	
Assessment	T1/T2[a]	T3	T1	T3	T1	T3	T1	T3	T2[a]	T3	T2[a]	T3	T2[a]	T3	T1	T3	T1	T3	T1	T3
Outcome indicator																				
HbA1c																				
Mean (mmol/mol)	48.3	49.4*	56.2	54.7*	48.3	50.2*	48.5	50.1*	51.2	55.0*	49.8	49.9	49	50.4*	53.0	51.6*	50.1	49.3*	50.5	51.0*
% of patients ˂53 mmol/mol	76.6	74.9	42.3	50.2*	76.4	66.9*	73.0	66.7*	65.2	50.7*	70.1	69.1	72.8	71.9	56.2	61.7	69.9	66.8*	66	63.2*
% of patients >69 mmol/mol	0.8	1.7	14.3	11.7*	1.2	1.8	2.5	2.8	5.5	10.1*	2.3	2.4	0.9	4.4	8.7	6.8	4.8	3.1*	5.3	4.7*
Systolic blood pressure																				
Mean (mmHg)	140	139	140	137*	139	139	141	140*	137	136	141	140*	138	139	144	140*	140	137*	141	139*
% of patients <140 mmHg	47.4	52.0	47.6	58.2*	52.6	52.5	42.9	46.0*	54.1	56.2	44.9	46.6*	54.3	50.4	39.3	52.2*	48.3	61.7*	45.2	51.3*
BMI																				
Mean (kg/m^2)	29.71	29.73	29.32	29.26	29.48	29.35*	30.21	30.15*	29.29	29.17	29.61	29.53*	28.98	28.97	30.02	29.69*	30.09	30.04	29.93	29.86*
% of patients <25 Kg/m^2	15.2	15.9	18.9	20.6*	16.4	18.0	14.3	15.7*	19.3	20.0	17.5	18.0	19.7	18.6	12.7	14.2	13.0	14.3	15.3	16.8*
% of patients >30 Kg/m^2	42.4	43.9	37.6	37.3	40.9	39.4	45.9	45.2	37.7	37.8	40.4	40.0	34.1	34.8	43.8	41.5	45.0	43.7	43.5	42.7*
Kidney function																				
% of patients with	–	–	–	–	–	–	–	–	–	–	–	–	–	–	–	–	–	–	–	–
Clearance >60 ml/min (MDRD)																				
% of patients with microalbuminuria	–	–	–	–	–	–	–	–	–	–	–	–	–	–	–	–	–	–	–	–
% of patients with proteinuria	–	–	–	–	–	–	–	–	–	–	–	–	–	–	–	–	–	–	–	–
Lipid profile																				
Mean LDL (mmol/l)	2.6	2.5*	2.6	2.4*	2.3	2.3	2.6	2.4*	2.7	2.5*	2.6	2.5*	2.7	2.6	2.5	2.5	2.6	2.1*	2.6	2.4*
% of patients with LDL <2.5 mmol/l	49.0	57.8*	47.8	60.0*	59.9	62.2	46.4	55.8*	43.6	48.9*	50.3	53.4*	42.0	42.0	52.4	51	49.2	71.5*	48.2	58.6*

Mean HDL (mmol/l)	1.3	1.3	1.2	1.3*	1.2	1.3*	–	–	1.2	1.2	1.4	1.4	1.3	1.3	1.3	1.3	1.1	1.2*	1.2	1.3*
Mean triglycerides (mmol/l)	1.6	1.5*	1.7	1.6*	1.8	1.8	1.9	1.8*	2.0	1.9	1.7	1.7*	1.7	1.7	1.7	1.6	1.6	1.5*	1.8	1.7*
Mean total cholesterol (mmol/l)	4.6	4.5*	4.6	4.4*	4.4	4.4	4.7	4.5*	4.8	4.6*	4.7	4.6*	4.8	4.8	4.5	4.5	4.3	4.0*	4.6	4.4*
% of patients with total	48.0	55.6	47.6	57.2*	57.7	57.5	42.9	53.0*	41.0	44.7*	45.6	49.6*	41.4	35.7	50.8	51.4	57.4	73.1*	46.8	56.2*
Cholesterol <4.5 mmol/l																				
Smoking																				
% of smokers among patients	–	10.5	–	14.7	–	14.7	–	18.6	–	14.5	–	15.6	–	23.8	–	13.5	–	18.2	–	16.4
With known smoking behaviour																				
% of quitters	–	–	–	–	–	–	–	–	–	–	–	–	–	–	–	–	–	–	–	–
Complications																				
% of patients with foot problems	–	–	–	–	–	–	–	–	–	–	–	–	–	–	–	–	–	–	–	–
% of patients with eye problems	–	–	–	–	–	–	–	–	–	–	–	–	–	–	–	–	–	–	–	–
% of patients with any complications	–	–	–	–	–	–	–	–	–	–	–	–	–	–	–	–	–	–	–	–

From Struijs et al. [36]

*Significant ($P < .05$).

[a]T1 values not known for care groups 1, 6, 7 and 8 (except blood pressure and BMI for group 1), hence T2 values reported (final value in second year after implementation) and differences with T3 assessed; not included in totals

patients interviewed judged the cooperation and coordination to be either good or excellent. The providers perceived improved quality and more patient-centredness [38]. The adherence to care standards (CS) improved from 79 % to 89.2 % during the period 2010–2013 [34]. This positive trend was transferred into high levels of patient satisfaction and their involvement in treatment [34].

Conclusions

The limited evidence for a positive impact of bundled payments under the Dutch health system has led to discussions over whether the current methodological approaches are sophisticated enough to differentiate between differences due to bundled payments compared with other influences of health-care reform that could be superimposed [39]. Moreover, interactions of other secular factors (e.g., regional, national or local trends and characteristics) make it difficult to assign outcomes to the influence of bundled payments alone. As Struijs et al. [39] point out, new methods are needed to distinguish between the effects of the core elements of the payment reform, the core elements of the provider-led entities and the core elements of the health-care delivery transformations. Such analyses could inform the global debate over how to implement integrated care. For example, Busetto et al. [40] argue in favour of mixed methods studies. Overall, while the Dutch approach to integrated care, using a bundled payment system with a mixed payer approach, has created a limited improvement in integration, there is no evidence that the approach has reduced morbidity and premature mortality: and it has come at an increased cost.

References

1. Björnberg A. Euro health consumer index 2014. Health Consumer Powerhouse Ltd; 2015.
2. Mahon M, Fox B. US health system ranks last among eleven countries on measures of access, equity, quality, efficiency, and healthy lives – the commonwealth fund 2014 [05/15/2016]. Available from: http://www.commonwealthfund.org/publications/press-releases/2014/jun/us-health-system-ranks-last.
3. van den Berg M, Heijink R, Zwakhals L, Verkleij H, Westert G. Health care performance in the Netherlands: easy access, varying quality, rising costs. Eurohealth. 2010;16(4):3.
4. Schölkopf M, Pressel H. Das Gesundheitswesen im internationalen Vergleich: Gesundheitssystemvergleich und europäische Gesundheitspolitik. 2., aktualisierte und erweiterte Auflage, rev. Ausg ed. Berlin: MWV Medizinisch Wissenschaftliche Verlagsgesellschaft; 2014
5. Organisation for Economic Co-Operation and Development (OECD). Health at a glance 2013 – OECD indicators 2013 [05/15/2015]. Available from: http://www.oecd-ilibrary.org/docserver/download/8113161e.pdf?expires=1445258459&id=id&accname=guest&checksum=B2A1378438D4D53DB27F2A5CE6B6174A.
6. van Roojen M, Goedvolk R, Houwert T. A Vision for the Dutch health care in 2040 – towards a sustainable, high-quality health care – a report from the World Economic Forum prepared in cooperation with McKinsey & Company Amsterdam2013 [05/15/2016]. Available from: http://www.mckinsey.com/global-locations/europe-and-middleeast/netherlands/en/latest-thinking.
7. International Diabetes Federation. IDF diabetes atlas. 6th ed. Brussels: International Diabetes Federation; 2013.
8. Shaw JE, Sicree RA, Zimmet PZ. Global estimates of the prevalence of diabetes for 2010 and 2030. Diabetes Res Clin Pract. 2010;87(1):4–14.
9. American Diabetes Association. Economic costs of diabetes in the U.S. in 2012. Diabetes Care. 2013;36(4):1033–46.
10. Zhang P, Zhang X, Brown J, Vistisen D, Sicree R, Shaw J, et al. Global healthcare expenditure on diabetes for 2010 and 2030. Diabetes Res Clin Pract. 2010;87(3):293–301.
11. Slocum TA. Thematic cartography and geographic visualization. 3rd ed. Upper Saddle River: Pearson/Prentice-Hall; 2009.
12. Lynch R, Altenburg-van den Broek E. The drawbacks of Dutch-style health care rules: lessons for Americans. Backgrounder. Washington, DC: The Heritage Foundation; 2010.
13. Daley C, Gubb J. Healthcare systems: The Netherlands: CIVITAS; 2013 [05/15/2016]. Available from: http://www.civitas.org.uk/research/health/health-systems/.
14. Gowling A. Dutch health insurers squeeze health providers: IAM EXPAT; 2013 [05/15/2016]. Available from: http://www.iamexpat.nl/read-and-discuss/expat-page/news/dutch-health-insurers-squeeze-providers.
15. Gowling A. Dutch doctors strike to protest health insurance amendment 2014 [05/15/2016]. Available from: http://www.iamexpat.nl/read-and-discuss/

expat-page/news/dutch-doctors-strike-health-insurance-change.
16. Clark B. Dutch health insurance premiums set to rise in 2015 2014 [05/15/2016]. Available from: http://www.iamexpat.nl/read-and-discuss/expat-page/news/dutch-health-insurance-premiums-rise-2015#sthash.cRkDlxco.dpuf.
17. Health Insurance Information Centre. Compare health insurances 2015 [05/15/2016]. Available from: http://www.zorgverzekering.org/eng/compare/.
18. MedTech Europe. The Netherlands: market-based reform n.d. [05/15/2016]. Available from: http://www.reforminghealthcare.eu/economist-report/some-roads-ahead-innovative-approaches-in-five-west-european-countries/the-netherlands-market-based-reform.
19. Government of the Netherlands. Health insurance – standard health insurance n.d. [05/15/2016]. Available from: https://www.government.nl/topics/health-insurance/contents/standard-health-insurance.
20. Koenraadt B. Healthcare insurance in the Netherlands: an overview 2014 [05/15/2016]. Available from: http://www.iamexpat.nl/read-and-discuss/expat-page/articles/healthcare-insurance-in-the-netherlands-overview.
21. Struijs JN, Baan CA. Integrating care through bundled payments – lessons from The Netherlands. N Engl J Med. 2011;364(11):990–1.
22. de Wildt JE, Leusink GL, Beek GJ. Nulmeting zorggroepen: Een beschrijvend onderzoek van de karakteristieken. Utrecht: LVG; 2008.
23. Struijs J. Integrating care by bundled payments: lessons from the Netherlands: Rijks Instituut voor de Volksgezondheid en Milieu; 2012 [05/15/2016]. Available from: http://www.kingsfund.org.uk/sites/files/kf/jn-struijs-integrated-care-netherlands--kingsfund-sept12.pdf.
24. Ham C, Zollinger-Read P. What are the lessons from the USA for clinical commissioning groups in the English National Health Service? Lancet. 2012;379(9811):189–91.
25. Luft HS. Becoming accountable-opportunities and obstacles for ACOs. N Engl J Med. 2010;363(15):1389–91.
26. Bertko J, Effros R. Analysis of bundled payment. RAND Corporation; 2010 [05/15/2016]. Available from: http://www.rand.org/pubs/technical_reports/TR562z20/analysis-of-bundled-payment.html.
27. Washington State Hospital Association. Integrated delivery systems. n.d. Available from: http://www.wsha.org/files/62/Gov_Board_Manual_integrated.pdf.
28. Struijs JN. Experimenting with a bundled payment system for diabetes care in the Netherlands – the first tangible effects. Bilthoven: National Institute for Public Health and the Environment (RIVM) 2010 RIVM-rapportnummer: 260224002.
29. Taakgroep Programma Diabeteszorg. Diabeteszorg Beter – rapport van de Taakgroep Programma Diabeteszorg. The Hague: Ministerie van Volksgezondheid, Welzijn en Sport; 2005.
30. Nederlandse Diabetes Federatie. NDF Voedingsrichtlijn Diabetes 2007.
31. Elissen A, Duimel-Peeters IGP, Spreeuwenberg C, Vrijhoef HJM, Nolte E. The Netherlands. In: Nolte E, Knai C, editors. Assessing chronic disease management in European health systems – country reports. 39th ed. Copenhagen: World Health Organization; 2015.
32. Raaijmakers LGM. Diabetes care and the introduction of a new standard in the Netherlands – a closer look from the perspectives of health care professionals and patients. Dissertation. Maastricht: Maastricht University; 2014.
33. Nederlandse Diabetes Federatie. NDF Zorgstandaard – diabetes type 2 volwassenen. 2015 [05/15/2016]. Available from: http://www.zorgstandaarddiabetes.nl/type-2/.
34. Raaijmakers LG, Kremers SP, Schaper NC, de Weerdt I, Martens MK, Hesselink AE, et al. The implementation of national action program diabetes in the Netherlands: lessons learned. BMC Health Serv Res. 2015;15:217.
35. de Bakker DH, Struijs JN, Baan CB, Raams J, de Wildt JE, Vrijhoef HJ, et al. Early results from adoption of bundled payment for diabetes care in the Netherlands show improvement in care coordination. Health Aff (Millwood). 2012;31(2):426–33.
36. Struijs JN, de Jong-van Til J, Lemmens L, Drewes H, de Bruin S, Baan C. Three years of bundled payment for diabetes care in the Netherlands. Bilthoven: National Institute for Public Health and the Environment (RIVM); 2012.
37. Struijs JN, Mohnen SM, Molema C, de Jong-van Til JT, Baan CA. Effects of bundled payment on curative health care costs in the Netherlands – an analysis for diabetes care and vascular risk management based on nationwide claim data, 2007–2010. Bilthoven: National Institute for Public Health and the Environment (RIVM); 2012.
38. Busse R, Stahl J. Integrated care experiences and outcomes in Germany, the Netherlands, and England. Health Aff (Project Hope). 2014;33(9):1549–58.
39. Struijs JN. Payment reform and integrated care: the need for evaluation. Int J Integr Care. 2013;13:e056.
40. Busetto L, Luijkx KG, Vrijhoef HJ. Implementation of integrated care for type 2 diabetes: a protocol for mixed methods research. Int J Integr Care. 2014;14:e033.

12 Integrated Diabetes Care in Sweden

Helmut Wenzel, Stefan Jansson, and Mona Landin-Olsson

Basic Principles of the Swedish Health-Care System

The Swedish health-care system is a form of the "Beveridge model," with a strong orientation towards subnational levels, i.e., municipalities and regions. Thus, the responsibility is shared between the central government, county councils ("landsting" in Swedish) and municipalities ("kommuner" in Swedish). The Health and Medical Service Act regulates the responsibilities of the different actors, giving the local governments more freedom in this area [1]. The role of the central government is to establish principles and guidelines, and to set the political agenda for health and medical care. This is primarily achieved through laws and ordinances or by reaching agreements with the Swedish Association of Local Authorities and Regions (SALAR), which represents the county councils and municipalities [2]. Figure 12.1 shows the make-up of the organisation, and the financial flows.

In principle, the central government sets the health-care policies, whereas the local governments organise the delivery of services to ensure that their own residents receive the medical care they need [3]. Health care is mainly tax funded; this applies at Government level as well as to the levels of the county councils and the municipalities. The latter also levy proportional income taxes on the population to cover the services that they provide [4]. Therefore, the county council tax, supplemented by a government grant, is the main means of financing the health-care system. In addition, small user fees are paid at the point of use. Long-term care for the elderly is financed and organised by the municipalities. Each county council and region is governed by a political assembly, whose representatives are elected for 4 years in general elections [5]; Anell [4] gives a detailed overview on the financial flow.

Swedish health care is also characterised by its universal access and both visits and prescriptions of drugs are heavily subsidised meaning that virtually all people can get help with their medical problems. The Ministry of Health and Social Affairs is primarily responsible for drafting health policy legislation. It also works with the county councils and municipalities to determine how to best finance and deliver health care to the citizens of Sweden [6]. It supervises 25 agencies, of which

H. Wenzel (✉)
Health Economist, Konstanz, Germany
e-mail: hkwen@aol.com

S. Jansson
Department of Family Medicine, Brickebacken Primary Health Care Center, Örebro, Sweden
e-mail: Stefan.jansson@regionorebrolan.se

M. Landin-Olsson
Department of Endocrinology, Lund University Hospital, Lund, Sweden
e-mail: Mona.landin-olsson@med.lu.se

D. Simmons et al. (eds.), *Integrated Diabetes Care*, DOI 10.1007/978-3-319-13389-8_12

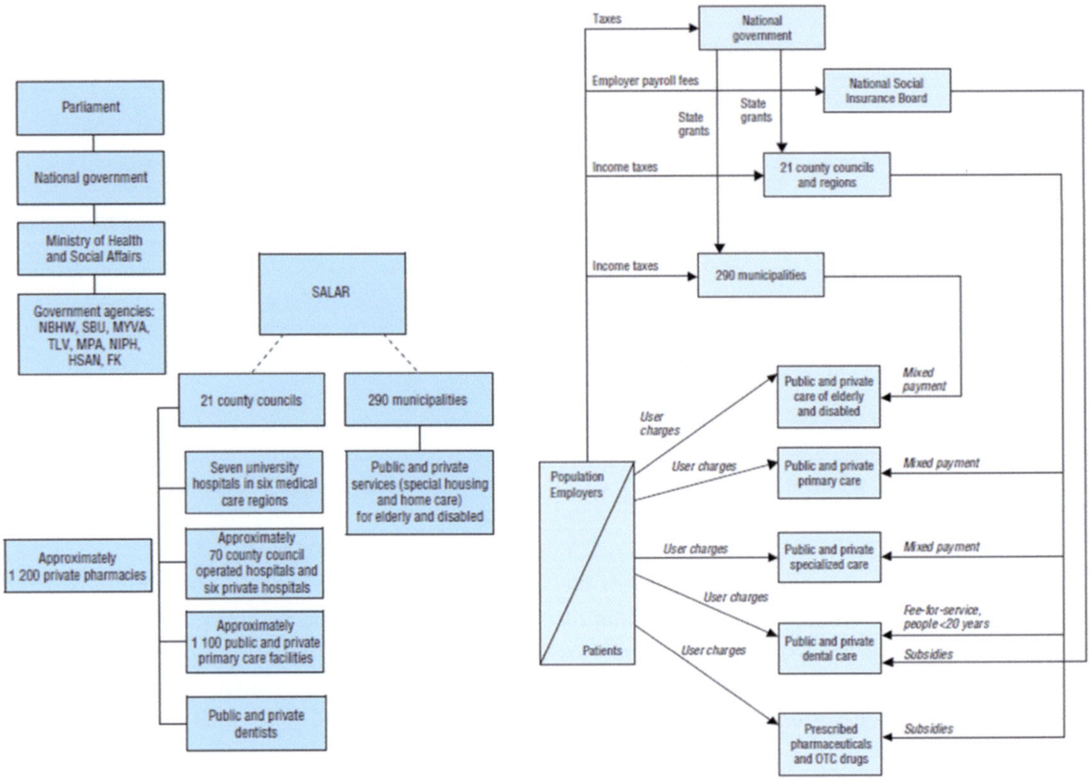

Fig. 12.1 Organisation of the Swedish Health-Care System and Financial Flows (Used with permission from Anell et al. [4])

11 are directly involved with health care at the national level. These are: The National Board of Health and Welfare, The Health and Social Care Inspectorate, The Public Health Agency, The Swedish Agency for Health and Care Services Analysis, The Swedish Agency for Health Technology Assessment and Assessment of Social Services, The Swedish eHealth Agency, The Medical Products Agency, The Dental and Pharmaceutical Benefits Agency, The Medical Responsibility Board, Apoteket AB, and The Social Insurance Agency [7]. The central government provides funding, and distributes money and resources to each of the agencies, mentioned above and establishes the general role of each; the agencies are then free to act independently, deciding on their own how to address particular issues.

Sweden is divided into 290 municipalities and 21 county councils (Fig. 12.1). Nine of the county councils: Gävleborg, Halland, Jämtland, Jönköping, Kronoberg, Skåne, Västra Götaland, Örebro and Östergötland – as well as the Gotland municipality – are called regional councils and have assumed responsibility for regional development from the state. There is no hierarchical relation between municipalities, county councils and regions. Around 90 % of the work of Swedish county councils concerns health care, but they also deal with other areas such as culture and infrastructure.

The municipalities are responsible for care for the elderly in the home or in special accommodation, i.e., nursing homes. Their duties also include care for people with physical disabilities or psychological disorders and providing support and services for people released from hospital care as well as for school health care. Chronic diseases that require monitoring and treatment, and often life-long medication, place significant demands on the system [8].

In this way, the health system is highly decentralised and organised; however, this does lead to variation in care provision. Primary and secondary care are funded and delivered at county level. Municipalities are responsible for nursing and residential homes as well as home care and other social services [9]. This, along with other issues, leads to fragmented care. For example, Åhgren identifies three major causes: *decentralisation*, which leads to rather independent processes, a *high degree of specialisation*, driven by medical development, and *professional organisation*, which means that nurses and doctors focus on their part of the care process for which they are responsible. Aiming for common health-care goals has a low priority [10].

Expenditure and Evaluation of the System

In 2013 Sweden spent the equivalent of 4,904 USD per capita on health – whereas the Organisation for Economic Co-operation and Development (OECD) average was at 3,453 USD, with 84 % of the expenditure coming from public sources. Both numbers are above the OECD average [11]. Compared with the OECD average of 73 %, Swedish Government spending has one of the highest proportions of public expenditure among OECD countries. Similarly high proportions can be found in the Netherlands (88 %), Norway (85 %) and Denmark (84 %) [11]. Health spending as a proportion of Gross Domestic Product (GDP), as an indicator for affordability, grew from 7.4 % in 2000 to 11 % in 2013; the corresponding OECD average in 2013 was 8.9 % [11, 12]. Health expenditure in the Netherlands, as a percentage of GDP, increased from 7.4 % in 1980 to 11.9 % in 2011 [13, 14]; in Sweden it was 10.6 % in 2011. In Germany the comparable numbers rose from 9.8 % in 2011 to 11.1 % in 2014; in Switzerland the share was 11.1 % in 2013, and it was 16.4 % in 2013 in the USA [12].

Interpreting this time series (i.e., share of GDP) needs caution: increasing rates could be due to increased spending, as well as due to a reduction in overall GDP, e.g., as a consequence of the so-called economic crisis (especially in 2008) [15].

Performance of the System: The OECD Health Care Quality Reviews

The OECD Health Care Quality Indicators project, initiated in 2002, aims to measure and compare the quality of health service provision in the different countries, based on a set of quality indicators at the health systems level, which allows an assessment of the impact of particular factors on the quality of health services [16]. According to the Health Care Quality Review of 2013, the quality of health care in Sweden is generally good. Rates of avoidable hospitalisation for chronic conditions such as asthma (22.2 per 100,000 population) are among the lowest in the OECD (average 45.8) and long-term complications of diabetes including amputation rates among diabetic patients are all lower than the OECD average [17]. In the 2011 survey, 90 % of primary care patients in Sweden said the particular staff treated them respectfully. Sweden's quality registers, for tracking the quality of care that patients receive and the corresponding outcomes for several conditions, are among the most developed across the OECD [17].

Yet, the coordination of care for patients with complex needs is less good. Only one in six patients had contact with a physician or specialist nurse after discharge from hospital for stroke, again with substantial variation across counties. Fewer than half of patients with type 1 diabetes, for example, have their blood pressure adequately controlled, with a considerable variation (from 26 % to 68 %) across counties [17].

As with primary care, the governance structure around long-term care is divided. Municipalities are responsible for institutional care and nursing care in private homes, and county councils are responsible for the delivery and financing of medical care. There are few built-in incentives for coordination across these governance levels, or across the health and social care components of long-term care services.

Whereas central government has set out a holistic vision for care of the elderly, this has not successfully transformed to local implementation. Joint care planning, joint purchasing or bundled payments, which should help to integrate local health and long-term care services, are frequently absent. Consistently high levels of unnecessary hospitalisation for the elderly are a clear indicator of this fragmentation. For example, at 260 admissions per 100,000 people aged over 80, avoidable hospital admissions for uncontrolled diabetes in Sweden's elderly population are the sixth highest in the OECD, and about 1.5 times higher than in Denmark. On the other hand, the average length of stay in hospital after a myocardial infarction in Sweden is less than 5 days, which is among the lowest in the OECD, and a sign of efficiency [17].

Municipalities are often not adequately equipped to manage patients after hospital discharge. Home care services needs up to 5 days to reorganise their work, and allocate resources, to ensure a safe and convenient situation in the home after hospital stay. This situation leads to crowding in the hospitals, with many patients unable to leave the hospital, staying for social rather than medical reasons. Only around 20 % of primary care doctors in Sweden report that they receive the information necessary to manage a patient within 48 h after hospital discharge, compared to almost 70 % in Germany. Sweden's health and elderly care systems deserve their reputation as being among the best in the world. Yet, an ageing population with growing chronic conditions and requiring more complex health services are testing Sweden's ability to continue delivering high-quality care, according to a new OECD report. Sweden has a larger share of elderly people than most OECD countries: 5.2 % are over 80, compared to the average of 4.2 %. Spending on elderly care is 3.6 % of GDP, compared to an OECD average of 1.7 %. The country also has the highest number of care workers per capita, and they deliver care where it is generally most wanted - at home. Seven out of ten dependent elderly people receive care in their homes [17].

Coordination of care between hospitals, primary care providers and local authorities is becoming one of the biggest challenges to the continued quality of Sweden's health and social care system. This means, the central government will have to set out responsibilities very clearly, by developing standards, building the evidence base and sharing knowledge. For example, central authorities should be given a more defined role in assuring the quality of services by setting out *national quality standards*. Moreover, clear standards are needed to underpin the new intermediate care facilities being developed by municipalities. The information infrastructure must improve by developing new indicators of quality of care provided by GPs and elderly care services. Finding ways to link across different data sources is also necessary, to allow a complete picture of an individual's care to be built up [18].

Waiting times have long been a cause of dissatisfaction [19]. In an OECD ranking of 2011, Sweden was rated second worst [20]. Therefore, Sweden introduced a health-care guarantee in 2005. This means that all patients should be able to be in contact with a primary health care the same day they seek help, and have a doctor's appointment within 7 days. After an initial examination, no patient should have to wait more than 90 days to see a specialist, and no more than 90 days for an operation or treatment, once it has been determined what care is needed. If the waiting time is exceeded, patients are offered care elsewhere; the expenditures, including those for travelling, is then paid by their county council [8, 21] . Statistics from 2015 indicate that about eight out of ten patients see a specialist within 90 days and receive treatment or are operated on within a further 90 days. In 2013, 78 % felt they received the care they needed. In 2006, the figure was 74 % [8]. Most patients who appeal under the health-care guarantee and prioritised in the "queue" had acute conditions rather than medical problems as a consequence of an underlying chronic disease. Patients waiting for a hip replacement or a cataract surgery are cured after surgery and no life-long follow-up is needed. When such patients are prioritised, the long-term care for patients with chronic diseases is "crowded out," lowering their priority and risking worse outcomes. The health-care guarantee can therefore lead to longer intervals between check-ups, with difficulties in accessing health care if their pre-existing condition has deteriorated.

The OECD summarises "Sweden's generous health care system performs well on most quality indicators but like all other OECD countries, it faces a number of challenges...." (17 p. 13). Challenges are, for example, better coordination between primary, secondary care and community health services. There is now a greater interest in enabling patients to make choices and in encouraging quality-based competition between providers. Taking the consumer and patient's point of view, Powerhouse in their Euro Health Consumer Index 2014 stated that, in principle, "the Swedish healthcare services are excellent, but their ranked position is dragged down by the seemingly never-ending story of access/waiting time problems, in spite of national efforts such as Vårdgaranti (National Guaranteed Access to Healthcare); in 2014, Sweden dropped to 12th place with 761 points" (22 p. 5).

Chains of Care: The Swedish Approach to Integration

Between 2000 and 2011 several reforms were implemented, aiming at introducing the waiting-time guarantee, improving the transparency of quality comparisons between counties, addressing the national coordination of highly specialised care, fostering choice and privatisation in primary care. In 2008 the government also introduced a bonus payment to county councils that met national waiting-time targets [4].

However, the ever-increasing fragmentation in health care called for approaches to *integrate* the care of the various providers. Quality of care issues were the most important reason for developing "chains of care." These chains of care are "coordinated activities within health care, linked together to achieve a qualitative final result for the patient. A Chain of Care often involves several responsible authorities and medical providers" (10 p. 2). This means that a chain of care has to include all health care that is provided for a specific patient group within a county council, i.e., all health care produced within the catchments area of the county council in question. Consequently, patient flow within a hospital or within a primary care centre is not a chain of care [10]. Chains of care provide evidence-based health care and have to take into account clinical guidelines, e.g., agreements on the distribution of medical work between different providers of health care within a county council catchment area [10]. In other words, chains of care involve coordinating multidisciplinary care based on clinical guidelines. This approach is similar to the concept of "Managed Clinical Networks," which aims to bring together different health professionals and organisations and help them work in a more coordinated manner without restrictions [23]. Applying Fulop's typology these characteristics reflect more of a *virtual* clinical integration through contractual agreement than a real organisational integration [24]. This kind of virtual integration between commissioners and providers can often involve several responsible authorities and medical providers [10]. Commissioners set up the contractual agreements with providers which specify volume, cost, quality and method of delivery [24]. Chains of care may have a manager responsible for organising activities resources and finance. The two largest Swedish county councils have each developed more than 50 chains of care [9].

Although numerous chains of care have been established, appraisals have concluded that there is little evidence that significant change have been achieved [24]. Ham et al. [25] also conclude that studies show limited impact of chains of care. Moreover, they highlight the challenges, which result from overcoming professional and structural barriers to realise integrated care. Yet, others see some benefits such as a reduction in the number of hospital beds and other improvements in efficiency [26]. On the other hand, a number of problems were created, for example, a lack of physicians in nursing homes. Additionally, some resistance from GPs towards integration, the policy shift towards free choice for patients, and the competing demands of managing competition alongside collaboration have also caused challenges [26, 27]. Other obstacles include resistance among some health-care managers who are afraid of changes. Some authors also point to perceived threats to clinical autonomy; moreover, it is also expected that the differentiation of clinical functions, which comes from sub-specialism, could further contribute to fragmentation [28, 29]. For Curry et al. [24] this indicates limits of contractual integration, and emphasises the point that commissioners face major challenges in using their influence to create better integrated care.

For Åhgren the most frequently stated reason for this lack of success is the intense compartmentalisation of responsibilities between different professions and departments, while the responsibilities and power remain in the vertical organisational structure. Limited or even absent participation among some local authorities has also been perceived to be responsible for chains of care, which were developed, missing some activities throughout a patient's treatment [10]. To ensure or improve quality of care, county councils will continue to develop chains of care in spite of their doubts whether they have been successful in their development [10].

Åhgren et al. note that policy makers promoted two important changes in health care with a strong impact on the provision of unfragmented care: free patient choice in primary health care and mergers of hospitals and clinical departments. These decisions will also have an adverse effect on the development of integrated care. Moreover, they recommend putting more efforts into evaluation of integrated care solutions in order to provide a basis for a more rational decision-making and to replace political beliefs about the benefits of such policies with evidence [27].

Growing Burden of Diabetes

Sweden has a population of almost ten million people with an increasing life expectancy for women and men over the past decades, reaching 84 years for women and 80 years for men in 2013 and is estimated to be close to 89 for women and 87 years for men in 2060 [30]. The percentage of people above the age of 65 is now 19.6 % [31] and by 2060 it is estimated to be 25 % [32]. This development of a growing proportion of elderly will increase the pressure on the health-care system to change and be prepared to meet people in older age with different claims about their own health. Diabetes mellitus is no derogation from this development and the prevalence of diabetes is increasing, mostly due to people with diabetes living longer with the disease than previously [33]. Currently, the total diabetes prevalence in Sweden is estimated at 4.7 %, which is equivalent to almost 450,000 individuals [34].

Diabetes is essentially treated effectively by multidisciplinary teams consisting of doctors and diabetes nurses in collaboration with other professionals, i.e., dieticians, podiatrists, physiotherapists, psychologists (Fig. 12.2a, b). Regular follow-up of patients with type 1 diabetes are carried out in hospitals by specialist endocrinologists while type 2 diabetes patients are followed up in primary health-care centres (PHCC) by GPs. Much of the care given is closely assessed through the Swedish National Diabetes Register (NDR) with 100 % of specialist clinics and 95 % of PHCC reporting to the register. The reporting is not mandatory, but all clinics and PHCC are encouraged to do so. The Swedish Association for Diabetology initiated the NDR in 1996. The purpose of NDR is to endorse evidence-based development of diabetes care by offering up-to-date information about changes in the treatment of glycaemia and other risk factors, as well as diabetic complications. Data on quality indicators are continuously collected from different clinics and primary health-care centres. For every clinic/PHCC it is then possible to make comparison with other units in the region or on national level. Anyone can easily access all available data instantaneously by internet. This means that providers as well as patients can seek information about a certain diabetes care unit to compare the health care given there with other units. Moreover, the overall aim of NDR is to reduce morbidity and mortality and to conduct a cost-effective diabetes care while every participating unit is

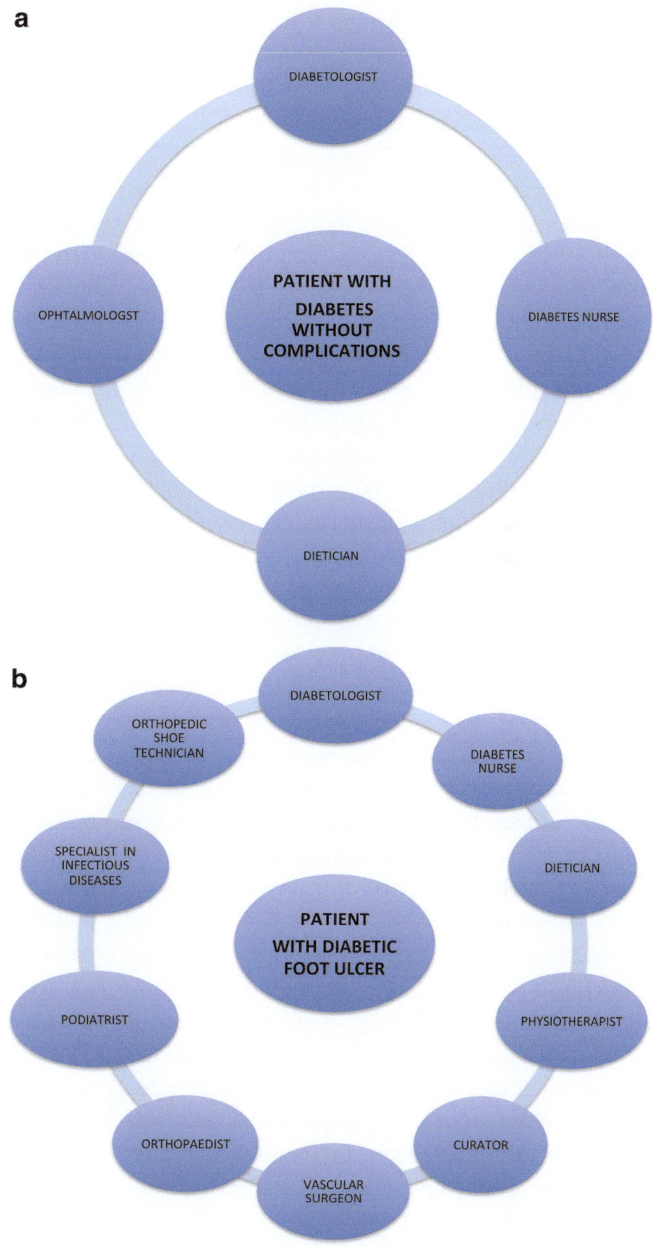

Fig. 12.2 (**a**, **b**) The care of the diabetic patient is more complex if more complications exist

interested in knowing how well they are doing in their care of people with diabetes.

Having a very high quality registry provides good opportunities to engage in a high-quality diabetes care. This is the probable main reason why Sweden turned out so well in a recent diabetes investigation among EU member states. The Euro Diabetes Index 2014 shows Sweden (936 points out of a maximum possible of 1,000; the highest score ever observed in a HCP Index) as the country with the best diabetes care delivery in Europe [22]. The secret of the high performance is probably "the art of knowing what you are doing." It was the only country out of 30 countries assessed that could provide data on all 28 indicators and areas, including prevention, case finding, range and reach of services, access to treatment and care, procedures and outcomes.

Organisation of Diabetes Care

Within each region / county council the care of patients with diabetes is divided. Patients with type 1 diabetes get their care at specialist clinics in hospitals and the majority of patients with type 2 diabetes in primary care. Patients with type 2 diabetes who have severe complications are referred to the Diabetes Clinics at the hospital. Approximately 10 % of all patients with type 2 continue their care at the hospital clinics. They are almost always on insulin in high doses often in combination with oral agents but despite massive medication many of these patients have difficulties to achieve metabolic balance. Patients with advanced complications such as foot ulcers, macroangiopathic manifestations and treatment with dialysis are also treated at the hospitals. Since these patients have multiple medical problems, the care has to be carried out in close collaboration with primary care and home health care. There is also a shared use of resources, where hospital doctors can refer patients with type 1 diabetes to primary health-care providers, e.g., if patients have asthma/chronic obstructive pulmonary disease, psychological disease or musculoskeletal disorders. Primary care physicians assess referrals and decide which profession will best take care of the patient, for example, a doctor, a counsellor or a physiotherapist. The specialist in the hospital can also write a referral to another specialist at another hospital in the region or to other hospitals outside the region for patients with type 1 diabetes. There may be patients who are in need of, for example, surgery, or other more specific treatments carried out only in some hospitals in the country.

In the majority of regions and county councils all records are electronic. Some county councils have the same electronic medical records (EMR) in primary and secondary care and therefore can electronically refer between each other. In other regions EMR can be read by all, but referrals between primary and secondary care have to be postal. For both doctors and nurses there are electronic decision supports at the point of care for some specified diseases. Some of these decision supports have been developed through cooperation between the profession and an authority, for instance sick leave. Guidelines for treating diabetes with different conditions and associated diagnoses are solely developed by the profession.

Different specialists provide education for GPs and nurses and in some cases even for community nurses. As an example, in the diabetes field, there is also a collaboration between diabetologists and some GPs who have deeper skills in diabetology in providing education for primary health-care providers, e.g., GPs and nurses specialised in diabetes. This education can be done "physically" as webinars or linked by video.

Diabetes and Pregnancy

Women with type 1 are informed early about pregnancy risks and advised to plan their pregnancies in advance. When pregnancy is detected the woman should be referred immediately to a specialised maternal diabetes team to ensure optimised metabolic control combined with intense obstetric management. Women with type 2 diabetes have contact with a midwife at the PHCC in the beginning of the pregnancy. During the rest of the pregnancy the women are followed up through local and regional treatment programmes, which differ in different parts of Sweden. For instance, in some regions, the diabetes care of women with type 1 diabetes and women with type 2 diabetes treated with oral antihyperglycaemic agents and/or insulin treatment is provided by the hospital maternal care unit through a multidisciplinary team of diabetologists, diabetes nurses and midwives (Fig. 12.3). All other contacts during the pregnancy are provided by the midwives at the PHCC. The treatment follows a standardised programme which varies in different regions of the country. A national care programme is under development. For women with type 2 diabetes, the follow-up continues at the PHCC according to a special care programme. The midwives are responsible

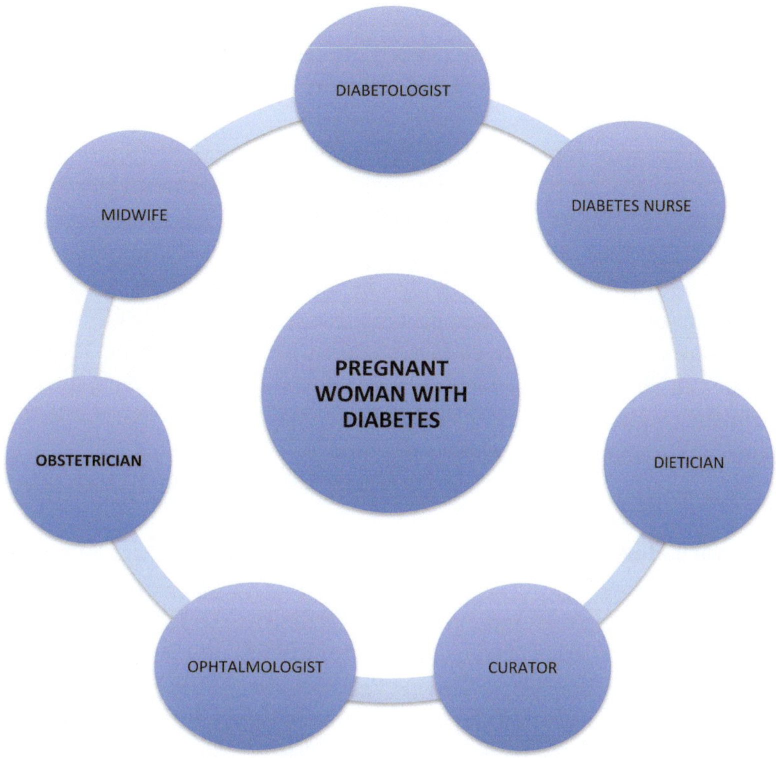

Fig. 12.3 Integrated and multi-professional care of women with type 1 diabetes and pregnancy

for the antenatal care, but diabetes nurses and GPs are also involved. Women are referred to a hospital for evaluation by a diabetologist. Women remain at the PHCC level as long as the glucose control is good according to the care programme. When insulin treatment needs to be started to optimise glucose control, the woman is then referred to the maternity care unit in the hospital. For women diagnosed with gestational diabetes mellitus (GDM) pregnancy care continues at the PHCC as long as glucose control is good. When glucose values deteriorate, care is transferred to the maternity unit at the hospital. All deliveries occur at a hospital. After pregnancy, the care continues as usual at the hospital unit for women with type 1 diabetes and at the PHCC for women with type 2 diabetes. Women who have had GDM during pregnancy are followed up according to a special care programme including visits to the PHCC annually to receive advice on healthy lifestyle, e.g., physical activity, diet, and to undergo an oral glucose tolerance test (OGTT) for the exclusion of incident diabetes.

Care at Municipalities

When patients with type 1 or type 2 diabetes need social services including short-term and long-term special housing (e.g., for the elderly and disabled), this becomes the municipalities' responsibility for providing care. The municipalities are also responsible for various types of domestic assistance for people living in their own housing. Many persons also receive home-based curative health care provided by nurses and auxiliary staff employed by the municipalities.

Primary Health-Care Level

For patients with type 2 diabetes, doctors in primary care write referrals to various units in the hospital for patients in need of different types of medical assistance, for instance orthotic shoes, eye examination, or if they need to be examined by, e.g., a neurologist or surgeon. Patients with more complex diabetes may need a "second opinion," and then the patient is referred to the diabetologist for assessment. Many of these patients use the hospital clinic as 'advisory', to obtain recommendations for their ongoing care. The patient will come back for follow-up and receive revised recommendations with certain time intervals but the main care is still given at the PHCC. Each PHCC also has a medical responsibility for patients living in nursing homes. Usually this means that primary care doctors make rounds once a week to the care accommodation. The round may involve both direct and indirect contact with the patient. The charge nurse at nursing homes is always present.

Primary Health-Care Changes

During the past years the structure of primary health care has been changed. Before 2010, patients were, by law, assigned to the PHCC in the geographic area in which the patient lived. The patients could apply to be listed at another PHCC outside the living area, for instance close to their job, but there was no guarantee that they would be listed there. In 2010 the Swedish government initiated "Health Choices," which allowed patient freedom in choosing the PHCC wherever they like. Most Swedish studies of such "freedom of choice systems" are built around having studied the change before and after the introduction of health-care choice. This makes it difficult to state whether a change in waiting times, for example, is an effect of health-care choice in itself, or an effect of some other health-care reform introduced by "The Swedish Agency for Health and Care Services Analysis" [35]. However, some conclusions from the reports are worth mentioning. Those who made an active choice of provider were more satisfied, although patients chose their health-care provider on the basis of proximity and reputation, not on medical results. The costs have remained under control, the effects on patient waiting times were small and the patients now live at a shorter distance from their medical centre. Finally, the "Vårdanalys" stated that there are deficiencies in knowledge about the effects of freedom of choice in terms of efficiency, medical quality and equality. The same authority concluded in another report in 2013 that there is a need for a more in-depth analysis of the various forms of health care and of possible inequalities based on socioeconomic factors rather than diagnosis of illness [36]. Studies regarding the effect of the reforms on the care of patients with diabetes are few but a recent study in 7,121 adult diabetes patients living in south of Sweden showed that continuity of care given by GPs in PHC decreased substantially after the reform. The decrease was independent of sex, type of diabetes, age, and income [37].

Type 1 Diabetes

Children defined as patients younger than 18 years are treated at 1 of the 43 Swedish Departments of Paediatrics. At the onset of the disease, the children are hospitalised for about a week. During the stay, the whole family is offered contact with both the diabetes team and the child psychiatry clinic. Parents are given up to 2 weeks of sick leave after leaving the hospital in order to adapt life to a child with diabetes. The hospital seeks contact with the child's school to inform and educate the school staff about the patient and his or her special needs. During the first year the diabetic child and the parents have several visits to the clinic and the diabetes team consisting of doctor, nurse and dietician. For continuous follow-up, the patient and his/her family have at least four visits per year when they meet both a doctor and a diabetes nurse. The patients with diabetes at the Paediatric Departments are seen by diabetes staff and registered in two registers. The first register, Better Diabetes Diagnosis (BDD), aims to provide the correct classification of the diabetes type by "human leucocyte antigens" (HLA) typing and testing for beta cell specific autoantibodies [38]. About 90 % of the children are classified as having Type 1 diabetes based on positive autoantibodies and a few percent receive a diagnosis of "Maturity Onset Diabetes of the Young" (MODY) [39]. Type 2 diabetes among children is very rare in Sweden. The departments also take part in a second register, a quality register called Swed-diab kids.

This register keeps track of the clinical performance for all Paediatric Clinics by registration of HbA1c and secondary complications. During recent years a significant improvement measured as a decrease in median and mean HbA1c has been observed across the whole Sweden. The mean HbA1c during 2015 was 57 mmol/mol which is the lowest value ever in the register [40]. In 2014, a majority, i.e., 52.2 % of the patients between 0 and 18 years had insulin delivered by continuous subcutaneous insulin infusion (CSII or insulin pump), [40] and an increasing proportion of the patients use continuous glucose monitoring (CGM). At the age of 18 years, the patient is transferred to the adult diabetes clinic at the hospital since patients with Type 1 diabetes are not referred to primary care.

When adults develop type 1 diabetes they are initially hospitalised for 3–5 days but referred to day care units as soon as possible. Insulin treatment is started immediately, and patients receive training in how to inject insulin and laboratory tests are carried out. The main purpose of the inpatient stay is to teach the person to manage insulin and learn to self-care. This education, as mentioned, is provided by diabetes nurses and is continued into outpatient care. Two weeks of sick leave is standard after discharge from hospital. After the initial inpatient care episode, the outpatient care starts, including fundal photography and meeting with the dietitian.

In some cases, when the patient needs intensive care, the care process can be followed by up to 10 days in hospital. In the first year, approximately six follow-ups occur, to primarily educate the patient about the disease and to manage their own care. These follow-ups include, e.g., laboratory tests, selection of insulin and the injection technique. At least two visits to the doctor and two visits to the diabetes nurse per year are recommended, but in practice, often only one visit per year to the physicians and diabetes nurses respectively takes place. The incidence of Type 1 diabetes in the age group 18–34 years. has almost doubled during the last decades, which is a similar trend to what has been observed among children [41].

About 22 % of patients aged between 18 and 21 years have insulin pumps but the usage varies largely in different parts of the country [42]. The remaining patients use either disposable or cartridge insulin pens. All patients with Type 1 diabetes are treated with insulin analogues for both basal and bolus doses. Retinal photos occur every other year and the pictures reviewed by an ophthalmologist. Foot inspections occur at least annually and help with shoes or insoles are given if needed. If complications occur, contact is established with the appropriate team in other departments such as cardiologist, vascular surgeon, orthopaedist or ophthalmologist. Pregnancies in women with Type 1 diabetes are treated at specialised maternity care units with a team of obstetricians, midwives and a diabetologist with experience with these women.

Almost all of patients with Type 1 diabetes receive care primarily from outpatient diabetes clinics in hospitals. Most diabetes clinics are organised within a hospital's medicine or endocrine unit and the diabetes care is managed by specialists in internal medicine or endocrinology/diabetology and by specialised nurses. In a broader perspective the diabetes care is often provided by multi-professional teams to allow the opportunity to meet different patient's specific needs. A diabetes team beyond physicians and diabetes nurses may include dieticians, podiatrists, counsellors, physiotherapists, specialists in vascular surgery and infectious diseases.

Diabetes nurses play an important role in diabetes care. These nurses are employed in both diabetes clinics and in the primary health-care services. Diabetes care includes different components, but one of the more important parts is patient-education, which is managed by diabetes nurses. The goal for such education is to teach patients to manage their own care on a daily basis and to recognise risk factors in order to maintain a good quality of life. Many hospital-based diabetes clinics and primary health-care clinics offer group-based patient-education. Consequently, specialised diabetes nurses responsible for patient-education must not only have specific diabetes knowledge, but must also have competence in adult learning approaches.

Type 2 Diabetes

Similar to many other developed countries, patients with type 2 diabetes are usually treated under primary health care. Only if severe complications arise is the care shifted to specialised clinics in hospitals. This is the case for about 10 % of the patients and these patients have the most expensive care due to costly treatment of for example foot ulcers and renal insufficiency. Uncomplicated patients continue at the PHCC with regular medical check-ups, usually through one visit per year to the general practitioners (GPs) and diabetes nurse respectively. The check-ups also include patient education provided by GPs and nurses. Patient education is given both individually and as group-based meetings four to six times in groups of six to eight patients. The latter are normally led by a diabetes nurse. The providers follow national standard guidelines from the National Board of Health and Welfare, updated February 2015. These guidelines contain a total of 140 recommendations, over 50 of which are of particular significance to the finances and organisation of the health service and to ensuring that people with diabetes receive a consistently high standard of care [43]. The NDR plays a key role in the assessment of diabetes care as it provides health-care professionals individualised information for each patient to help establish targets for, e.g., HbA1c. However, despite the findings of Euro Diabetes Index 2014, new research shows inequalities in terms of resource allocation and implementation of organisational features within Swedish diabetes care in primary health care [43, 44].

Summary

The Swedish health-care system has been built with a strong orientation towards subnational levels, i.e., municipalities and regions. The responsibility is shared between the central government, county councils and municipalities. Health care is mainly tax funded both at the Government level and at the level of the county councils and municipalities. The health system is highly decentralised and organised; this leads to variation in care provision. To overcome this, the government has created national guidelines for common diagnoses including diabetes. The health-care system is trying to combine decentralisation, a high degree of specialisation, and professional organisation in a system where common health-care goals can be maintained. To avoid fragmentation, "chains of care" have been identified to bridge different care givers.

Diabetes is managed by multidisciplinary teams consisting of doctors and diabetes nurses in collaboration with other professionals at primary or secondary care level. This means that virtually all patients with type 1 diabetes have their care given at hospitals while patients with type 2 diabetes are managed in primary care.

Diabetes care in Sweden is mainly decentralised to PHCCP but with close connection to both home care and specialised diabetes units at the hospitals. To maintain comparable quality across the country, Sweden has emphasised participation in the NDR with an annual quality registration. NDR enables comparison with other units and deviations from national goals are easily detected. EMR are used by the majority of care providers and are linked to the NDR as well as to other national registers. EMR are also used for referrals within or between county councils. For the most common diagnosis or complications Sweden has created quality indicators and all units shall try to achieve these goals. The most costly care takes place at the specialised units at the hospital where patients with severe complications are treated. These patients also have needs from primary care and home services. Coordination activities are needed to optimise resource use. For this purpose, chains of care have been developed and established in order to facilitate collaboration between different levels of care.

References

1. Rättsnätet. Hälso- och sjukvårdslag (1982:763) n.d. [05/15/2016]. Available from: https://www.notisum.se/Pub/Doc.aspx?url=/rnp/sls/fakta/a9820763.htm.

2. Sveriges kommuner och Landsting. Swedish Association of Local Authorities and Regions n.d. [05/15/2016]. Available from: http://skl.se/tjanster/englishpages.411.html.
3. Svensk författningssamling. Lag om ändring i hälso- och sjukvårdslagen (1982:763). 2009.
4. Anell A, Glenngard AH, Merkur S. Sweden health system review. Health Syst Transit. 2012;14(5):1–159.
5. Hanning M, Schmidt I. Peer Review Health System Performance Assessment (Brussels, 19–20 May 2014) – Sweden: ÖSB Consulting; 2014 [05/15/2016]. Available from: http://ec.europa.eu/social/keyDocuments.jsp?advSearchKey=Peer+Review+Health+System+Performance+Assessment+&mode=advancedSubmit&langId=en&policyArea=&type=0&country=12&year=2014.
6. N.N. The Swedish Health Care System – The Organization and Delivery of Care n.d. [05/15/2016]. Available from: http://fall09hpm101sweden.providence.wikispaces.net/The+Organization+and+Delivery+of+Care.
7. Government Offices of Sweden. Ministry of Health and Social Affairs 2014 [05/15/2016]. Available from: http://www.government.se/government-of-sweden/ministry-of-health-and-social-affairs/.
8. Swedish Institute. Health care in Sweden 2015 [05/15/2016]. Available from: https://sweden.se/society/health-care-in-sweden/.
9. Robertson H. Integration of health and social care. A review of literature and models. Implications for Scotland. Prepared for the RCN in Scotland. 2011.
10. Åhgren B. Chain of care development in Sweden: results of a national study. Int J Integr Care. 2003;3:e01.
11. OECD. How does health spending in Sweden compare? 2015 [05/15/2016]. Available from: http://www.oecd.org/els/health-systems/Country-Note-Sweden-OECD-Health-Statistics-2015.pdf.
12. OECD. Health Expenditure n.d. [11/27/2015]. Available from: http://www.oecd.org/els/health-systems/health-expenditure.htm.
13. Schölkopf M, Pressel H. Das Gesundheitswesen im internationalen Vergleich: Gesundheitssystemvergleich und europäische Gesundheitspolitik. 2. aktualisierte und erweiterte Auflage ed. Berlin: MWV Medizinisch Wissenschaftliche Verlagsgesellschaft; 2014. 300 S p.
14. OECD. Health at a Glance 2013 – OECD indicators. Paris: OECD Publishing; 2013.
15. OECD. Health at a glance 2015: OECD indicators. Paris: OECD Publishing; 2015.
16. Kelley E, Hurst J. Health care quality indicators project – conceptual framework paper OECD Health Working Paper No 23 – DELSA/HEA/WD/HWP(2006)3 OECD; 2006.
17. OECD. OECD reviews of health care quality: Sweden – executive summary, assessment, and recommendations. 2013.
18. OECD. Sweden has excellent health care but must improve care co-ordination – Press release 2013 [05/15/2016]. Available from: http://www.oecd.org/newsroom/sweden-has-excellent-health-care-but-must-improve-care-co-ordination.htm.
19. Bidgood E. Health care systems: Sweden & localism – an example for the UK? : Institute for the Study of Civil Society (Civitas); 2013 [10/5/2015]. Available from: http://civitas.org.uk/2013/10/22/new-report-the-merits-of-swedish-style-localism-for-improving-uk-healthcare/.
20. OECD. Waiting times. In: OECD, editor. Health at a Glance 2011: OECD Indicators: OECD Publishing; 2011.
21. Vogel H. Health Care Guarantee 2015 [05/15/2016]. Available from: http://www.1177.se/Other-languages/Engelska/Regler-och-rattigheter/Vardgaranti/.
22. Cebolla Garrofé B, Björnberg A, Yung Phang A. Euro Diabetes Index 2014 Health Consumer Powerhouse Ltd; 2014.
23. NHS Lanarkshire. Managed Clinical Networks 2009 [05/15/2016]. Available from: http://www.nhslanarkshire.org.uk/Services/MCN/Pages/default.aspx.
24. Curry N, Ham C. Clinical and service integration – the route to improved outcomes. London: The King's Fund; 2010.
25. Ham C, Curry N. Integrated care – what is it? Does it work? What does it mean for the NHS? London: The King's Fund; 2011.
26. Burgess L. Integration of Health and Social Care: International Comparisons 2012 [05/15/2016]. Available from: http://www.scottish.parliament.uk/ResearchBriefingsAndFactsheets/Factsheets/SB_12-48.pdf.
27. Åhgren B, Axelsson R. A decade of integration and collaboration: the development of integrated health care in Sweden 2000–2010. Int J Integr Care. 2011;11 Spec Ed:e007.
28. Åhgren B, Axelsson R. Determinants of integrated health care development: chains of care in Sweden. Int J Health Plann Manag. 2007;22(2):145–57.
29. Trägårdh B, Lindberg K. Curing a meagre health care system by lean methods – translating "chains of care" in the Swedish health care sector. Int J Health Plann Manag. 2004;19(4):383–98.
30. Statistiska centralbyrån. Life expectancy by sex 1960–2014 and forecast 2015–2060 2015 [05/15/2016]. Available from: http://www.scb.se/en_/Finding-statistics/Statistics-by-subject-area/Population/Population-projections/Population-projections/Aktuell-Pong/14505/Current-forecast/The-future-population-of-Sweden-20152060/273436/.
31. Statistiska centralbyrån. Sweden's Population by sex and age on 31/12/2014 2015 [Available from: http://www.scb.se/en_/Finding-statistics/Statistics-by-subject-area/Population/Population-composition/Population-statistics/Aktuell-Pong/25795/Yearly-statistics--The-whole-country/262459/.

32. Statistiska centralbyrån. Population by age 1960 och 2014 and forecasts 2060 2015 [05/15/2016]. Available from: http://www.scb.se/en_/Finding-statistics/Statistics-by-subject-area/Population/Population-projections/Population-projections/Aktuell-Pong/14505/Current-forecast/The-future-population-of-Sweden-20152060/273430/.
33. International Diabetes Federation. Sweden 2015 [11/24/2015]. Available from: http://www.idf.org/membership/eur/sweden.
34. Jansson SP, Fall K, Brus O, Magnuson A, Wandell P, Ostgren CJ, et al. Prevalence and incidence of diabetes mellitus: a nationwide population-based pharmaco-epidemiological study in Sweden. Diabet Med. 2015;32(10):1319–28.
35. Vårdanalys. The effects of freedom of choice in healthcare 2012 [05/15/2016]. Available from: http://www.vardanalys.se/Support/In-English/Reports1/The-effects-of-freedom-of-choice-in-health-care/.
36. Vårdanalys. Who has benefited from choice in healthcare? 2013 [05/15/2016]. Available from: http://www.vardanalys.se/Support/In-English/Reports1/Who-is-benefiting-from-choice-in-healthcare/.
37. Tillman C, Beckman A. Sämre läkarkontinuitet efter vårdvalet för patienter med diabetes. Lakartidningen. 2015; 112 pii: DFDZ.
38. Andersson C, Vaziri-Sani F, Delli A, Lindblad B, Carlsson A, Forsander G, et al. Triple specificity of ZnT8 autoantibodies in relation to HLA and other islet autoantibodies in childhood and adolescent type 1 diabetes. Pediatr Diabetes. 2013;14(2):97–105.
39. Carlsson A, Kockum I, Lindblad B, Engleson L, Nilsson A, Forsander G, et al. Low risk HLA-DQ and increased body mass index in newly diagnosed type 1 diabetes children in the better diabetes diagnosis study in Sweden. Int J Obes (Lond). 2012;36(5):718–24.
40. SWEDIABKIDS – Nationellt register för barn-och ungdomsdiabetes. Årsrapport 2014 2015 [01/17/2016]. Available from: https://swediabkids.ndr.nu/Documents/NDR-Child/AnnualReport-2014.pdf.
41. Rawshani A, Landin-Olsson M, Svensson AM, Nystrom L, Arnqvist HJ, Bolinder J, et al. The incidence of diabetes among 0–34 year olds in Sweden: new data and better methods. Diabetologia. 2014;57(7):1375–81.
42. Nationalla Diabetesregistret (NDR) – Registercentrum Västra Götaland. Årsrapport – 2014 års resultat 2015 [05/15/2016]. Available from: https://www.ndr.nu/#/arsrapport.
43. Socialstyrelsen. National Guidelines for Diabetes Care – support for governance and management 2015 [05/15/2016]. Available from: http://www.socialstyrelsen.se/publikationer2015/2015-4-12.
44. Swedish Association of Local Authorities and Regions (SALAR). Success factors in Swedish Diabetes Care 2015 [05/15/2016]. Available from: http://webbutik.skl.se/bilder/artiklar/pdf/5388.pdf?issuusl=ignore.

13 Integrated Diabetes Care for Adults with Diabetes: A Patient Organisation Perspective

Heather Bird and Bridget Turner

What We Mean by Integrated Care: A Patient Perspective

Integrated care is an approach that seeks to improve the quality of care for people with diabetes by ensuring that services are well coordinated around their needs. Integrating care around the needs of the person with diabetes must be about improving outcomes and – at a wider level – reducing the incidence of complications and the proportion of people who do not feel equipped to self-manage their condition. This can only be achieved by designing a system that focuses on the patient's perspective of care, enables healthcare professionals and people with diabetes to work in partnership and supports the individual to take control and self-manage their condition.

Integrated care is about maximising the value both healthcare professionals and people with diabetes get from the time they spend in routine consultation [1]. It is about making sure that people are supported and able to self-manage their condition and about people being able to access the right care as soon as they need to. Integrated diabetes care is underpinned by vertical structural integration between primary, community and specialist care services.

H. Bird (✉) • B. Turner
Diabetes UK, London, UK
e-mail: Heather.bird@diabetes.org.uk; Bridget.turner@diabetes.org.uk

The Need to Improve Outcomes for People with Diabetes in the UK

The need to improve outcomes for people with diabetes in the UK is clear.

There are currently 3.3 million people who have a diagnosis of diabetes in the UK [2]. Each year, 20,000 people die prematurely from diabetes [3]. It is responsible for more than 100 amputations a week, is the leading cause of preventable sight loss in people of working age and a major contributor to kidney failure, heart attack and stroke [4–6].

Too many people with diabetes are still not getting all the checks that they need. Too few are being offered or are accessing diabetes education to support self-management. Large numbers of people with diabetes have not received or had access to emotional or psychological support when needed [7].

We know that people living with diabetes face daily challenges managing their condition. Such as, diet and exercise, treatment-taking, psychological stress, education, illness and disability. We also know that people are not as engaged in their care as they might be. A study by the Royal College of General Practitioners (RCGP) found a lack of engagement in consultations, including a failure to attend follow-up appointments. It has also been found that up to 50 % of the medication prescribed for managing long term conditions is not taken, or is not taken as prescribed [8].

D. Simmons et al. (eds.), *Integrated Diabetes Care*, DOI 10.1007/978-3-319-13389-8_13

The English Health System: Understanding the Context for Integrated Care

The National Health Service (NHS) in the UK is publicly funded and free at the point of use. Health is a devolved responsibility within the UK. So, the structure of the service in England, Wales, Scotland and Northern Ireland is different. The following is an explanation of the English system.

Overall political responsibility rests with the Secretary of State for Health, supported by the UK Department of Health. There have been a number of reconfigurations, following the creation of the NHS in 1948. A "purchaser provider split" (i.e. service commissioning and provision were separated into different organisational structures) was introduced in 1991 to develop an internal market within the NHS [9].

Commissioning is the planning and purchasing of NHS services. Since 1991 it has been carried out by organisations acting as purchasers of services from healthcare providers. From 2013, NHS England has been commissioning primary care services, through its Area Teams. At a local level, 211 Clinical Commissioning Groups (CCGs) have responsibility for commissioning services across a range of clinical areas (hospital services, emergency and urgent care, ambulance services and community services) [10]. The CCGs report to NHS England, again through its Area Teams.

In the UK, diabetes care is delivered by a range of providers. There can be local variation in the way services are delivered but in general, people with diabetes will be registered with a general practitioner working in primary care. Primary care includes general practitioners and practice nurses. Access to specialist care is through referrals by general practitioners who serve as "gate keepers". Specialists work in multidisciplinary teams, with links to allied health services – such as podiatry – who may be based in a hospital or community setting. There are distinct funding streams for primary care, specialist care and sometimes community care services. Each organisation is responsible for their own finances and, in addition, regulation of services is at an organisation level rather than across a pathway of care [11].

The Need for Change

The boundaries between primary and specialist services are reinforced by payment systems, the physical location of healthcare providers and the separation of responsibility for the commissioning and provision of services [12]. This is particularly problematic for delivering integrated diabetes care because diabetes is such a complex condition and people need access to a range of healthcare professionals across specialist, community and primary care.

The need to join up health services across the National Health Service (NHS) to centre on the needs of patients rather than the needs of the system is well recognised in national policy. The NHS Mandate, issued annually by the Department of Health, challenges the NHS to improve the provision of care to ensure it is coordinated around the needs, convenience and choices of patients, rather than the interests of organisations that provide care [13]. This was more explicitly called for in The NHS Five Year Forward View. Published in October 2014, this is the vision for the NHS in England and explains the need for services to change to meet the needs of patients and be sustainable over the next 5 years. In particular, this document encourages local areas to dissolve traditional boundaries between primary, community and specialist services to improve the way care is delivered and enable clinicians to focus on delivering personalised care [14].

Supporting the Patient: The Importance of Supported Self-Management

The input and skills of healthcare professionals across primary, community and specialist care are essential to provide high quality care for people with diabetes, which meets their individual needs and enables them to be engaged in their own care. Integrated care is about making sure that the time people spend with healthcare professionals is joined up and it is clear to the individual how each aspect of care contributes to supporting them to live their life with diabetes well.

Part of this is about making sure that people are seen by the appropriate healthcare professional to manage their condition at the right time. For example, in general, people with Type 1 diabetes should have their care coordinated by a multi-disciplinary specialist team – which includes a consultant diabetologist [15]. Everybody with diabetes should have straightforward, rapid access to specialist care services based on needs.

It is also about making sure that the time a person with diabetes spends in consultation with a healthcare professional supports their ability to self-manage their condition. It is estimated that 99 % of diabetes care is self-management and, as outlined above, people living with diabetes face daily challenges [16]. Although, on average, people with diabetes spend approximately only 3 h a year with healthcare professionals (versus 8757 h of self-management) this time can be used effectively to support self-management [16]. This has most clearly been shown through the Year of Care pilot, which ran in three pilot sites, concluding in 2011 [1]. The Pilot ran for 3 years and focused on the delivery of routine care to make sure that the annual review appointment was transformed into a meaningful and constructive discussion between the person with diabetes and their healthcare professional. The pilot showed support for self-management to be an effective intervention in improving engagement among people with diabetes. In Tower Hamlets, as a pilot site in the Year of Care, care planning was implemented in 31 out of 32 practices, over 90 % of patients had an annual care and support planning review and patients reported that "involvement in care" rose from 52 % to 82 % over the course of the pilot [17]. In addition, in Tower Hamlets, the proportion of people achieving an HbA1c of less than 7.5 % steadily improved from 36 % to 55 % over the same time period. The pilot recognised that although the UK is comparatively successful in ensuring people with diabetes have an annual surveillance review, less than half of people with diabetes felt that this time was being maximised to facilitate discussion between them and clinicians that would support them to self-manage. The study therefore looked at how to use this time more effectively to make sure discussions focused on the needs of the person with diabetes and supported them in their day to day management of their diabetes [1].

Changing Attitudes to Focus on the Person with Diabetes

A key focus of the Year of Care was demonstrating the need for a fundamental change in the way healthcare professionals and people with diabetes interact with each other and the system to manage the individual's diabetes. The pilot showed that healthcare professionals must abandon the traditional approach to care delivery, where they are the primary decision maker, in favour of a partnership model, working with the person with diabetes [18]. At the same time, people with diabetes need to take an active role in determining their care and support needs. This is not straightforward, due to the diversity of need and the degree of engagement people with diabetes have said they want in their care, but it is essential in every case to improve individual outcomes [17]. The partnership approach should focus on identifying the individual's priorities and goals. It is about making healthcare relevant to the life and circumstances of the person with diabetes and identifying additional aspects of support, such as peer support, that can help to deliver the outcomes they want to achieve.

The 3 year pilot was split into two phases: feasibility and implementation. The Year of Care offered a practical approach that engaged staff at a practice level, and involved patients through participation events in pilot sites. Local engagement and ownership is key to implementing change but a challenge for the Year of Care was to ensure healthcare professionals embraced the philosophy of partnership working and did not just implement the practical steps involved in the new way of working, e.g. sending out test results prior to consultations, as an add-on to the existing approach. Ongoing training that reacted to this challenge was a central part of the Pilot [1].

Practices were incentivised to participate in the project and each site committed resources but no further extra funding was available. The Year of Care found the care planning approach to be cost neutral once it was up and running. This cost did not include the large amount of additional work that practices had to do to change the way they worked, and for introducing changes to the IT systems to properly support care planning [1].

At its conclusion, people with diabetes reported an improved experience of care and real changes in their self-management. Healthcare professionals also reported improved knowledge and skills, and greater job satisfaction [18].

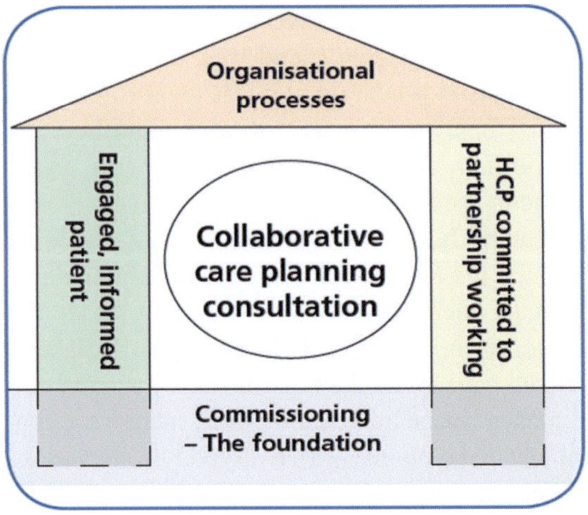

Fig. 13.1 The house of care framework (Used with permission from Year of Care: Report of findings from the pilot programme. June 2011. Year of Care Partnership. Diabetes UK/NHS Diabetes; 2011)

The Importance of the House of Care

The house of care is a metaphor introduced through the Year of Care to illustrate the fact that all parts of the system, people with diabetes and healthcare professionals must be aligned in support of the partnership approach to care [19]. See Fig. 13.1.

In the Year of Care pilot, the house of care initially explained the engagement needed for this but it has subsequently been applied much more widely as a framework, explaining how a whole system might adapt to deliver collaborative care planning to support integrated care [20]. Delivering the philosophy of the house of care requires localities to define and agree their model of care and approach to delivery, with complete commitment from all involved.

Commissioning all the aspects of the diabetes care pathway is the foundation in the house of care metaphor and provides the basis on which an integrated system can be implemented.

The Diabetes Care Pathway

The provision of integrated care for people with diabetes must be underpinned by access to all aspects of the diabetes care pathway [21].

Commissioners should work together to make sure that all aspects of the diabetes pathway are being delivered by the appropriate provider, with well-defined referral pathways between services. Within an integrated diabetes pathway local services should have clear protocols for who does what and what services are provided where. Within the full pathway of diabetes care, as outlined below, care pathways and referral pathways for particular aspects of care, such as diabetes foot care, should be defined to enable delivery of the right care, in the right place and at the right time. Figure 13.2 illustrates the care pathway for diabetes.

Although the various services that make up the pathway are constant, how the pathway is delivered in each locality can vary and should be defined in a local model of care. All areas in the UK should have a well-defined model of diabetes care. Broadly, a model of care describes the way health services are configured [22]. It can be applied to health services delivered in a provider or organisation, within a team or across a whole local system of care. For diabetes, it will need to set out the care to be commissioned and delivered by provider organisations – defining who does what, where and how. In any configuration, effective delivery must be underpinned by partnership

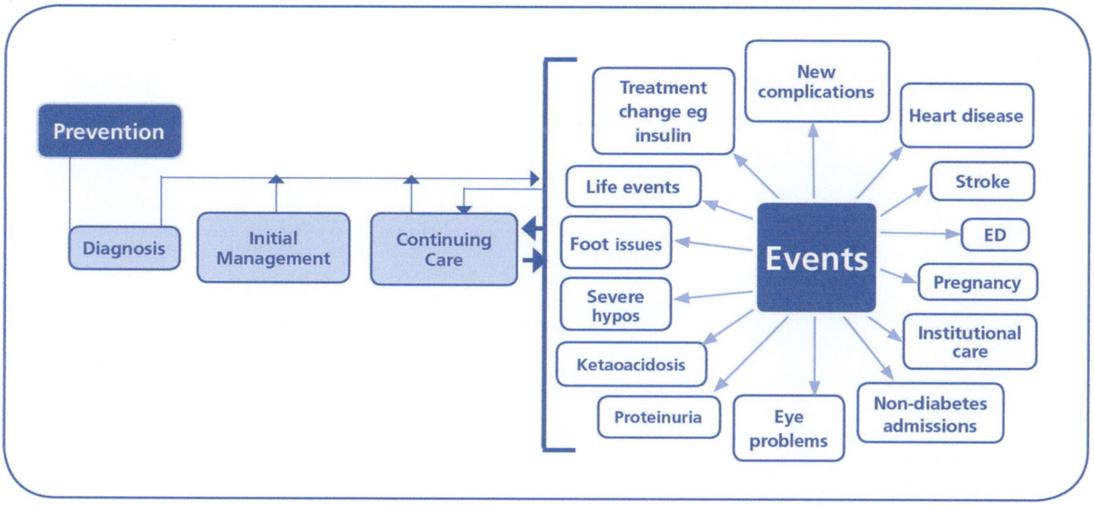

Fig. 13.2 The diabetes care pathway (Used with permission from Year of Care: Report of findings from the pilot programme. June 2011. Year of Care Partnership. Diabetes UK/NHS Diabetes; 2011)

working between generalists and specialists to support and deliver care whether it is provided in a general practice, in a community setting or in the hospital.

The National Clinical Director for obesity and diabetes in England has produced a Diabetes Sample Service Specification Fig. 13.3 [23]. This outlines the provision of high quality care for all those with diabetes and, as appropriate, differentiates the care needs of adults with Type 1 diabetes (T1DM) and those with Type 2 diabetes (T2DM). It describes all the services needed to provide a complete care pathway for people with diabetes, including those with the long-term complications of diabetes. It also meets the National Institute for Health and Care Excellence's (NICE) Quality Standard for diabetes (QS6), which defines clinical best practice in the delivery of diabetes care [24].

As well as making sure that all the components of the pathway are in place commissioners must make sure the appropriate support for delivery is commissioned. This includes ongoing training and education to assure staff competency in diabetes as well as training for healthcare professionals to enable them to work in partnership with people with diabetes through care planning. It is also about making sure that the methods and processes are in place to facilitate integrated care [25].

Supporting Integrated Care Through the Integration of Systems and Processes

The diabetes community in the UK have identified five integration enablers that must be in place to support the delivery of integrated diabetes care [26]. Within the house of care framework four of the enablers are organisational processes and local infrastructure which need to be in place to support the development of integrated care focused on the individual with diabetes, through care planning (at the centre of the house). This left and right walls of the house need to be in place to deliver care planning whereby engaged and informed individuals and carers and healthcare professionals are committed to partnership working [19].

The five distinct but mutually reinforcing integration enablers are:

1. Integrated IT
2. Aligned finances and responsibility
3. Care planning
4. Clinical engagement and leadership
5. Robust clinical governance [26]

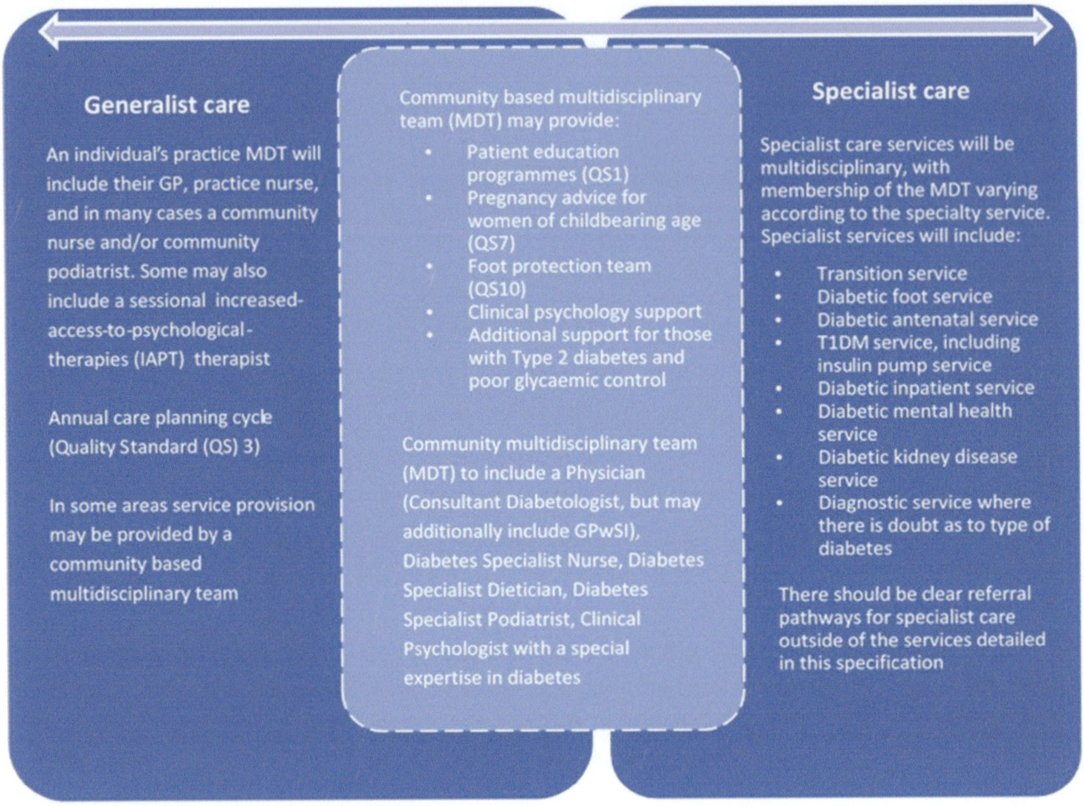

Fig. 13.3 The diabetes sample service specification (Used with permission from Valabhji J). [23]

Integration Enablers to Facilitate Integrated Care

Wherever possible, localities should make sure all the enablers are in place. Although they can be introduced independently and drive some improvement, it is evident that they are mutually reinforcing so the ability of an area to provide integrated care is further enhanced when the enablers are developed at the same time to support the delivery of integrated care.

Where these enablers are in place to support the delivery of integrated diabetes care, early evidence suggests patient experience is improved and the cost efficiency of the service increased. Derby introduced a new model of delivering diabetes care in 2009 – commissioned by the Primary Care Trust (the body responsible for commissioning at the time). This was driven by the enthusiasm for change of GPs and consultant diabetologists locally. The redesign saw care delivery supported by a single IT system and a single budget. Evaluation of this model found that in the first 6 months, there was a reduction of mean length of inpatient stay from 11 to 6.5 days in patients with a primary diagnosis of diabetes from participating GP practices compared with the same time period 12 months previously.

Formal feedback was obtained from patients annually using a questionnaire which explored their experiences in the service using a 5 point score with 5 being excellent and 1 poor. The questionnaire was administered to 50 users in 2012. The process was repeated in 2013, but this time the survey was administered by users instead of administrators. The results were similar. Overall:

- 85 % rating the service as excellent or very good
- 70 % felt that the service was excellent or very good compared with their previous care
- 80 % felt the waiting time between referral and first appointment was excellent or very good.
- 90 % felt that the service was able to help them with the problem they were referred with
- 95 % stated they would recommend the service to another person with diabetes.

Understanding the Five Enablers

Integrated IT Systems

Why Integrated IT Is Important

In 2013, National Voices (a coalition of health and social care charities) was commissioned by NHS England to produce "a narrative for person-centred coordinated care" [27]. This document is focused on understanding what integrated care looks like from a patient perspective, and uses a series of "I" statements to do this. In this, patients stress the importance of being able to tell their story once, without needing to repeat themselves across the system [27]. A culture change to remove boundaries between organisations and encourage meetings and dialogue between clinicians goes some way to facilitate this. Optimal information sharing, however, should be underpinned by an information system that provides clinicians across primary, community and specialist care with a patient's clinical record regardless of setting.

Integrated IT: In Practice

The ideal is for all providers in a pathway to use the same system. For example, in the Derby model all GP practices and the hospital in Derby use SystmOne (TPP). There can be initial frustrations with this, as clinicians must get consent from patients to share their data and the necessary data sharing and governance structures need to be introduced. However, once the system is fully established clinicians can see a patient's records, regardless of whether their previous appointment was in primary or specialist care, to optimise care and make the referral process more efficient [28].

An information system, where GPs and specialists can see the same record, can be used to automatically identify and target "at risk" patients [29]. This is the approach being used in Wolverhampton. Wolverhampton has developed a system focused on delivering integrated diabetes care for many years, which supports the development of primary care led diabetes services. Specialist care is delivered in partnership with primary care to meet the clinical needs of the patient. The model of care is based on self-care through education, patient centeredness and empowerment. As part of their model of care, the Clinical Commissioning Group (CCG) (explained earlier in this chapter) as the relevant commissioning body has introduced a central portal (Graphnet's Care Centric Portal). This is used to extract data from 49 GP practices. These data are fed into the trust's Diabeta3 system and a locally developed algorithm stratifies patients according to risk [30]. Patients are rated against the NICE recommended nine diabetes care processes (Table 13.1) and based on their risk status for micro and macro vascular complications of diabetes they are flagged as red, amber or green. The results are then used to decide where care should be provided to that patient along the pathway and what should be done to improve care for that particular person [30]. Using data in this way allows the clinicians to operate outside of the constraints of the system, enabling them to identify patients most at need and enable treatment at an early point and in the right setting, removing delays

Table 13.1 Nine care processes

1. Blood glucose level measurement
2. Blood pressure measurement
3. Cholesterol level measurement
4. Retinal screening
5. Foot and leg check
6. Kidney function testing (urine)
7. Kidney function testing (blood)
8. Weight check
9. Smoking status check

in referral and looking to reduce emergency admissions.

Aligned Finances and Responsibility

Defining Who Does What

Clearly defining responsibility for all aspects of service delivery is essential for delivering the full diabetes care pathway. The pathway should be clearly defined in the model of care, and the infrastructure supporting the delivery of care should ensure that all clinicians are able to deliver against national standards. As illustrated by the Diabetes Sample Service Specification, the specific care needs of people with Type 1 diabetes should be drawn out in the configuration of services [23]. As stated above, in general, support for people with Type 1 should be coordinated by a multi-disciplinary diabetes specialist team. The team can be based either in hospital or in a community setting. This is because managing Type 1 diabetes is complex and requires significant expertise, and there can be serious consequences if things go wrong [15]. At the same time people with complex Type 2 diabetes will also need timely access to specialist care. The ongoing care of people with Type 2 diabetes is generally provided by GPs with clear systems in place for call and recall, regular review and referral when necessary.

A common feature that has preceded change in areas that have looked at improving the delivery of diabetes care across the whole pathway is an unacceptable variation in the quality of care (particularly across primary and community care) and a lack of consistency in the delivery of services.

In Portsmouth, for example, the diabetes clinical lead at Portsmouth Hospital, a GP with special interest in diabetes and the commissioning managers developed a proposal for change. The initiatives focused on clarifying the role of the consultant diabetologist in the delivery of diabetes care. The model of care defines who does what within the system and is widely known as the "super six". The "super six" are the areas of diabetes care that it was agreed must be managed by consultant specialists [31]. This saw the consultants focus on super-specialist areas of diabetes care in the hospital and refer all other care, which is was felt did not need to be managed exclusively by specialists, to community and primary care. This model is based on an increased role for primary care in the management of diabetes, and required the engagement of GP practices within the local area. For this approach to work it is essential that all healthcare professionals have the skills, clinical support and infrastructure necessary to be able to provide high quality diabetes care. Under the new alignment, the diabetologists in Portsmouth were given two functions: to continue in their role as deliverers of specialist care; and a new function as healthcare professional educators [32]. All the GP practices involved in the "super six" initiative have virtual access to consultant support (telephone and email) and each practice is visited by a diabetes specialist nurse and consultant biannually to deliver training and support as needed. This is accompanied by a programme of accredited training [33]. There are indications that clinical outcomes have improved since 2011 when the new service model was introduced. For example, the hospital's diabetic hypoglycaemia admissions fell from 224 to 198 between 2011/2012 and 2013/2014 [34].

In North West London, a pilot was started in 2011 aimed at improving the delivery of diabetes care and care for older people in North West London. This pilot focused on better coordinating good practice to enable clinicians to work efficiently across provider boundaries. Investment was made in IT and the model of care introduced a stratification process which segments people with Type 2 diabetes according to need and refers them to the appropriate part of the system. The multidisciplinary group structure provides GPs with direct access to specialist knowledge – links which had previously not been made – to discuss complex cases and develop their skills [35]. Over three quarters of professionals surveyed, as part of the evaluation of the pilot, reported that this new structure "enhanced inter-professional working and levels of professional knowledge" [36]. No outcomes data have been released.

The Role of Payment Systems in Supporting the Delivery of Care

The implementation and use of payment systems must support the delivery of services as explained in the local model of care. In a traditional model of diabetes care the rigid divide between primary and specialist care is exacerbated by the provision of funding. For example the tariff system used in England, to pay for activity in specialist care, can create incentives for one part of the system to "hold on" to patients who might be better treated elsewhere. This system was originally introduced to incentivise providers to increase elective activity and reduce waiting times. Whilst it has been effective for improving access to planned care, it is not so well suited to achieving the continuity of care needed to facilitate integrated care [37].

Going forward, a key commitment in The NHS Five Year Forward View is a central focus on introducing "national flexibilities in the current regulatory, funding and pricing regimes to assist local areas to transition to better models of care" [13]. Within the current constraints of payment systems, however, there is an acceptance that the providers involved need to focus on the needs of the whole health economy rather than their own organisation.

Using Payment Systems to Support Integrated Care: In Practice

- Derby introduced a new NHS organisation, which held a pooled budget to deliver diabetes care based on historical prices across the care pathway [28].
- North West London had a set budget to support the delivery of their pilot project. This budget was used to compensate providers for the time spent working on additional features of the pilot. For example, GPs were paid for the time spent attending multi-disciplinary group meetings and putting together care plans [38].
- Portsmouth, Derby and Wolverhampton have introduced a locally enhanced service payment which is paid to GP practices to incentivise attendance at diabetes training courses and interaction with the diabetes specialist team to attain endorsement as a GP practice with an interest, and high level of competency, in the delivery of diabetes care [28].

Care Planning

Through the Year of Care pilot, care planning has been shown to be an effective way of engaging people with diabetes and healthcare professionals in a way of working which effectively supports the individual's ability to self-manage [1].

Care planning is a continuous process in which clinicians and patients work together to agree goals, identify support needs, develop and implement action plans and monitor progress [18]. People with diabetes should have active involvement in the care planning process of deciding, agreeing and owning how their diabetes will be managed [1].

For care planning to be truly collaborative, the person with diabetes must be engaged in the process and allowed time to think about his/her own priorities. In Wolverhampton the care planning process is initiated through a questionnaire sent to patients prior to their annual review appointment, which includes a list of questions for them to consider and identify their priorities. This is discussed at their consultation and an action plan based on this is designed in collaboration with the clinician to inform their ongoing care [39].

Clinical Engagement and Leadership

Engaging the Right People in Designing a Model of Care

To maximise the chances of the model of diabetes care meeting the needs of people with diabetes and healthcare professionals all relevant stakeholders (Table 13.2) should be engaged collaboratively in discussion at an early point. The North West London integrated care pilot clearly illustrated the central importance of this [40]. The initial meeting to develop the ICP was attended by the Chief Executive of Imperial Hospitals NHS Trust, diabetologists, diabetes leads, commissioners, representatives of Central

London Community Healthcare Trust, GP leads, psychiatrists, Diabetes UK and Age UK. Chief executives and senior managers gave the pilot their backing from an early point, giving clinicians the financial and managerial support necessary to enable them to better focus the model of diabetes care on the needs of people with diabetes. The trust chief executives were particularly supportive of the diabetologists spending time away from the hospital to work more closely with colleagues across the pathway [41].

Getting Clinicians Support

One of the most significant challenges for North West London was getting clinicians from all providers involved and supportive of the pilot. Initially, clinicians were concerned about the challenges the pilot posed to their position and current way of working. These concerns were gradually overcome as an external chair was appointed to lead the pilot and bring people together on equal terms. The number of clinicians attending the meetings to develop the pilot steadily grew as people got to know one another and unite behind the aim of improving the service for people with diabetes (41).

Engaging People with Diabetes

In the initial developmental discussions about the pilot, people with diabetes were represented by Diabetes UK. As the pilot developed it was agreed that people with diabetes must have a direct role throughout the structure of the pilot to help determine priorities such as education and training needs. People with diabetes were therefore included on all the groups and an additional patient and users committee was established to discuss the progress of the pilot as a whole [41].

Table 13.2 Initiating change: who to involve

Local diabetes network, to include:
People with diabetes and groups representing them
Healthcare professionals from the full range of relevant specialties
From primary, specialist and community care
CCG clinical lead
Area Team representative
Additionally:
Senior managers (inc. hospital chief execs)
Trust finance managers
Trust IT leads
Medicines management
Existing network (e.g. SCN) representatives

Clinical Governance

What Is Clinical Governance and Why It Is Important

Clinical governance is a system through which NHS organisations are accountable for continuously improving the quality of their services and safeguarding high standards of care by creating an environment in which excellence in clinical care will flourish [42].

Implementing a clear and effective clinical governance structure helps to align the ambitions of clinicians with those of commissioners and most importantly with people with diabetes. An integrated system which removes barriers between care providers and overcomes perverse financial incentives allows services and the people involved to align and take shared responsibility for a single goal [42].

Implementing Clinical Governance

In Derby and North West London establishing a structure of clinical governance for their respective initiatives was core in their drive to improve. They took different approaches to this, reflecting the scale and complexity of the project.

In the Derby model a clinical board structure has been established to oversee the model of care. The board has responsibility for ensuring the quality of the service delivered to patients. As a new NHS organisation was set up as a company limited by shares in Derby, the two shareholders (the group of GP practices and the Derby Hospital NHS Trust) were directors of the board. The directors had responsibility for holding the board to account for delivery of the commissioned service specification and the financial state of the company. In addition to the directors, the clinical board is made up of consultant diabetologists, GPs, practice nurses, diabetes specialist nurses, dietitians, service managers, consultant ophthalmologist and people with diabetes. An additional patient board meet every 2 months to discuss how to improve the service [28].

Conclusion

Integrated care must be about improving the way diabetes care is delivered to better meet the needs of people with diabetes.

Healthcare systems are complex and improvement requires leadership to orchestrate all the "… items, people and processes to work together toward a common purpose" [43]. Achieving integrated care needs the full commitment of commissioners and providers to work together, in partnership with people with diabetes to realign the system.

In many areas of the UK progress is being made, through different approaches to delivery, design and support. It is challenging but change needs to be driven locally to make sure people with diabetes have access to a whole system pathway of care, which provides excellent ongoing management and rapid access to specialist services when required. This must be underpinned by the structural integration enablers of shared information systems; aligned finances and responsibility, clinical engagement and leadership and robust clinical governance. Clinicians and people with diabetes need to be engaged as equal partners in the management of diabetes through the ongoing care planning process.

References

1. Year of care partnership. Year of care: report of findings from the pilot programme. Diabetes UK/NHS Diabetes; 2011. Available from: http://www.yearofcare.co.uk/key-documents.
2. Health and Social Care Information Centre. Quality and Outcomes Framework (QOF) 2013–14. London: HSCIC; 2014.
3. Health and Social Care Information Centre. National Diabetes Audit 2012–13. Report 2: complications and mortality. London: HSCIC; 2015.
4. Health and Social Care Information Centre. National Diabetes Audit 2011/12: the Information Centre for Health and Social Care Hospital Episode Statistics 2007/8–2011/12. London: HSCIC; 2013.
5. Liew G, Michaelides M, Bunce C. A comparison of the causes of blindness certifications in England and Wales in working age adults (16–64 years). 1999–2000 with 2009–2010. BMJ Open. 2014;4:e004015.
6. Morrish NJ, Wang SL, Stevens LK, Fuller JH, Keen H. Mortality and causes of death in the WHO multinational study of vascular disease in diabetes. Diabetologia. 2001;44 Suppl 2:S14–21.
7. Health and Social Care Information Centre. National Diabetes Audit 2012–13. Report 1: care processes and treatment targets. London: HSCIC; 2014.
8. Mathers N, Roberts S, Hodkinson I, Karet B. Care planning: improving the lives of people with long term conditions. London: Clinical Innovation and Research Centre; 2011.
9. UK Parliament. Health Committee. Commissioning 1948–2010 [internet]. 2010. Available from: http://www.publications.parliament.uk/pa/cm200910/cmselect/cmhealth/268/26805.htm.
10. Holder H, Thorlby R. The new structure of the NHS in England [internet]. 2013. Available from: http://www.nuffieldtrust.org.uk/talks/slideshows/new-structure-nhs-england.
11. NHS England. Understanding the new NHS. London: BMJ; 2014.
12. Ham C, Dixon J, Chantler C. Clinically integrated systems: the future of NHS reform in England. BMJ. 2011;342:d905.
13. Department of Health. The NHS mandate. London: Department of Health; 2014.
14. NHS England. The NHS five year forward view. London: NHS England; 2014.
15. Diabetes UK, Association of British Clinical Diabetologists. Care coordination for adults with Type diabetes. London: Diabetes UK; 2015. Available from: https://www.diabetes.org.uk/About_us/What-we-say/Specialist-care-for-children-and-adults-and-complications/Adults-with-type-1-diabetes/.
16. Roberts S. Working together for better diabetes care. UK: Department of Health (UK); 2007.
17. Eaton S, Roberts S, Turner B. Delivering person centred care in long term conditions. BMJ. 2015;350:h181.
18. Coulter A, Roberts S, Dixon A. Delivering better services for people with long term conditions. Building the house of care. London: The King's Fund; 2013.
19. Coalition for collaborative care [internet]. Available from: http://coalitionforcollaborativecare.org.uk/aboutus/house-of-care/.
20. NHS Improving Quality [internet]. Building the house of care – the house of care toolkit. Available from: http://www.nhsiq.nhs.uk/improvement-programmes/long-term-conditions-and-integrated--care/long-term-conditions-improvement-programme/house-of-care-toolkit.aspx.
21. Department of Health. National service framework for diabetes. London: Department of Health; 2001.

22. Queensland Government. Queensland health. Changing models of care framework. 2000.
23. Valabhji J. Diabetes sample service specification [internet]. NHS England. 2014. Available from: www.diabetes.org.uk/integrated-diabetes-care.
24. National Institute for Care and Health Excellence. Diabetes in adults quality standard. 2011. Available at: http://publications.nice.org.uk/diabetes-in-adults-quality-standard-qs6/quality-statement-6-insulin-therapy.
25. Shaw S, Rosen R, Rumbold B. What is integrated care? London: Nuffield Trust; 2011.
26. NHS Diabetes. Best practice for commissioning diabetes services: an integrated care framework. London: NHS Diabetes; 2013.
27. Department of Health. Integrated care and support: our shared commitment. London: Department of Health; 2013.
28. Diabetes UK. Improving the delivery of diabetes care through integration. London: Diabetes UK; 2014.
29. Ham C, Imison C, Goodwin N, Dixon A, South P. Where next for the NHS reforms? Making the case for integrated care. London: The King's Fund; 2011.
30. Todd R. Wolverhampton shares info on diabetics. Digitalhealth.net. 24 February 2014 Sect. News. Available from: http://www.digitalhealth.net/news/EHI/9246/wolverhampton-shares-info-on-diabetics.
31. Kar P. The "super six" for the acute trust; all else for primary care? Pract Diabetes. 2011;28(7):308–9.
32. Kar P. The Super Six model of diabetes care: two years on. Diabetes Prim Care. 2013;15:211–5.
33. Cummings M. Professional education programme [internet]. Available from: http://www.porthosp.nhs.uk/departments/Diabetes-and-Endocrinology/professional-education-programme.htm.
34. Robertson R, Sonola L, Honeyman M, Brooke B, Kothari S. Portsmouth and South East Hampshire diabetes service. London: King's Fund; 2014.
35. Greaves F, Pappas Y, Bardsley M, Harris M, Curry N, Holder H, Blunt I, Soljak M, Gunn L, Majeed A, Car J. Evaluation of complex integrated care programmes: the approach in North West London. Int J Integr Care. 2013;13:e006.
36. Bardsley M, Smith J, Car J. Evaluation of the first year of the Inner North West London Integrated Care Pilot. 2013. Nuffield Trust. Int J Integr Care. 2013;13:1–11.
37. Ham C, Smith J, Eastmure E. Commissioning integrated care in a liberated NHS. London: Nuffield Trust; 2011.
38. NHS NW London. Integrated care in North West London. 2012 Feb. Available from: http://www.nuffieldtrust.org.uk/sites/files/nuffield/daniel_elkeles_integrated_care_in_nw_london_290212.pdf.
39. Wolverhampton Diabetes Centre [internet]. My diabetes plan. Available from: http://www.wdconline.org.uk/downloads/education/MyDiabetesMyPlan.pdf.
40. Steeden A. The integrated care pilot in North West London. Lond J Prim Care. 2012;5:8–11.
41. Vize R. Integrated care: a story of hard won success. BMJ. 2012;344:e3529.
42. Scally G. Clinical governance and the drive for quality improvement in the new NHS in England. BMJ. 1998;317:61.
43. Langley G, Moen R, Nolan K, Nolan T, Norman C, Provost L. The improvement guide: a practical approach to enhancing organizational performance. New York: Wiley; 2009.

14 Training for Diabetes Integrated Care: A Diabetes Specialist Physician Perspective from the English NHS

Anne Dornhorst

The provision of healthcare is challenging for everyone, the politicians, the providers, the workforce as well as the patients on the receiving end. The provision of education for the healthcare workforce is equally challenging for the politicians, the universities, the training and regulatory bodies and the trainees on the receiving end. Clearly the medical workforce of tomorrow should be trained to meet the challenges of delivering a sustainable high quality healthcare system of the future. Currently in the UK there is a miss-match between what the healthcare policies require and what the workforce is actually being trained for. The specialist training for the long-term conditions, for which diabetes is one, is a good example of this miss-match. The last 5 years in the UK and England, in particular, has seen seismic changes in the healthcare landscape including how the education of its workforce is funded. Health Education England (HEE) has, since 2015, been an autonomous national body responsible for the education and training of the NHS healthcare workforce, and is overall responsible for commissioning under and postgraduate medical education. Supporting education and training for integrated care is a priority for HEE. HEE delegates the training and education programmes, both clinical and non-clinical, to 13 Local Education and Training Boards (LETBs) within 13 separate areas in England [1].

In the United Kingdom the Secretary of State for Health, a cabinet minister in the UK elected government has financial control and oversight of NHS delivery and performance; however, since 1998, this has been largely restricted to England. Today the majority of non-English related NHS policy is devolved from the UK parliament to its member parliaments, or assemblies, in Scotland, Wales and Northern Ireland, leaving the Department of Health (DH) responsible for health and adult social care policy mostly in England. The principals of the NHS that pledges a comprehensive health service, available to all with access based on clinical need, not an individual's ability to pay, remains a fundamental tenet across all four UK health systems [2].

In late 2014 NHS England published their 5-year forward plan for the NHS [3]. Central to this plan was commissioning new models of integrated care that would promote different providers including GPs, hospital consultants and social care to work more closely together to allow more non-elective healthcare to move out of secondary care back into the community and reduce unnecessary hospital admissions. A drive shared across all political parties. However, current medical training is not aligned to this. For example, the current Certificate in Endocrinology and Diabetes, awarded on a multiple choice

A. Dornhorst (✉)
Department of Diabetes and Endocrinology, Imperial College Healthcare NHS Trust, Hammersmith Hospital, London, UK
e-mail: a.dornhorst@imperial.ac.uk

D. Simmons et al. (eds.), *Integrated Diabetes Care*, DOI 10.1007/978-3-319-13389-8_14

examination of best of 5 of 200 questions and a prerequisite for completion of higher specialist training in diabetes, includes only 10 questions relevant to integrated care [4]. While the training curriculum does cover delivery of diabetes care (Table 14.1), this knowledge can all be acquired solely through reading not actual exposure to integrated care, and currently represents a very small fraction of the total curriculum [5].

Overall undergraduate and speciality postgraduate medical training today has little exposure to the different community healthcare teams working across a local population. This lack of community exposure and hospital centric focus has resulted, not surprisingly, in a negative perception among trainees and consultants on community work, with hospital based consultant posts being considered more prestigious to community based posts. Going forward, undergraduate and postgraduate medical training will need to change as will the perception around community work if integrated care as envisaged by the 5-year forward plan, is to flourish. The concept that postgraduate medical training and workforce planning need to be intimately interwoven with health service policy and delivery is not new and was emphasised by Sir Professor John Took in 2008 in his report on Modernising Medical Careers [6].

In the UK from the selection of medical students through to higher speciality training and the revalidation process of doctors to practise, there is no one unifying professional body responsible. There are eight main bodies involved in the regulation, commissioning and delivery of medical education and training, each representing multiple members (Table 14.2). All represent the interests of their respective membership and some with conflicting interests around supporting integrated care.

The General Medical Council (GMC) is an independent regulatory organisation responsible for setting standards for the delivery of undergraduate and postgraduate training including the final Certificates of Completion of Training (CCT), the universal requirement for all GPs and consultants, in any specialty, be it diabetes, respiratory or other specialty, to obtain to work within the UK [7].

To date the GMC has not been involved in the content of either the undergraduate or postgraduate training programmes. The content of the undergraduate curriculum is the responsibility of the 34 different UK undergraduate medical schools, all members of the Medical Schools Council. Although all medical schools do offer some community-based teaching in their curricula, the time spent and emphasis on cross-organisation and cross-discipline training, community placements and population health varies among the medical schools [8]. As a generalisation, undergraduate teaching is given predominantly by university lecturers and hospital consultants, with little experience in chronic disease management in the community. A significant percentage of undergraduate clinical placements are timetabled in the hospital environment. There also remains a real financial dis-

Table 14.1 Aspects of endocrinology and diabetes curriculum of Joint Royal Colleges of Physicians diabetes and endocrinology Training Board (JRCPTB) relating to the management of delivery of diabetes care

1. The factors which influence commissioning diabetes care within the NHS
2. Which aspects of diabetes care can be appropriately delivered in different clinical settings
3. The role of information technology in integrating care across different providers
4. The role of diabetes networks and advisory groups in the organisation of care

Table 14.2 Organisations responsible for the regulation, commissioning and delivery of medical education and post graduate training in the UK

1. The General Medical Council (GMC)
2. The Medical Schools Council (MSC)
3. Education England (HEE)
4. NHS Education Scotland (NES) l the Northern Ireland Medical and Dental Training
5. Northern Ireland Medical and Dental Training Agency (NIMDTA)
6. The Conference of Postgraduate Medical Deans of the UK (COPMeD)
7. Wales Deanery
8. The Academy of Medical Royal Colleges (AoMRC)

incentive for universities and their university hospitals to actively encourage clinical placements in the community as this would result in lost income. University hospitals are Local Education Providers (LEPs) and receive tariffs for education and training for each undergraduate placement from the Local Education and Training Boards (LETBs), which in turn receive their money through HEE. These tariffs would be lost if more clinical placements took place in the community. Currently a tariff for an annual clinical placement is in excess of £33,000 [9].

For the profile of undergraduate teaching on chronic disease management in the community to increase requires not only more out of hospital based clinical placements, but for the assessment of population health to be part of the final qualifying exams. The Medical Schools Council Assessment Alliance (MSCAA) a partnership of its members has already agreed to include a proportion of finals examination questions from a shared question bank. Potentially the MSCAA could play a role in supporting integrated care by mandating its inclusion into all curricula and final assessment exams [10].

There is a significant focus from HEE and the individual LETBs to support medical workforce planning and educational commissioning that fosters doctors to meet the changing needs of and ageing population with complex health needs and high expectations. There is a real appreciation by the LETBs that there will need to be fundamental changes in postgraduate training to equip medical physicians for integrated care and recognition that current training is not doing this.

The first 2 years of postgraduate medical education and training after qualifying, are undertaken in a foundation programme that provide a generic training to bridge the transition from medical school into specialist and general practice training. Both the GMC and the LETBs assess these educational programmes for the standards of training they provide. Placement opportunities are in broad specialty areas with opportunities to work in both primary and secondary care settings. Integrated care was widely referred to in the Health Education England *Broadening the Foundation Programme* report of 2014 [11]. This report recommended a greater amount of training during these first 2 years to be undertaken in community-based settings, anticipating the need for the next generation of foundation doctors to be better equipped to provide integrated care. A major recommendation from this report was that at least 80 % of foundation doctors should undertake a community placement or an integrated placement starting in August 2015. A view echoed in the 2014 Shape of Training report [12].

The responsibility of postgraduate speciality training after the foundation years is dissolved to the different medical royal colleges, faculties and specialty associations to deliver the curricula and to assess trainees' competencies. For example, diabetes speciality training is the responsibility of the Joint Royal Colleges of Physicians Endocrine and Diabetes Training Board (JRCPTB) [13].

The GMC involvement and influence on curriculum content as well as training standards may increase following two major reports in the last 3 years. Firstly, the publication on the *Shape of Training Review* by Professor Greenaway's in 2013 [12], an independent review commissioned by the four UK governments sponsored in part by the GMC, reported what changes were required in medical postgraduate training to meet the future healthcare needs across the UK. The report came up with 19 recommendations. Although these continue to be hotly debated, changes to medical training are likely to follow. This will equip tomorrow's medical specialist to be better suited to work in integrated care settings. This will include closer training with GPs and other healthcare professionals to deliver out of hospital speciality care at a population level in the community. Another one of the 19 recommendations of this report was for more subspecialty training to be undertaken following qualification as a doctor. The GMC is in favour of credentialing; however, who exactly would pay for and accredit this extension to training remains unclear. Potentially training in integrated care for the long-term conditions both for general practitioners and hospital specialists could become a recognised post CCT credential [12].

The second factor that might lead to the GMC having a greater influence on the core medical curriculum is it support for a national licensing examination to be taken by all graduates and doctors wishing to work in the UK, with 2021 being the provisional date for its implementation. Such an exam could support integrated care by including greater focus on the nature of multidisciplinary team-work, the impact of differing UK health systems and the interface between acute and primary healthcare and social care [14].

Currently, following foundation training, those trainees wishing to pursue a career in one of the 27 medical specialties enter a 2 year core medical programme in which they rotate through generic medical disciplines before a competitive selection process during year 3 of their post graduate training (ST3) into one of the specialist training programmes. These specialty training programmes are usually an additional 4–5 years of training. Those wishing to pursue a career as a general practitioner, enter 3 years of GP Specialty Training (GPST) that normally includes 18 months in an approved training practice with a further 18 months in approved hospital posts.

The Royal College of General Practitioners (RCGP) has been a long-term champion of integrated care [15]. The Shape of Training report concentrates on medical as opposed to general practice training. It proposes expanding the number of trainees working purely in general medicine to 3 rather than 2 years before entering specialist training, and to continue with a commitment to general medicine throughout their specialty training. Current funding for these training years is paid half by the LETBs with the other half from the hospital trusts for clinical service. While there is a general acceptance that there needs to be a balance between training and clinical service along with greater integrated work, there is reluctance among the different speciality Royal College training boards and speciality medical societies to shorten or dilute speciality training.

For LETBs to commission a specialist training post that supports integrated care, training placements will need be outside of the acute setting and be able to provide suitable training experiences. Placements that span the acute sector, community and private/voluntary sector organisations will require training programme directors and educational supervisors, at a local level, who meet the GMC standards for training. This may initially be difficult to establish in organisations that are unfamiliar with training. Certain specialities, such as respiratory medicine, have, through their speciality society the British Thoracic Society (BTS), developed a curriculum for integrated respiratory physician training [16, 17]. Other speciality societies, including those involved with diabetes training, have yet to develop a curriculum for integrated care. The BTS Working Group on Integrated Respiratory Care recognises it is essential in the future for all specialist trainees to have some experience of primary care at least once during their training, probably twice a year and late in the course of their training. The BTS acknowledges, in the future, the roles of consultant involvement in respiratory care is likely to increase to include supervision of community sleep services, reviews of those dying from airway disease and provision of medical input into and care for those with idiopathic pulmonary fibrosis.

While exposure to community work during training is available in other medical specialties, including diabetes, this exposure is extremely patchy and other specialty curricula could learn from the proactive endorsement the respiratory specialty society, BTS, has given to specialty training in integrated care. Diabetes UK, the UK's leading diabetes charity, has widely supported integrated care as the way forward in their 2014 published report on the subject; however, this report failed to address the needs for professional medical training to deliver such care, and the on going training consultants in diabetes would need to support out of hospital services [18]. While this report had the endorsement of the Association of British Clinical Diabetologists (ABCD), the national organisation of Consultant Physicians in Britain who specialise in Diabetes (the increasingly influential body) has remained lukewarm concerning integrated care concentrating more on the role of consultant diabetologists as specialty hospital based [19]. The ABCD has representation on the RCP training and Specialist Certificate Exam Board Specialist training Committee boards and is in a very strong position to influence change in diabetes postgraduate training if it so wished. While the ABCD do acknowledge a role for consultants to provide specialist leadership for the local health economy in designing a high quality and cost-effective integrated model of diabetes care, the training required to do this has not yet been addressed. This contrasts with the emphasis on diabetes educational training for all healthcare professionals in primary care and the need for clinical up skilling the workforce that has come from general practice and the Diabetes UK Primary Care Network [20] and Primary Care Diabetes Society [21]. For true integrated care in diabetes and the other long term condition specialties to work, the education and training needs for both general practitioners and hospital specialists need to be more closely aligned.

The Royal Colleges, both the RCP and the Royal College of General Practitioners, have a pivotal role in supporting integrated care, for all specialities. Not only through the RCP speciality training boards but also through on going educational programmes and support for those consultants involved in community care. The RCP through its Advisory Appointments Committees (AAC) is involved in scrutinising consultant job plans and the appointment process of most consultant posts in the England. They are also working with medical staffing departments to make them compliant with British Medical Association guidelines. The RCP continues to have a representative on most medical consultant interviews. The RCP should take a lead from the respiratory society, the BTS, which has published a generic job plan for community consultant.

For new diabetes and other speciality consultant posts that have a community component, and an increasing number do, the RCP is well placed to ensure that there is a balance between community and hospital work, that a newly appointed consultant is supported by the hospital specialist team to guarantee that they have the skills necessary, there is access to continual professional development and appropriate time set aside in the job plan for supporting the professional activities (SPAs) necessary *to underpin direct clinical care work*. The SPAs for a community consultant post will differ from those in a traditional hospital based consultant job plan but are equally as important (Table 14.3).

Table 14.3 Supporting professional activities

1. Continuing professional development
2. Local clinical governance activities
3. Multidisciplinary training
4. Formal teaching
5. Management
6. Appraisal
7. Job planning
8. Audit
9. Research

At the very core of integrated care is working across primary and secondary care. Advertised consultant appointments that are purely in the community are not the way forward as this just replaces one form of working in *silos* for another. The RCP Advisory Appointments Committees should not sanction such posts and should strongly encourage the host institution holding the contract to be an NHS trust, preferably a hospital NHS trust. A major reason for this is that if the contract for the community specialist service is not re-commissioned or is commissioned by a non-NHS private provider, the consultant would still hold an NHS contract with the hospital. This is important as this has implications for pensions and other employment benefits. Again the RCP is in a strong position to actively encourage this when approving consultant posts.

The royal colleges are also well placed to raise the clinical profile and stature around integrated care by hosting faculty with expertise in integrated care within their colleges and supporting research and educational conferences on integrated care. These programmes could include programmes in leadership skills required for consultants in these roles. At the end of the day it will be action not purely words that will dictate the success and implementation of high quality integrated care clinical services. Action around education is key to this success.

References

1. https://hee.nhs.uk
2. https://www.gov.uk/government/uploads/system/uploads/attachment_data/file/480482/NHS_Constitution_WEB.pdf
3. https://www.england.nhs.uk/wp-content/uploads/2014/10/5yfv-web.pdf
4. https://www.mrcpuk.org/sites/default/files/documents/sce-endocrinology-and-diabetes-blueprint_0.pdf
5. http://www.jrcptb.org.uk/sites/default/files/2010%20Endo%20%26%20Diabetes%20%28amendment%202012%29.pdf
6. http://www.medschools.ac.uk/AboutUs/Projects/Documents/Final%20MMC%20Inquiry%20Jan2008.pdf
7. UK. http://www.gmc-uk.org/about/role.asp
8. Lee SW, et al. The current provision of community-based teaching in UK medical schools: an online survey and systematic review. BMJ Open. 2014;4(12):e005696.
9. https://www.gov.uk/government/uploads/system/uploads/attachment_data/file/390006/2015-16_Tariff_guidance_-_DRAFT_-_web_version.pdf
10. http://www.medschools.ac.uk/Pages/default.aspx
11. https://www.hee.nhs.uk/sites/default/files/documents/Broadening%20the%20foundation%20report.pdf
12. http://www.shapeoftraining.co.uk/static/documents/content/Shape_of_training_FINAL_Report.pdf_53977887.pdf
13. http://www.jrcptb.org.uk/specialties/endocrinology-and-diabetes-mellitus
14. http://www.gmc-uk.org/information_for_you/25688.asp
15. http://www.rcgp.org.uk/policy/rcgp-policy-areas/~/media/Files/Policy/A-Z-policy/General_Practice_and-the_Integration_of_Care%20_An_RCGP_Report.ashx
16. https://www.brit-thoracic.org.uk/document-library/delivery-of-respiratory-care/integrated-care/role-of-the-respiratory-specialist-in-the-integrated-care-team-june-2014/
17. www.jrcptb.org.uk/sites/default/files/2010%20Respiratory%20Medicine.pdf
18. https://www.diabetes.org.uk/Documents/About%20Us/What%20we%20say/Integrated%20diabetes%20care%20(PDF,%20648KB).pdf
19. http://www.diabetologists-abcd.org.uk/home.htm
20. https://www.diabetes.org.uk/Professionals/Professional-groups/Primary-Care-Network/
21. http://www.pcdsociety.org

Diabetes Integrated Care: Are We There Yet?

15

David Simmons, Helmut Wenzel, and Janice C. Zgibor

Introduction

The preceding chapters describe a plethora of definitions of, and perspectives on, integrated care and diabetes integrated care, including a multitude of components that are thought to be important in the running of "the system." There are common elements, but also aspects, which differ significantly. Some have been associated with tangible clinical benefits, others less so.

Each chapter describes the growth in numbers with diabetes and its complications, the persisting under-performance in the clinical systems to optimise clinical assessment and metabolic control, maximise self-care (an accepted key feature of quality diabetes care) and treat detectable tissue damage early. The patient perspective is well described in Chap. 13, detailing the breadth and depth of non-engagement and lack of articulation between different parts of the English National Health Service: surely experiences of patients well beyond the United Kingdom. The scale of the epidemic described for Africa in Chap. 6 is particularly concerning: clearly we need affordable, population based approaches for preventing diabetes, and to ensure that those who do develop diabetes have a better quality of life, are less likely to develop complications and do not die prematurely. Diabetes integrated care sounds as though it should be a major part of the solution, but is it?

Our chapters show that integrated care for people with diabetes has now been tested in a range of settings and with a variety of approaches. So, can we now say "yes, we are able to roll out diabetes integrated care systematically?" Are we, as suggested in the recent Royal College of Physicians report [1], still dependent on local personal relationships between primary and secondary care rather than a framework which will work in most areas? Or do we need to re-invent the diabetes care wheel repeatedly, depending on whether the lead specialists, lead GPs and other health professionals "get on." We would suggest not, but implementing diabetes integrated care is certainly neither simple nor easy. Finally, should we be looking at more creative and innovative ways to improve diabetes care by more systematically integrating the services and expertise of others including pharmacists and peer support facilitators, and for those under more medically-centred systems, nurses and diabetes educators?

D. Simmons (✉)
School of Medicine, Western Sydney University, Sydney, New South Wales, Australia
e-mail: Da.simmons@westernsydney.edu.au

H. Wenzel
Health Economist, Konstanz, Germany
e-mail: hkwen@aol.com

J.C. Zgibor
Department of Epidemiology and Biostatistics, College of Public Health, University of South Florida, Tampa, FL, USA
e-mail: jzgibor@health.usf.edu

D. Simmons et al. (eds.), *Integrated Diabetes Care*, DOI 10.1007/978-3-319-13389-8_15

There are other initiatives globally not described in these chapters, which we also draw upon to help define where we are, and perhaps what we need to do to implement diabetes integrated are more widely. These include the Australian Diabetes Care Project (DCP) (Table 15.1) [2] and the work of Kaiser Permanente and other US providers, particularly since the introduction of the Affordable Care Act [3]. There are also many smaller "front line" approaches designed to integrate care around individuals with additional needs, such as recurrent diabetic ketoacidosis (DKA) with a combined diabetes specialist service case manager-mental health approach [4] and among rural indigenous people [2]. The former included a diabetes specialist dietitian with approval to manage continuous subcutaneous insulin infusion (pump) therapy and carrying out some aspects of social work, while the latter including a dedicated Aboriginal Health Worker. These provide examples of how diabetes integrated care can benefit from broader skills and broader membership. One thing that is clear is that there are some fundamentally different perspectives on diabetes integrated care and what it involves. We therefore commence this chapter with a fundamental dichotomy – is diabetes integrated care an entity to be developed in itself (i.e., a front line diabetes approach) or should it be simply a product of a system carefully crafted by the health system masters (i.e., waiting for the wider system to become "integrated")?

We then describe the components of diabetes integrated care systems reported to date, and compare how and whether different diabetes integrated care approaches dealt with them. The validity of the methods for evaluation is crucial of course, so we make a few comments on how the different projects have been assessed. We finalise by trying to build up to suggested foundations for functioning and sustainable diabetes integrated care.

Table 15.1 The diabetes care project (DCP): Australia's national cluster randomised control trial of primary care coordination of diabetes care

The components of the DCP [2]:
1. An integrated information (IT) platform for general practitioners, allied health professionals and patients. But not specialists
2. Continuous quality improvement (CQI) processes informed by data-driven feedback within primary care
3. Flexible funding for primary care, allocated based on patient risk stratification.
4. Quality improvement support payments linked with a range of patient population outcomes
5. Funding for care facilitation, provided by dedicated Care Facilitators
Study cost: A$33.4 million over the period 2011–2014
Intervention groups
1. Group 1 IT platform and CQI processes (i.e., no funding changes)
2. Group 2 all five components
3. Control group
Study population
184 general practices and 7781 people with diabetes enrolled over 6 months
18 months intervention
Included type 1 and type 2 diabetes
Outcomes
1. Group 2: HbA1c dropped 0.2 %, systolic blood pressure (1 mmHg), LDL cholesterol (0.06 mmol/l), waist circumference (0.4 cm) care-plan take-up, completion of recommended "annual cycles of care," and allied health visits (educator, podiatrist, dietitian) improved
2. Group 1: increased care plan take-up
3. No relationship between health care need and the amount of chronic disease funding received
4. Having a care plan or completing an annual cycle of care did not influence metabolic control
5. Significant increase in cost per person, no significant decrease in costs of hospitalisation
Comment
No significant clinical improvements
More expensive
Hypoglycaemia not considered in the risk stratification
Specialists excluded from the payment system-only GP and allied health Medicare item numbers included

Top Down or Front Line Approaches?

The improvements in care (at least for some patients, for a period of time) that are possible with policy changes, such as the Affordable Care Act in the USA [3] and the Quality Outcomes Framework [5] in the UK reflect the reality that diabetes care (including self-care) does not sit alone, but is part of total health and social care systems, and indeed, overall society. This generates an immediate dichotomisation of perspectives that goes to the heart of the diabetes integrated care debate:

- Is the way to improve diabetes care through a top down approach, i.e., change the broader health system and diabetes care will inevitably be optimised as a result OR
- Is the way to improve diabetes care through a "front line" approach that defines each component of care, related barriers to component optimisation and finds holistic ways to address them

The former reflects a more managerial policy, public health perspective, often encapsulated by the think tanks (e.g., Kings Fund [6]) and accounting firms (McKinsey [7, 8]), while the latter reflects a more grounded, clinical perspective. What we can see from the chapters in this book is that both perspectives are needed: an integrated approach! We know clearly that there are significantly different perspectives between patient, primary care and secondary care [9]. The paradox that we are dealing with is that in spite of health professionals wanting the best for their patients on a patient by patient basis, the way that individuals and institutions are organised and paid, directly influences the clinical decisions that are made. In South Africa (Chap. 6), it was reported that "many…. programs concentrate on *cost-savings* rather than *patient service utilization* and *improved clinical outcomes*." Furthermore, the ease with which the "best" decision can be made, directly determines what action is taken: the more time/effort required, the less likely that it will take place. A simple skeletal representation of the paradox is as follows (Fig. 15.1).

Naturally, optimising personal care and the provider/purchaser-commissioner budget may be aligned, but this is where diabetes poses substantial problems from a health system point of view:

- *This year vs the future*: The majority of adverse diabetes outcomes (e.g., stroke, myocardial infarction, blindness, amputation, end stage renal failure) are many years in the future, so a system based on this year's budget will often not prioritise the future (with harms predicted by, e.g., HbA1c, blood pressure).
- *Cost attribution*: Even for these adverse "diabetes" outcomes, other clinical factors contribute to the end result. This is even more the case for, e.g., infections, falls and other conditions which are more common or more expensive with diabetes. As a result of this complexity, attribution to diabetes may not be so obvious to those seeking ways to minimise expenditure. It has previously been shown in England that the population attributable fraction of the excess hospitalisation costs from diabetes is approximately 40 % [10], comprising excess admission and readmission rates, length of stay, and cost of stay.
- *Cost impact of drugs*: Payment for drugs can range from personal, insurance and government subsidised budgets. Evidence for reducing future health costs is complex and time consuming to collect and the pharmaceutical companies themselves decide the final price of the drugs. In England, drugs may be shown to improve quality of life at an acceptable cost when benchmarked against other drugs (through NICE), but might still not be taken up because of the cost impact on local budgets: budgets held by the same primary care practitioners who are managing the people with diabetes.
- *Separation of ambulatory and inpatient budgets*: Payment for ambulatory diabetes care, which is essentially the preventative part of diabetes care, usually sits in a different budget to the inpatient budget where the big expenses are. Increasing real funding for ambulatory diabetes care for possible reductions in hospitalisation in the future is hard to "sell" as the perspective that "if you have a bed you will fill

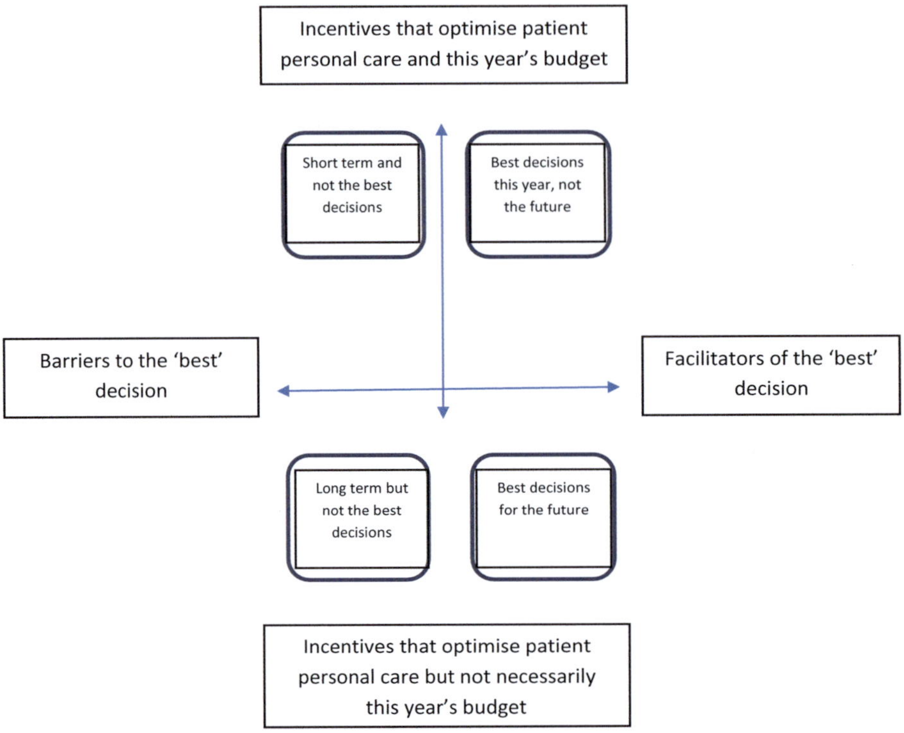

Fig. 15.1 How optimisation of care and annual budgeting can compete in diabetes

it" is common among commissioners. Furthermore, good evidence for reducing hospitalisation through diabetes integrated care is limited, although the South African and Hong Kong models do show that it is possible: of course this will depend upon context and starting point.

- *Obstruction to referral to a more specialist service*: There is ample evidence [11, 12] where clinicians own, and profit from, other services (e.g., laboratory, radiology), that referral rates are increased, often inappropriately (although showing this on a case by case basis can be difficult). Under the English NHS, the converse exists, where GPs, either holding health budgets, or receiving payments for maintaining health budgets [13], reduce their referrals to more specialist care. While this may be appropriate in many cases, it may result in delays and avoidance of referrals, even when specialist care is likely to be of benefit.
- *Qualitative impacts*: There is a mantra that fragmentation of care and reductions in continuity of care are likely to harm the quality of care [14], but hard evidence is difficult to obtain.

So, the payment, funding or commissioning system can clearly be a major determinant of the quality of care around the person with diabetes. The problems outlined above, suggest that any health system that fails to take account of the need to integrate the payment system from both an immediate and long term perspective, must be at greater risk of their diabetes integration attempts failing and/or being unsustainable. The Derby example (Chap. 8) shows that even when the immediate payment system is merged at the provider level, and benefits have accrued, sustainability is not assured unless vertical integration has occurred. Similarly, the East Cambs and Fenland approach (Chap. 7) tried to address each care component, but the insufficient movement in vertical integration was the likely cause of the lack of effect or sustainability. The "bundled care" and "chains of care" in the Netherlands (Chap. 11) and Sweden (Chap. 12) have tried to link providers in different ways, but neither seems to have reduced cost.

Essentially, the "front line approach" seems to be required to ensure that the strategy is grounded in clinical best practice, but the overarching framework of the health economy needs to support an integrated approach within, and potentially, beyond diabetes. As the changes to governance and commissioning are substantial, it may be more acceptable to change the whole system – on the other hand, the details are such that an integrated care pilot within diabetes should be attractive if those involved appreciate the complexity of what is required to create an integrated system.

Components of Diabetes Integrated Care

Although the patient is often appropriately placed in the centre of policy diagrams to reflect "patient centred care," in fact, from a clinical perspective, outcomes depend upon the patient-health care professional (HCP) interaction. This relationship is strengthened through consideration of factors outlined in the American Diabetes Association/European Association for the Study of Diabetes position statement which include risks or side effects associated with treatment, disease duration, life expectancy, important comorbidities, vascular complications, patient attitude and expected treatment efforts, and resources and support system [15]. At the Veterans (Chap. 2), this is called the patient-doctor dyad. The importance of this relationship is emphasised in the chronic care model [16–20].

Figure 15.2 summarises pictorially, the components of diabetes integrated care included in the chapters in this book. The figure places the patient-HCP dyad in the centre, but, of course, both "patient" and HCP sit within their own context: the former in relation to their family, mental (including motivational and spiritual) and "socio-economic" health, and the latter within the health system.

As per Fig. 15.1, both patients and HCP's have to work with facilitators and obstructions to optimal diabetes care and self-care. Obstructive components sit within the barriers to diabetes care framework described in Chap. 7 (East Cambs and Fenland initiative). Many of the facilitators of the best patient decisions also facilitate best clinical practice. However, the health care professional sits upon a range of systems facilitators (or otherwise) within a context that can promote a population based approach to health (goals of population based outcomes, finance, shared clinical governance) or otherwise (organisational finance, separate clinical governance).

Table 15.2 compares the context of each of the approaches described in this book, and adding the Australian DCP, a trial of integrated care components in a fragmented health system [2]. Two successful front line (micro) approaches (managing UK patients with repeat diabetic ketoacidosis [21] and managing patients within an Australian Aboriginal Health Service [22] are also included.

Table 15.3 compares the components within each of the approaches. There are clearly a number of common factors and several that differ between successful and less successful models.

Data and Its Interpretation

Success in these models is usually described in terms of hospitalisation (including, e.g., DKA, amputation, cardiovascular disease events, hypoglycaemia, eye disease, renal disease, all cause), metabolic outcomes (e.g., HbA1c), health costs and access to complex care. Some have described patient related outcomes, quality of life and other staff satisfaction, but the methodology and biases have often not been open to scrutiny. There are some methodological issues that suggest that many of those with positive results may be illusory and reflect the pre-existing landscape and/or wider changes, particular to that locality. It is important to note that these do not in any way denigrate the models described, simply that benefits may not be as large as described.

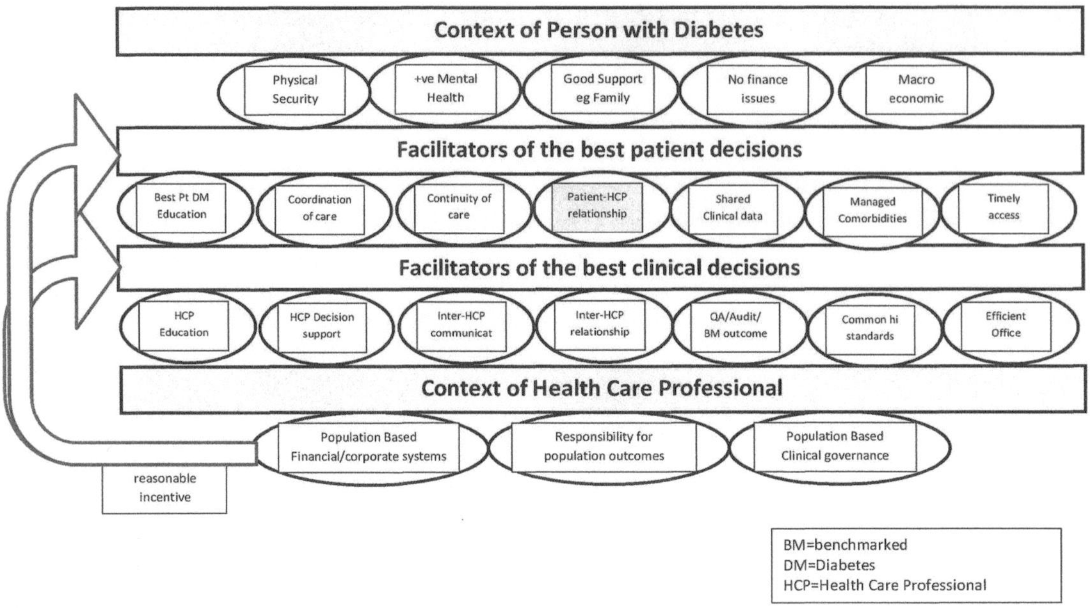

Fig. 15.2 Components of diabetes integrated care placed within the patient-health care professional dyad and the barriers to diabetes care framework: the four slice sandwich

Secular Trends

The reported "success" of intermediate diabetes clinics run by English General Practitioners with a Special Interest led to extension of the model to other areas. This was finally tested in a randomised controlled trial as described in Chap. 9 (Warwickshire) and shown to be a more costly model with no real benefit for patients or the system. Similarly in East Cambs and Fenland, the 1 year results suggested major reductions in hospitalisation and costs in practices participating fully in the integrated care initiative, compared with those who "engaged" later [9]. However, once the trends in neighbouring areas and among those without diabetes were accounted for, it became clear that the benefits originally reported were actually due to wider hospitalisation reductions, not just in those with diabetes. Studies of hospitalisation/hospital costs that do not compare with rates in the non-diabetic population need to be interpreted with caution. The Affordable Care Act in the USA provides a natural experiment in which the role of insurance coverage, provider incentives and outcomes can be evaluated, although it may be too early to tell.

Relativity and Starting Points

Kaiser Permanente is often described as a great diabetes success story in the USA due to its higher than peer levels of, e.g., HbA1c testing [23]. However, in the 2015 HEDIS data, levels of testing, metabolic control achieved and complication rates show quality metrics lower than the English NHS, in spite of the problems with the latter [23]. Furthermore, HbA1c rates above 9 % remain at approximately 20 %, in Southern California [24] or 19 % in Northern California [25], a level much higher than that in the UK [7], and nearly abolished in an Aboriginal Medical Service [22]. Similarly, the Super Six model, an approach with commendable primary care based interventions, has been lauded as a success, as a result of reductions in patients with, e.g., amputations. However, these complications were in the bottom quartile of performance for these outcomes in England [26] and hence improvement would be expected with the additional diabetes resources invested into the area. Amputation rates remain higher than the national average, in spite of a less heterogenous population than in many other parts of England [27]. Studies showing

Table 15.2 Comparison of different contexts within which the models of diabetes integrated care sit

	US-Vet	SF	UPMC	HK	SA	ECF	Derby	Cov-W	Ger	NL	Swe	DKA-P	A-DCP	Rumba
CF National $ /capita 2011 [33]	8508	8508	8508	–	–	3405	3405	3405	4495	5099	3925	3405	3800	3800
Coordinated [33] care CF-Rank	6/11	6/11	6/11	–	–	1/11	1/11	1/11	10/11	5/11	11/11	1/11	4/11	4/11
Outcomes														
Hospitalisation	?[b]	?[b]	↓[a]	↓[a]	↓40 %[a]	↑[c]	↓[a]	?[b]	↓[a]	?[b]	↔[b]	↓[a]	↓[a]	?[b]
Glycaemia+ (e.g., HbA1c)	↓0.6 %[a]	↓[a]	↓[a]	↓[a]	↓1.5 %[a]	↔[b]	↓[a]	RCT ↔ IT 0.8 %[b]	?[b]	↑[c]	↔[b]	↓[a]	↓0.2 %[b]	↓[a]
Costs	Productivity↑[a]	↔[b]	?[b]	↓[a]	↓[a]	?[b]	↓[a]	↑[c]	↓[a]	↑[c]	↔[b]	↓[a]	↑[c]	?[b]
Access to complex spec care	↑[a]	?[b]	↔[b]	↑[a]	↑[a]	↓[c]	↑[a]	1st? IT yes[b]	?[b]	↓[c]	↔ easy[b]	↑[a]	↔[b]	↑[a]
HCP context														
Funder	Federal Govt	Local Govt	Insured Govt	Govt	Insured	Govt	Govt	Trial/Pilot	Insured	Insured	Govt	Govt	Govt	Govt
Defined population	Veterans	Low income	Members	Capitated	Members	Capitated	Capitated	Capitated	Members	National	Regional	>1 DKA admit	Capitated	Indigenous
Levels covered	2°	1°-I	1°-I	2° :90 % of all DM	1°-I-2°	1°-I-2°	1°-I-2° 70 %DM	I	1°-I-2°	1°-I-2°	1°-I-2°	2°	1°-I	1°-I-2°
Organisations leading	Hospital	GP	GP+ hospital	Hospital	Specialist	CS	JV	Specialist	JV	GP	Local Govt	Hospital	GP	AHS+ hospital
Number of employers	1	1	1	1	Multiple	Multiple	1	1	Multiple	Multiple	1	1	Multiple	2
Financial governance	Single	Single	Single	Single	Single	Multiple	Shared	Single	Shared saving	Multiple	Single	Single	GP	AHS+ hospital
Service management	Single	Single	Single	Single	Within provider	Multiple	Single	Single	Multiple	Multiple	Single	Single	GP	GP+ specialist
Clinical governance	Single	Single	Single	Single	Within provider	Within provider	Shared	Shared	Shared	Within provider	Within provider	Within provider	Within provider	Within provider
Information governance	Single[b]	Single[b]	Single[b]	Single[b]	Some shared[b]	Within provider[c]	Shared[a]	Single[b]	Shared[a]	Within provider[c]	National/ internal[b]	Within provider[c]	Within provider[c]	Within provider[c]
$ Incentives	No	Yes	Yes	No	No	QoF	QoF	QoF	Shared saving	Profit	No	No	Yes multiple	No

Key: Levels = *1°* Primary, *2°* Secondary, *I* intermediate, *CF* Source: Commonwealth Fund [8] *QoF* Quality Outcomes Framework, *IT* IT/Education based pilot project, *JV* Joint Venture

[a]Good/improved between primary and secondary care

[b]maybe-unclear

[c]worse/not included

Table 15.3 Comparison of the content of different models of diabetes integrated care

	US-Vet	SF	UPMC	HK	SA	ECF	Derby	Cov-W	Ger	NL	Swe	DKA-P	A-DCP	Rumba
Patient factors														
Continuity of care	Yes[a]	Yes[a]	yes[b]	Yes[a]	Yes[a]	Yes[a]	Yes[a]	No[b]	Yes[a]	Yes[a]	Recently reduced[c]	Yes[a]	Yes[a]	Yes[a]
Team working	Yes[a]	Yes[a]	yes[c]	Yes[a]	Yes[a]	Partly[b]	Yes[a]	Partly[b]	Yes[a]	Yes[a]	Yes[a]	Yes[a]	Yes not specialist[b]	Yes[a]
Overcoming patient barriers	Personalised care[a]	Team care[a]	yes[c]	Yes[a]	Personalised care[a]	Yes[a]	Yes[a]	No[c]	Some[b]	No[c]	Some social[b]	Yes[a]	No[c]	Yes[a]
Co-morbidity	Yes[a]	Yes[a]	No[c]	No-GP only[c]	No-GP only[c]	1°-yes[b]	Partly[b]	No-GP only[c]	Partly[b]	No[c]	No[c]	Yes[a]	No[c]	Yes[a]
Mx articulation						2°-no[b]								
Pt Co-payment	Some[b]	Yes[c]	Yes[c]	Yes[c]	No[a]	No[a]	No[a]	No[a]	No[a]	Yes[c]	Yes[c]	No[a]	Partly[b]	No[a]
Patient education	Yes[a]	Yes[a]	Yes[a]	Yes[a]	Yes[a]	Yes[a]	Yes[a]	Yes[a]	Yes[a]	Yes[a]	Yes[a]	Yes[a]	Yes[a]	Yes[a]
Case management	Dyad[a]	Yes[a]	yes[c]	No[c]	No[c]	No[c]	No[c]	No[c]	No[c]	No[c]	No[c]	Yes[a]	Care facilitators[b]	No[a]
Peer support	No[b]	Yes[a]	No[b]	Yes[a]	No[b]	No[b]	No[b]	No[b]	No[b]	No[b]	No[b]	No[b]	No[b]	No[b]
Patient e-records	No[c]	Yes[a]	yes[c]	No-but reports[b]	No[c]	No[c]	No[c]	No[c]	No[c]	No[c]	No[c]	No[c]	Yes[a]	No[c]
HCP factors														
Electronic health records	Yes[a]	Yes[a]	yes[c]	Yes[a]	Yes[a]	No[c]	Yes[a]	Yes[a]	Yes[a]	No[c]	National data[b]	No[c]	Yes[a]	No[c]
Electronic communication	Yes[a]	Yes[a]	yes[c]	Yes[a]	No[c]	No[c]	Yes[a]	No[c]	?[b]	No[c]	No[c]	No[c]	No[c]	No[c]
Referral p' ways risk stratification	Yes[a]	Some[b]	Some[b]	Yes[a]	Yes[a]	Yes partly[b]	Yes[a]	Yes[a]	Yes[a]	Maybe[b]	T1-2°[a] T2 1°[a]	Yes[a]	Yes[a]	Yes[a]
Guidelines	Yes[a]	Yes[a]	Yes[a]	Yes[a]	Yes[a]	Yes[a]	Yes[a]	Yes[a]	Yes[a]	Yes[a]	Yes[a]	Yes[a]	Yes[a]	Yes[a]
HCP Decision support	No[c]	No[c]	yes[b]	Yes[b]	Regular audit[b]	Joint reviews[a]	Yes[a]	No 1st[b] Yes 2nd[b]	No[c]	No[c]	Yes[a]	Yes[a]	Yes[a]	Yes[a]
HCP education	No[c]	No[c]	Yes[a]	Yes[a]	Yes[a]	Yes[a]	Yes[a]	Yes[a]	No[c]	No[c]	No[c]	Yes[a]	Yes[a]	Yes[a]
Diabetes														
Prevention	No[c]	No[c]	No[c]	Yes[a]	No[c]	No[c]	No[c]	No[c]	Yes[a]	No[c]	No[c]	No[c]	No[c]	No[c]

Care facilitators coordinated but did not deliver care

Key: Levels = *1°* Primary, *2°* Secondary, *I* intermediate, *CF* Source: Commonwealth Fund [33], *QoF* Quality Outcomes Framework, *IT* IT/Education based pilot project, *JV* Joint Venture

[a]Good/improved between primary and secondary care

[b]maybe-unclear

[c]worse/not included

improvement from a low baseline do not necessarily provide a best practice model, but perhaps a change from a system that required improvement. Was it the greater resource, a change in leadership or the new model or a mixture of all: without well conducted randomised controlled trials (which are probably impossible), we will not know.

HbA1c Changes

Several projects report improvements in HbA1c, however, to show improvements in mean or proportion with better control in an area with worse than average glucose control does not necessarily denote improvements due to integrated care. More importantly, improvements in HbA1c, without reports of hypoglycaemia rates and weight gain, may be associated with worse outcomes as suggested from the ACCORD trial [28]. However, moving the population to better control by following a patient-centred approach should minimize the likelihood of adverse outcomes.

Future Changes

Surely, what is intended with any new approach is to create a sustainable approach to improved population based diabetes management, not just within primary care and within secondary care, but with all aspects working well together and properly articulated. It is here that the Super Six model is of particular concern. Notwithstanding its exemplary close collaboration between GP and specialist services, a model that prevents access to the specialist team by patients with type 1 diabetes (besides those with "poor glucose control," youth or continuous subcutaneous insulin infusion therapy), those with rare forms of diabetes and those with difficult to control type 2 diabetes is unlikely to produce long term benefit to patients and create sustainably low hospitalisation rates. Type 1 diabetes management in particular, requires experience in assessing, e.g., hypoglycaemia, hypoglycaemia unawareness, alternative diagnoses, and wider life impacts and behaviours. It is not credible to expect these skills across primary care, and most patients with type 1 diabetes continue to have substantial glycaemic variation even with a "good" HbA1c and are at high risk of premature death [29]. However, given differential access to specialty care, support for primary care through technology or other mechanism may provide a solution.

What Facilitates Diabetes Integrated Care

Figure 15.2 shows the large number of enablers and components for integrated care; taken from the models described, these include the need for integrated information technology systems, aligned finances and responsibility, care planning and robust clinical governance. However, the key to integrated care remains the relationships between patients and the different health care provider. The elements of this are discussed next.

Activated and Informed Patients

Most of the models attempt to activate and inform patients about their diabetes. This may be through access to their own electronic records as in Warwickshire or under the House of Care approach described in Chap. 13, where patients had access to their results. The role of social media and other electronic approaches to information and participation are yet to be fully explored and remain an exciting area for development. Conversely, peer support, so effectively used in both San Francisco and Hong Kong, appears to be an important mechanism to improve self-management and avoid hospitalisation in some patients.

Activated and Informed Health Care Professionals

Rao (Chap. 2) raises an important point that where a single clinician takes responsibility, the resulting personalised care might be a key factor in achieving metabolic outcomes, rather than simply prospective measurement of metabolic status. The House of Care reported improved knowledge and skills, and greater job satisfaction among HCPs [30]. Prior research by Pringle et al showed that the patients of GPs with an interest in diabetes had significantly better glycaemic control [31].

Team/Collaborative Care

Being within the same organisation does not mean that integrated working is inevitable, but looking at Table 15.2, would certainly appear to be an important facilitator. Co-location and concurrent team working has been suggested to be a key factor in the achievement of the Derby, Veterans and Pittsburgh UPMC outcomes. Mapping and planning the joint work, with clear definition of outcomes, process and roles, was also crucial to improving the efficiency of the care provided. The Veteran's chapter provides a step by step guide for those wishing to improve their own approach to care. One wonders to what extent the fact that all HCPs are regional employees, i.e., have the same employer, contributes to Sweden being the country with the best diabetes care delivery in Europe (936 points out of a maximum possible of 1000: the highest score ever observed in the Euro Diabetes Index 2014 [32], in spite of relatively limited integration (according to the Commonwealth Fund [33]).

Where HCPs are not within the same organisation (and even if they are), it is clear that training for integrated working should be implemented [34].

Clinical Engagement and Leadership

Different health systems and different aspects of heath have different leadership models. Diabetes UK have emphasised that whoever is leading, time and resource need to go into engaging clinicians to create a collaborative and constructive culture between those with diabetes and health care professionals and between the different health sectors. A culture of collaboration and a population based outcomes approach is unlikely to be "natural" in a market or competitive system, and part of the leadership training that is required for those involved in governance/management and leadership should be built upon this philosophy, when patients with diabetes are involved [1]. Similarly, the Royal College of Physicians [1] have emphasised the need for "a shared vision across organisations and professions, built around the user's perspective and supported by an ongoing process for co-design, continued stakeholder engagement and improvement." The bottom line is that diabetes integrated care in a population will not occur by chance currently, but will initially need investment in local leadership training and engagement frameworks. This must recognise the time constraints among many of those involved.

Evaluation and Feedback

The Warwickshire approach (Chap. 9), included Diabetes Manager, a tool not only providing real time feedback to improve decision-making, but allowing benchmarking with peers. Decision support was associated with a 37 % improvement in HbA1c in meta-analyses [34], Such an approach is not new in diabetes, and was part of the Diabcare movement over 20 years ago [35] and is a regular part of, e.g., the UPMC quality improvement efforts.

What Obstructs Diabetes Integrated Care

The importance of the perverse incentives that can be embedded in the reimbursement system is well described in Chap. 2 (veterans), Chap. 3 (Pittsburgh) and Chap. 7 (East Cambs and Fenland). In the former, the system obstructed a "contemporaneous and synchronised" multidisciplinary approach and promotes increased volumes of activity (but neither quality nor outcomes) activity. In the latter, the reimbursement system systematically blocked joint working and promoted box ticking rather than effective care. Under both, there remained practitioners dedicated to "best practice," but this was in spite of the reimbursement system. The Royal College of Physicians [1] also describe "short-term service contracts, funder-provider split, competing organisational budgets, activity-based tariff, inadequate resources, continual organisational change, inadequate training, poor management support from acute trusts and the lack of an evidence base for ensuring sustainable, effective services" as barriers to integrated care. The Center for Medicare and Medicaid Services (CMS) has instituted meaningful use criteria to improve quality, safety efficiency and to reduce health disparities [36]. CMS provides payment incentives as certain meaningful use parameters are adopted. While CMS funded 12 sites to evaluate the impact of meaningful use, these results are not yet available for diabetes measures.

Models of Clinical and Corporate Governance

If leadership, financial and governance structures are the upstream factors that obstruct diabetes integrated care (even before we get to the hardware, software, patient and health care professional factors), what are the governance models that are available? The Veterans, UPMC, and Kaiser are single organisations, so all components of their systems come under a single governance and management framework. All responsibility lies with a single entity. However, in most cases, multiple organisations (e.g., GPs, hospitals, community services, private providers) may be involved. In Cambridgeshire, the King's Fund [37] was commissioned to describe the advantages and disadvantages of the various governance models available in a setting where a single entity was not possible (Table 15.4).

Table 15.4 Governance models

Model	Advantages	Disadvantages
Virtual network	Inexpensive	Little potential for progression to focus on system-wide decision-making through informal lines of communication
	Uncomplicated	Dependent upon individual relationships
	Potential for cost savings	Unclear accountability
Hub and spoke model	Uncomplicated and intuitive model of delivery	Limits communication flows
	Allows easy entry of new provider organisations	Centralisation of expertise may create professional divide
	Clear lines of accountability	Lack of joint ownership might exacerbate traditional divides
Managed clinical network	Transparent decision-making processes	Potential inconsistency with espoused government policy (i.e., reduction of quangos)
	Dedicated management function	Cost and resource implications
	Clear lines of accountability	Possible additional bureaucracy
Equal partner network	Local stakeholders are receptive	Possibility of bureaucratic approach to decision-making (slowing down progress)
	Potential to allow more systematic approach to patient safety and clinical effectiveness	Cost and resource implications
	Builds on good relationships	
Legally binding joint venture	Establishment of a single, clear framework for clinical governance	Cost implications
	Could facilitate single vision and culture (not guaranteed)	Could be bureaucratic
		Possible conflict with emergent government policy
		Wouldn't necessarily lead to integrated care
		Could damage existing good relationships

Used with permission from Kings Fund. Consultancy Report: Partnership for Sustainable Health Care Development: Options paper for approaches to governance and clinical governance for an integrated care approach to diabetes. Final Report. London: October, 2010 [37]

Whereas the Derby model was a legally binding joint venture, most of the other models used in England have been virtual networks.

Is There a Tension Between Access to Quality Diabetes Care and Paying for Diabetes Care?

The cost of medications and devices has been known to be a significant barrier to self-care for many years [38]. However, costs remain a major barrier to care where out of pocket expenses remain significant. The International Diabetes Federation Europe analysed access to quality diabetes care in 47 countries of the European Region [39] based upon availability, access and affordability. Whereas availability reports the presence of products in a country that meet the needs, accessibility describes physical access to products, including access to prescribers and education. Affordability depicts the way of paying for products and care, especially reimbursement of the health care system and out-of pocket payments [39]. Naturally the situation varied from region to region. Nevertheless, the survey identified several problems that are directly or indirectly linked to the financing of care.

Budgetary constraints and austerity measures (Portugal, Spain, Greece) are especially a problem in southern European countries. Half of the countries that were included in the survey reported scarcity and supply problems (availability). More than one third of the respondents of those countries also reported increasing difficulties in getting their prescription. They encountered delays of up to several months to see their healthcare professional, or because there are no healthcare professionals close to where they live (accessability). The economic and financial crisis aggravates these issues. This is predominantly true for Mediterranean countries, such as Greece and Portugal, where local healthcare centres have had to reduce their staff or have simply closed down due to austerity measures [39]. Overall, the study also identified a general lack of access to continuous diabetes education for people living with diabetes, their families and healthcare professionals in all the countries surveyed. Furthermore, due to dependency on subsidized or free diabetes medicines and devices, many people either have to pay for their own treatment or just do without. People with diabetes in Spain reported spending on average 428 USD per year in 2013 [39] (300 euros) on their diabetes medicines and devices. This is, in turn, about 1.9 % of the median disposable monthly income in 2011 (1.265 euros per month [40]). In 2013, people with diabetes in Poland reportedly spent around 560 USD per year (about 400 euros) for their treatment; this is 3.6 % of the Household Net Adjusted Disposable Income [39]. In Bulgaria, Russia and Azerbaijan, people reported having to spend well over 821 euros a year up to 1200 euros [39].

What Would Ideal Diabetes Integrated Care Look Like? One or Many Variants?

We would suggest that while a diabetes integrated care approach may vary in its implementation depending on local relationships and leadership, the components are very clear. We list these in Table 15.5 with some of the ways they can be implemented.

Sustainability and Replication

Although the Pittsburgh Veterans integrated team model improved clinical outcomes and productivity, it has reportedly not been replicated elsewhere.

Wider Benefits

Besides the total health system learning and tools that can arise from implementing diabetes integrated care, the Hong Kong approach (Chap. 5), demonstrates the phenomenal research benefits that can accrue. As a result of the diabetes

Table 15.5 Blueprint for an integrated diabetes care service

Empowered/enabled/activated and informed patients	Education, access to electronic records, HCP telephone support, nominated "diabetes care promoter" or care lead/care manager, peer/health coach support/case management
All skills represented in the organisation, all HCPs competent at their level	All members of the team work at the top of their competency (not just license/certification as much of the world has often moved on from this training)-Ongoing HCP education
Clarity over roles and limitations and easy access to others for advice	Mapping and planning the joint work, with clear definition of outcomes, process and roles, was also crucial to improving the efficiency of the care provided. Chapter 2 provides a step by step guide for those wishing to improve their own approach to care. Similar re-engineering of work flow occurred in Hong Kong
Primary care support by specialists	In the "Super six" model and in the East Cambs and Fenland model, payments were made for specialists not only to see patients but to support primary care including:
	Virtual clinics (case-based discussions)
	Database reviews to discuss individual patients with regards to targets, hospitalisation, referrals
	Reviews of audits completed by the GP practice on diabetes care
	Educational sessions on areas of diabetes management of the practice's choice
	Patient reviews (in conjunction with GPs or practice nurses)
All information and communication shared readily-Information management optimised	Electronic communication, electronic records
Methods to overcome clinical inertia	Benchmarking, audit, decision support, QA, use of different health disciplines
Aligned finance-no disincentives	Link hospital costs with ambulatory costs-single budget for pts with diabetes. As for incentives-jury is still out
Single organisational governance/management structure even if made up of more than one organisation	Single organisation, joint venture, Hub and Spoke model, probably not network models
Endocrinologist/diabetes specialist leadership or joint venture model	The successful models integrating primary and secondary care were either led by specialists or were joint venture models
Leadership clearly defined and supported	..and trained
Nuts and bolts in place	Define risk categories, targets and wider guidelines, e.g., education, drugs, self-monitoring, support, diet, lifestyle and, e.g., palliative care, mental health, complications management
Define minimum visit/care expectations	As per the Veterans in the USA and Paediatrics/Transition under Best practice tariff in the UK
Define pathways	T1DM = is specialist in nearly all models
	T2DM = largely primary care but including a range of disciplines
	Other specialist = pre-pregnancy, antenatal, postpartum, inpatient, emergency, renal, foot, ?eye, cardiovascular, rare forms of diabetes
	Morbid obesity and type 2 diabetes: medical or surgical?
Importance of using the data for not only improving care but advancing knowledge through research (Hong Kong)	Electronic database-complementary epidemiological, social science and health economic (and health informatics) expertise

integrated care system and databases that have been developed, the Hong Kong team have been able to generate important new knowledge relating to the epidemiology of diabetes, the genetics of diabetes and testing different clinical assessments and interventions. Their approach has also generated biobanks and patient pipelines into clinical trials. Their JADE programme has also been able to support other health systems. A further benefit of the integrated care approach has been to assist with workforce planning, another key strategic component of maintaining a quality health system.

The Two Cinderellas of Diabetes Integrated Care

There remain two "Cinderellas" of diabetes care that few of the diabetes focussed models of care appear to address: integration with mental health services and with diabetes prevention.

The DKA prevention case management model [41] included a substantial and operational integration between the diabetes specialist service and the mental health services. While many primary and secondary care services have staff trained in, e.g., motivational interviewing, and can offer mental health first aid, few appear to be integrated seamlessly with mental health services. While this could be said for many co-morbidities, there are good examples of other wider integrated team working (e.g., multidisciplinary foot teams, obesity teams).

Prevention of type 2 diabetes is the other important issue that appears to continue to remain generally outside the remit of diabetes care. Hong Kong does have its nurse-led OPAL programme, the evaluation of which is keenly awaited. Many would see diabetes prevention as in the domain of public health and primary care and primary care is, of course, a key component of diabetes integrated care. However, there are growing aspects where those with diabetes may be able to facilitate prevention [42] and where those needing prevention are not being followed up adequately in primary care.

Conclusion

The creation of a local health system that can integrate primary, secondary and community diabetes care, sharing the work while getting the best from each, would seem to be an obvious and relatively simple and sensible way forward. We have shown in this book that while this can work, it is neither simple nor straightforward. Integration will require its own resource. Health systems are too complex for integration to happen just because it is good/best practice.

We provide individual components that appear to be required for successful integrated care. Some, such as integrated IT systems, may need to come later; other components, such as achieving a registered population and aligned financial incentives may take some time and substantial facilitation, but this should not stop a stepwise approach across each local health economy. Governments should move to systems that will facilitate integration, and away from the market systems that appear to increase cost and reduce the quality of diabetes care.

References

1. Hussain S, Dornhorst A. Integrated care – taking specialist medical care beyond the hospital walls. London: Royal College of Physicians; 2015.
2. Australian Department of Health. Evaluation report of the diabetes care project. Canberra, Australia; 2015.
3. Office of the Legislative Counsel. Compilation of patient protection and affordable care act 2010. Available from: http://housedocs.house.gov/energycommerce/ppacacon.pdf
4. Randall L, Begovic J, Hudson M, Smiley D, Peng L, Pitre N, et al. Recurrent diabetic ketoacidosis in inner-city minority patients: behavioral, socioeconomic, and psychosocial factors. Diabetes Care. 2011;34(9):1891–6.
5. Health & Social Care Information Centre. Quality and Outcomes Framework (QOF) (2014) [05/15/2016]. Available from: http://www.hscic.gov.uk/media/15053/QOF-Publication-Consultation-Results-2014/pdf/QOF_Publication_Consultation_Results_2014.pdf
6. Alderwick H, Ham C, Buck D. Population health systems: going beyond integrated care 2015 [05/15/2016]. Available from: http://www.kingsfund.org.uk/sites/files/kf/field/field_publication_file/population-health-systems-kingsfund-feb15.pdf

7. De Smet A, McGurk M, Vinson M. Unlocking the potential of frontline managers. New York: McKinsey & Companies; 2009. [05/15/2016]. Available from: http://www.mckinsey.com/business-functions/organization/our-insights/unlocking-the-potential-of-frontline-managers.
8. McKinsey & Company. How companies manage the front line today: McKinsey survey results (2010) [05/15/2016]. Available from: http://www.mckinsey.com/business-functions/organization/our-insights/how-companies-manage-the-front-line-today-mckinsey-survey-results
9. Simmons D, Lillis S, Swan J, Haar J. Discordance in perceptions of barriers to diabetes care between patients and primary care and secondary care. Diabetes Care. 2007;30(3):490–5.
10. Simmons D, Wenzel H. Diabetes inpatients: a case of lose, lose, lose. Is it time to use a "diabetes-attributable hospitalization cost" to assess the impact of diabetes? Diabet Med. 2011;28(9):1123–11230.
11. Relman AS. Dealing with conflicts of interest. N Engl J Med. 1985;313(12):749–51.
12. Schaffer W, Holloman F. Consultation and referral between physicians in new medical prac-tice environments. Ann Intern Med. 1985;103:600–5.
13. Simmons D, English P, Robins P, Craig A, Rush A. Should diabetes be commissioned through multidisciplinary networks, rather than practice based commissioning? Primary Care Diabetes. 2011;5(1):39–40.
14. Shih A, Davis K, C SS, Gauthier A, Nuzum R, McCarthy D. Organising the U.S. Health Care Delivery System for High Performance. The Commonwealth Fund (2008) [05/12/2016]. Available from: http://www.commonwealthfund.org/usr_doc/Shih_organizingushltcaredeliverysys_1155.pdf
15. Inzucchi SE, Bergenstal RM, Buse JB, Diamant M, Ferrannini E, Nauck M, et al. Management of hyperglycemia in type 2 diabetes, 2015: a patient-centered approach: update to a position statement of the American Diabetes Association and the European Association for the Study of Diabetes. Diabetes Care. 2015;38(1):140–9.
16. Wagner EH, Austin BT, Von Korff M. Improving outcomes in chronic illness. Manag Care Q. 1996;4(2):12–25.
17. Wagner EH, Austin BT, Von Korff M. Organizing care for patients with chronic illness. Milbank Q. 1996;74(4):511–44.
18. Wagner EH, Bennett SM, Austin BT, Greene SM, Schaefer JK, Vonkorff M. Finding common ground: patient-centeredness and evidence-based chronic illness care. J Altern Complement Med. 2005;11 Suppl 1:S7–15.
19. Wagner EH, Austin BT, Davis C, Hindmarsh M, Schaefer J, Bonomi A. Improving chronic illness care: translating evidence into action. Health Aff (Millwood). 2001;20(6):64–78.
20. Wagner EH, Glasgow RE, Davis C, Bonomi AE, Provost L, McCulloch D, et al. Quality improvement in chronic illness care: a collaborative approach. Jt Comm J Qual Improv. 2001;27(2):63–80.
21. Savage MW, Dhatariya KK, Kilvert A, Rayman G, Rees JA, Courtney CH, et al. Joint British Diabetes Societies guideline for the management of diabetic ketoacidosis. Diabet Med. 2011;28(5):508–15.
22. Simmons D. Impact of an integrated approach to diabetes care at the Rumbalara Aboriginal Health Service. Intern Med J. 2003;33(12):581–5.
23. NCQA. Comprehensive diabetes care (n.d.) [05/13/2016]. Available from: http://www.ncqa.org/report-cards/health-plans/state-of-health-care-quality/2015-table-of-contents/diabetes-care
24. Permanente K. Measuring care quality: Southern California Region. Rockville: Kaiser Permanente; 2015.
25. Permanente K. Measuring care quality: Northern California Region. Rockville: Kaiser Permanente; 2015.
26. NHS. The Information Centre. National Diabetes Audit: PCT summary. Year 2009/10 (n.d.) [05/15/2016]. Available from: http://www.hscic.gov.uk/catalogue/PUB06517/nati-diab-audi-pct-lhb-eng-scen-port-pct-rep.pdf
27. Diabetes Specialist Centre. Pattern review and outcomes from SMBG data in primary care. An evaluatuion of communication and technology support. Diabetes Voice Summer 2014(26).
28. Action to Control Cardiovascular Risk in Diabetes Study Group. Effects of intensive glucose lowering in Type 2 diabetes. N Engl J Med. 2008;358(24):2545–59.
29. Huxley RR, Peters SA, Mishra GD, Woodward M. Risk of all-cause mortality and vascular events in women versus men with type 1 diabetes: a systematic review and meta-analysis. Lancet Diabetes Endocrinol. 2015;3(3):198–206.
30. Coulter A, Roberts S, Dixon A. Delivering better services for people with long term conditions. Building the house of care. London: The King's Fund; 2013.
31. Pringle M, Stewart-Evans C, Coupland C, Williams I, Allison S, Sterland J. Influences on control in diabetes mellitus: patient, doctor, practice, or delivery of care? BMJ Br Med J. 1993;306(6878):630–4.
32. Cebolla Garrofé B, Björnberg A, Yung Phang A. Euro diabetes index 2014. Health Consumer Powerhouse Ltd; 2014.
33. Davis K, Stremikis K, Schoen C, Squires D. Mirror. Mirror on the wall, update: how the U.S. Health Care System compares internationally. The Commonwealth Fund; 2014.
34. Tricco AC, Ivers NM, Grimshaw JM, Moher D, Turner L, Galipeau J, et al. Effectiveness of quality improvement strategies on the management of diabetes: a systematic review and meta-analysis. Lancet. 2012;379(9833):2252–61.
35. Piwernetz K. DIABCARE Quality Network in Europe – a model for quality management in chronic diseases. Int Clin Psychopharmacol. 2001;16 Suppl 3:S5–13.
36. US Department of Health & Human Services. EHR Incentives & Certification [05/24/2016]. Available

from: https://www.healthit.gov/providers-professionals/meaningful-use-definition-objectives
37. Kings' Fund. Consultancy report: partnership for sustainable health care development: options paper for approaches to governance and clinical governance for an integrated care approach to diabetes. Final report. London; October 2010.
38. Simmons D, Peng A, Cecil A, Gatland B. The personal costs of diabetes: a significant barrier to care in South Auckland. N Z Med J. 1999;112(1097):383–285.
39. International Diabetes Federation Europe. Access to quality medicines and medical devices for diabetes care in Europe; 2013.
40. OECD – OECD. Stat. Income distribution and poverty: median disposable income at current prices (n.d.) [05/12/2016]. Available from: http://stats.oecd.org/Index.aspx?DataSetCode=IDD
41. Simmons D, Hartnell S, Watts J, Ward C, Davenport K, Gunn E, et al. Effectiveness of a multidisciplinary team approach to the prevention of readmission for acute glycaemic events. Diabet Med. 2015;32(10):1361–7.
42. Murray NJ, Gasper AV, Irvine L, Scarpello TJ, Sampson MJ. A motivational peer support program for type 2 diabetes prevention delivered by people with type 2 diabetes: the UEA-IFG feasibility study. Diabetes Educ. 2012;38(3):366–76.

Index

D. Simmons et al. (eds.), *Integrated Diabetes Care*, DOI 10.1007/978-3-319-13389-8